Pulmonary and Respiratory Diseases and Disorders

nova
Medicine & Health
New York

Pulmonary and Respiratory Diseases and Disorders

Understanding and Treating Acute Pulmonary Embolism
James K. Edwards (Editor)
2022. ISBN: 979-8-88697-149-1 (Softcover)
2022. ISBN: 979-8-88697-398-3 (eBook)

Chronic Obstructive Pulmonary Disease: From Diagnosis to Treatment
Jaber S. Alqahtani, PhD (Editor)
2022. ISBN: 979-8-88697-333-4 (Hardcover)
2022. ISBN: 979-8-88697-396-9 (eBook)

Interstitial Lung Disease: From Diagnosis to Treatment
Roberto G. Carbone, MD, FCCP (Editor)
Francesco Puppo, MD (Editor)
Keith Wille, MD, MSPH (Editor)
Pallav Shah, MD (Editor)
2022. ISBN: 978-1-68507-926-0 (Hardcover)
2022. ISBN: 979-8-88697-068-5 (eBook)

A Clinical Manual of Sarcoidosis
Vikas Pathak, MD (Editor)
Shambhu Aryal, MD (Editor)
2022. ISBN: 978-1-68507-681-8 (Hardcover)
2022. ISBN: 978-1-68507-782-2 (eBook)

Pulmonary Vascular Disorders
Francesco Puppo, MD (Editor), Roberto G. Carbone, MD, FCCP (Editor), Victor F. Tapson, MD, FCCP, FRCP (Editor)
2021. ISBN: 978-1-53619-458-6 (Hardcover)
2021. ISBN: 978-1-53619-553-8 (eBook)

More information about this series can be found at https://novapublishers.com/product-category/series/pulmonary-and-respiratory-diseases-and-disorders/

Antonio M. Esquinas
and Takatoshi Kasai
Editors

Obstructive Sleep Apnea in Pulmonary Critical Care

Essential Ventilatory Approach

nova
Medicine & Health
New York

https://doi.org/10.52305/MUQS3774

NOTICE TO THE READER

The Publisher has taken reasonable care in the preparation of this book but makes no expressed or implied warranty of any kind and assumes no responsibility for any errors or omissions. No liability is assumed for incidental or consequential damages in connection with or arising out of information contained in this book. The Publisher shall not be liable for any special, consequential, or exemplary damages resulting, in whole or in part, from the readers' use of, or reliance upon, this material. Any parts of this book based on government reports are so indicated and copyright is claimed for those parts to the extent applicable to compilations of such works.

Independent verification should be sought for any data, advice or recommendations contained in this book. In addition, no responsibility is assumed by the Publisher for any injury and/or damage to persons or property arising from any methods, products, instructions, ideas or otherwise contained in this publication.

This publication is designed to provide accurate and authoritative information with regards to the subject matter covered herein. It is sold with the clear understanding that the Publisher is not engaged in rendering legal or any other professional services. If legal or any other expert assistance is required, the services of a competent person should be sought. FROM A DECLARATION OF PARTICIPANTS JOINTLY ADOPTED BY A COMMITTEE OF THE AMERICAN BAR ASSOCIATION AND A COMMITTEE OF PUBLISHERS.

Library of Congress Cataloging-in-Publication Data

Names: Esquinas, Antonio M., editor.
Title: Obstructive sleep apnea in pulmonary critical care: essential ventilatory approach / editors, Antonio M. Esquinas, MD, PhD, FCCP, FAARC, Intensive Care Unit Hospital Morales Meseguer, Murcia, Spain;
Director, International School of Non-Invasive Ventilation; Director International Non Invasive Ventilation Expert of College, Takatoshi Kasai, MD, Department of Cardiovascular Medicine, Juntendo University Graduate, School of Medicine, Tokyo, Japan.
Identifiers: LCCN 2023021932 (print) | LCCN 2023021933 (ebook) | ISBN 9798886978582 (hardcover) | ISBN 9798886978919 (adobe pdf)
Subjects: LCSH: Respiratory emergencies. | Sleep apnea syndromes. |
Respiratory intensive care. | Intensive care units--Equipment and supplies. | Respirators (Medical equipment)
Classification: LCC RC735.R48 O27 2023 (print) | LCC RC735.R48 (ebook) |
DDC 616.2/09--dc23/eng/20230606 LC record available at https://lccn.loc.gov/2023021932
LC ebook record available at https://lccn.loc.gov/2023021933

Published by Nova Science Publishers, Inc. † New York

To our patients and their families

Contents

Preface

There is a significant prevalence of OSA disease in the current population with a great impact on the development of complications when these patients require hospital admission. The status of this patients is more vulnerable in critical situations when they require invasive or non-invasive ventilatory support in intensive care units or serious surgical procedures. In many of these cases, the development of infectious or non-infectious complications aggravates the prognosis. In these situations, precise knowledge of the pathophysiological aspects and the development of preventive actions and early treatment are required as it acts in the most vulnerable phase of this disease.

This book describes all the actions that are required as well as possible scenarios that the hospitalized patient with OSA may require.

The book has been structured from the analysis of epidemiology, comorbidities, Pharmacological data, and a description of all the Ventilatory Management Options (High Flow Nasal Oxygen in Sleep-Disordered Breathing, Invasive Mechanical Ventilation), details of essential aspects in Monitoring in Critical Care and a whole analysis of situations such as Hypercapnic. OSA and COPD: The Overlap Syndrome, Asthma. Overlap Syndrome: Concept and Ventilatory Modes, Severe Acute Pneumonia, Acute Heart Failure, Neurological Diseases, Interstitial Lung Diseases: Pathophysiology and Treatment.

We have analyzed an essential aspect such as weaning Mechanical Ventilation, extubation Period: Clinical and Practical Implications and all the situations of greatest risk in Anesthesiology-Perioperative Medicine (Pathophysiology, Diagnosis and Treatment).

Finally, it has been considered that it is essential to complete this study with a design of how to carry out the preparation of these patients in the discharge from Intensive Care Unit, determinants in Mortality and Outcome, Telemedicine: Clinical and social Life Effects.

We hope that this book may help in the complexity of OSA in critical care.

Antonio M. Esquinas, MD, PhD, FCCP
International Fellow AARC. Fellow NIV
Murcia, Spain

Takatoshi Kasai, MD, PhD
Tokyo, Japan

Chapter1

Epidemiology

Giovanni D'Agostino, MD
and Annachiara Marra*, MD, PhD
Department of Neurosciences, Reproductive and Odontostomatological Sciences, University of Naples "Federico II," Naples, Italy

Abstract

Obstructive sleep apnea (OSA) is a chronic condition characterized by at least five obstructive events (apneas and hypopneas) per hour during sleep due to an intermittent, complete, or partial, upper airway obstruction. OSA is related to various diseases determining an admission to intensive care unit (ICU) and poor outcome. Some articles have shown increased risk of poor outcomes and higher mortality and higher risk of admission to ICU in patients with hypercapnic acute respiratory failure with OSA compared to non-OSA patients. Thus, there is the necessity of earlier diagnosis for OSA patients in ICU and earlier treatment to improve the outcome. Their management in ICU must be individualized to increase the odds of discharge and to avoid the complications. The aim of this chapter is to describe the OSA in intensive care unit, its prevalence and what kind of complications OSA patients have.

Keywords: comorbidities, intensive care unit, hypercapnic acute respiratory failure, mortality, obstructive sleep apnea, outcome

* Corresponding Author's Email: dottmarraannachiara@gmail.com.

In: Obstructive Sleep Apnea in Pulmonary Critical Care
Editors: Antonio M. Esquinas and Takatoshi Kasai
ISBN: 979-8-88697-858-2

Introduction

Obstructive sleep apnea (OSA) is nowadays considered as one of the most frequent chronic diseases, with multi-organ consequences and a high societal burden. OSA is characterized by at least five obstructive events (apnoea and hypopnoea) per hour during sleep due to an intermittent, complete, or partial, upper airway obstruction. Most of the time, the respiratory events are associated with snoring, oxygen desaturations and brief arousal from sleep with a BMI ≥ 40 kg/m2. The global prevalence of OSA in the middle-aged population is above 20% [1]. This prevalence has substantially increased over the last few decades owing to the parallel epidemics of obesity and type 2 diabetes [2]. OSA prevalence is even higher in patients suffering from cardiovascular diseases, reaching 50% in hypertension, arrhythmia, or stroke patients [3].

The combination of OSA and morbid obesity might be associated with some specific frailties and a relatively high risk of cardiovascular and metabolic comorbidities, along with an increased risk of mortality.

OSA patients often present multiple comorbidities, such as obesity, diabetes, hypertension, ischemic heart disease, heart failure and/or stroke, which are also frequently the underlying causes for intensive care unit (ICU) admission [4-7]. Sleep disordered breathing has also been identified as a common contributing cause of hypercapnic respiratory failure in obese patients admitted to the ICU [8]. In addition, patients with OSA often have co-morbidities, such as chronic obstructive pulmonary disease (COPD) and asthma [9], and these would aggravate and complicate the pulmonary conditions when OSA patients develop acute respiratory failure [10].

The prevalence of OSA in the ICU population has been reported as being between 7.8% and 10.3% according to two retrospective American surveys [11, 12]. OSA prevalence certainly appears to differ from one ICU to another depending on the predominant ICU activity (i.e., surgical versus medical, pediatric neurological or trauma oriented ICU). In a study the physician-reported prevalence of OSA of only 5.6% reflects a massive under-diagnosis of OSA in ICU patients [7] while, studies implementing polysomnographic assessment of ICU survivors reported a much higher OSA prevalence [13, 14]. A study assessing the prevalence and severity of OSA in patients surviving acute hypercapnic respiratory failure (AHRF) in the ICU by sleep studies, observed a much higher than expected prevalence of moderate to severe OSA and severe OSA for both COPD and non-COPD groups[14]. For patients admitted and surviving acute hypercapnic respiratory failure the prevalence of

OSA increases to 65%% [13, 14]. Extensive data have demonstrated that undiagnosed OSA syndrome is associated with an increased risk of poor outcomes and higher mortality in the postoperative period [15, 16].

Patients presenting with OSA at ICU admission were older, with a higher BMI and a larger number of comorbidities than non-OSA patients [17].

The most common reasons for first-time ICU admission in critically ill OSA patients were cardiovascular events, followed by respiratory events, cerebrovascular events, and infectious events [18]. Hang et al., [18] found that the clinical variables of the patients admitted due to respiratory, cerebrovascular, and cardiovascular events showed no significant differences in age, gender, BMI, apnoea-hypopnoea index (AHI), mean oxygen saturation (SaO_2), minimum (SaO_2), laboratory data, length of ICU stay and in-hospital and two-year mortality rate. However, patients admitted due to respiratory events had significantly higher APACHE II scores, lower arterial blood gas pH levels and higher PaCO2 than patients admitted due to cardiovascular and cerebrovascular events. There was no difference in short- and long-term mortality but patients admitted due to respiratory had a significantly higher incidence of requiring NIV after extubation and higher ICU readmission rates [18].

Obese patients admitted to an ICU require more complex management and those with OSA often need continuous positive airway pressure (CPAP) treatment [19].

OSA is known to be associated with renal decline [20, 21] and it has been reported that OSA is linked with a higher risk of acute kidney damage in critically ill patients [22]. Also, sleep apnea and deterioration in sleep quality might impair immune responses and protection against infections [23]; e.g., for influenza patients with exacerbation OSA was a significant contributor to the reasons for ICU admission [24]. Moreover, OSA patients are more sensitive to opioids developing central apneas after extubation [25]. Intravenous fluid loading also influences OSA severity [26]. Taken together, these reports advocate that, as for obese individuals, the detection of underlying OSA should impact ICU management.

Combining OSA with other comorbidities may be associated with an effect on the impact of hospital-free survival [14]. A retrospective observation designed to identify novel risk factors associated with readmission after hospitalization for acute exacerbation of COPD identified sleep apnea among other comorbid conditions, as a novel risk factor for readmission [27].

It has been assumed that OSA patients have increased morbidity and mortality when admitted to an ICU. A study found that OSA patients were more likely to require ICU transfer and intubation or noninvasive positive pressure ventilation after surgery [28].

Recently, studies are being focused on the association between OSA status and the prognosis of critically ill patients, but with controversial results [7, 11]. One found that OSA was associated with decreased mortality [11] but the other did not identify such benefit [7]. A retrospective cohort study by Lin et al., found that compared with those without OSA, patients with OSA had a significantly lower risk of ICU- and in-hospital mortality [17]. After adjusted for age, gender, weight, SAPS II scores, sequential organ failure assessment (SOFA) score, comorbidities, and laboratory tests, OSA was still associated with decreased risk of mortality, which indicated that OSA itself might be a protective factor for mortality. Several factors could explain the protective effect of OSA in critical care patients. First, in this study, patients without OSA were older and had higher SAPS II scores, indicated that patients without OSA had greater severity of illness.

Second, long-term adaptation to hypoxia might cause ischemic preconditioning due to the nocturnal cycles of hypoxia-reoxygenation, which might alleviate the acute stress response and protect the cardiocirculatory system against infarction and further ischemic insults [29]. Furthermore, the mobilization, proliferative and angiogenic capacities of endothelial progenitor cells were heightened in patients with OSA, indicating that vascular endothelial cell repair might also be involved in the mechanism of cardiovascular protection [30]. Another mechanism by which OSA might reduce mortality was the development of coronary collaterals. OSA might promote angiogenesis through oxidative stress and upregulation of vascular endothelial growth factor in patients with coronary artery disease, which might trigger the development of coronary collaterals and improve blood supply to the heart [31].This adaptive change in the cardiovascular system might increase myocardial oxygen and reduce cardiovascular risk among patients with serious illnesses [32].

The prevalence of OSA in patients with severe Coronavirus Disease 2019 (COVID-19) has been subject of debate [33]. A study by Maas et al., found a prevalence of 6.3% in patients with COVID-19 in their cohort from the USA [34]. This is in concordance with the results of Voncken et al., [35], as well as with estimations of the worldwide prevalence of OSA between 3 and 7%.

There is a strong association of OSA with increased mortality in COVID-19 patients. A brief report studying 4,668 COVID-19 patients from an electronic patient registry from New England, USA, showed an increased all-cause mortality rate (11.7%) compared with controls (6.9%) [36]. Maas et al.,

[34] showed that OSA was associated with increased risk for hospitalization (OR 1.65) and respiratory failure (OR 1.98).

Several pathophysiological mechanisms may help to explain the increased mortality risk in COVID-19 patients with OSA. One frequently suggested mechanism is an increased risk of aspiration. This theory is supported by an overall higher incidence of pneumonia in OSA patients [37]. The mechanism may be related to laryngeal sensory dysfunction, laryngeal adductor reflection attenuation, impaired cough reflexes (during REM sleep) and/ or gastroesophageal reflux, which have all been described in patients with OSA [38]. In addition, gasping is a common phenomenon in patients with OSA and gasping may predispose to aspiration of virus particles [39]. Furthermore, also other mechanical problems in OSA contribute to less effective ventilation treatment, including a higher risk of difficult intubation and non-invasive ventilation may be less effective due to the intermittent airway obstruction episodes [40]. In addition, higher levels of inflammatory markers have been reported in OSA patients compared to patients without OSA. This could increase the risk for overproduction of prompt response proinflammatory cytokines which could increase chances of developing Cytokine Storm Syndrome (CSS) [41].

Conclusion

Patients with OSA in ICU represent a big challenge. Known OSA is not demonstrated to be an independent risk factor for adverse outcomes in ICU patients.

References

[1] Ogna A., Tobback N., Andries D., Preisig M., Vollenweider P., Waeber G., Marques-Vidal P., Haba-Rubio J., Heinzer R. Prevalence of sleep-disordered breathing in the general population: THE HypnoLaus study. *Lancet Respir. Med.* (2015) doi:10.1016/S2213-2600(15)00043-0.

[2] Reilly, J. J., El-Hamdouchi, A., Diouf, A., Monyeki, A. & Somda, S. A. Determining the worldwide prevalence of obesity. *The Lancet* (2018) doi:10.1016/S0140-6736(18)30794-3.

[3] Shahrokh Javaheri, Ferran Barbe, Francisco Campos-Rodriguez, Jerome A. Dempsey, Rami Khayat, Sogol Javaheri, Atul Malhotra, Miguel A. Martinez-Garcia, Reena Mehra, Allan I. Pack, sevolod Y. Polotsky, Susan Redline, Virend K. Somers.

Sleep Apnea: Types, Mechanisms, and Clinical Cardiovascular Consequences. *Journal of the American College of Cardiology* (2017) doi:10.1016/j.jacc.2016.11.069.

[4] Zamarron, C., Vanesa García Paz & Riveiro, A. Obstructive sleep apnea syndrome is a systemic disease. Current evidence. *European Journal of Internal Medicine* (2008) doi:10.1016/j.ejim.2007.12.006.

[5] Reutrakul, S. & Mokhlesi, B. Obstructive Sleep Apnea and Diabetes: A State of the Art Review. *Chest* (2017) doi:10.1016/j.chest.2017.05.009.

[6] [Richards, K. C., Anderson, W. M. D., Chesson, A. L. & Nagel, C. L. Sleep-related breathing disorders in patients who are critically ill. *J. Cardiovasc. Nurs.* (2002) doi:10.1097/00005082-200210000-00005.

[7] Sébastien Bailly, Louis-Marie Galerneau, Stéphane Ruckly, Alexandre Seiller, Nicolas Terzi, Carole Schwebel, Claire Dupuis, Renaud Tamisier, Bernard Mourvillier, Jean-Louis Pepin, Jean-François Timsit. Impact of obstructive sleep apnea on the obesity paradox in critically ill patients. *J. Crit. Care* (2020) doi:10.1016/j.jcrc.2019.12.016.

[8] BaHammam, A., Syed, S. & Al-Mughairy, A. Sleep-related breathing disorders in obese patients presenting with acute respiratory failure. *Respir. Med.* (2005) doi:10.1016/j.rmed.2004.10.021.

[9] Karachaliou, F., Kostikas, K., Pastaka, C., Bagiatis, V. & Gourgoulianis, K. I. Prevalence of sleep-related symptoms in a primary care population - Their relation to asthma and COPD. *Prim. Care Respir. J.* (2007) doi:10.3132/pcrj.2007.00045.

[10] Fletcher, E. C., Shah, A., Qian, W. & Miller, C. C. "Near miss" death in obstructive sleep apnea: A critical care syndrome. *Crit. Care Med.* (1991) doi:10.1097/00003246-199109000-00011.

[11] Bolona, E., Hahn, P. Y. & Afessa, B. Intensive care unit and hospital mortality in patients with obstructive sleep apnea. *J. Crit. Care* (2015) doi:10.1016/j.jcrc.2014.10.001.

[12] Jean, R. E., Gibson, C. D., Jean, R. A. & Ochieng, P. Obstructive sleep apnea and acute respiratory failure: An analysis of mortality risk in patients with pneumonia requiring invasive mechanical ventilation. *J. Crit. Care* (2015) doi:10.1016/j.jcrc.2015.03.016.

[13] Arnaud W. Thille, Ana Córdoba-Izquierdo, Bernard Maitre, Laurent Boyer, Laurent Brochard, Xavier Drouot. High prevalence of sleep apnea syndrome in patients admitted to ICU for acute hypercapnic respiratory failure: a preliminary study. *Intensive Care Medicine* (2018) doi:10.1007/s00134-017-4998-3.

[14] Dan Adler, Jean-Louis Pépin, Elise Dupuis-Lozeron, Katerina Espa-Cervena, Roselyne Merlet-Violet, Hajo Muller, Jean-Paul Janssens, Laurent Brochard. Comorbidities and subgroups of patients surviving severe acute hypercapnic respiratory failure in the intensive care unit. *Am. J. Respir. Crit. Care Med.* (2017) doi:10.1164/rccm.201608-1666OC.

[15] Matthew T. V. Chan, Chew Yin Wang, Edwin Seet, Stanley Tam, Hou Yee Lai, Eleanor F. F. Chew, William K. K. Wu, Benny C. P. Cheng, Carmen K. M. Lam, Timothy G. Short, David S. C. Hui, Frances Chung, Postoperative Vascular Complications in Unrecognized Obstructive Sleep Apnea (POSA) Study

Investigators. Association of Unrecognized Obstructive Sleep Apnea with Postoperative Cardiovascular Events in Patients Undergoing Major Noncardiac Surgery. *JAMA - J. Am. Med. Assoc.* (2019) doi:10.1001/jama.2019.4783.

[16] Ana Fernandez-Bustamante, Karsten Bartels, Claudia Clavijo, Benjamin K. Scott, Rachel Kacmar, Kenneth Bullard, Angela F. D. Moss, William Henderson, Elizabeth Juarez-Colunga, Leslie Jameson. Preoperatively Screened Obstructive Sleep Apnea is Associated with Worse Postoperative Outcomes Than Previously Diagnosed Obstructive Sleep Apnea. *Anesth. Analg.* (2017) doi:10.1213/ANE.0000000000002241.

[17] Lin, P., Li, X., Zhang, J. & Liang, Z. Association between obstructive sleep apnea and reduced mortality in critically ill patients: A propensity score-based analysis. *Int. J. Gen. Med.* (2021) doi:10.2147/IJGM.S330752.

[18] Hang L. W., W. Chen, S. J. Liang, Y. C. Lin, C. Y. Tu, H. J. Chen, K. L. Chiu. Clinical characteristics and outcomes of patients with obstructive sleep apnoea requiring intensive care. *Anaesth. Intensive Care* (2010) doi:10.1177/0310057x1003800315.

[19] Lee, C. K., Tefera, E. & Colice, G. The effect of obesity on outcomes in mechanically ventilated patients in a medical intensive care unit. *Respiration* (2014) doi:10.1159/000357317.

[20] Oreste Marrone, Salvatore Battaglia, Paschalis Steiropoulos, Ozen K Basoglu, John A. Kvamme, Silke Ryan, Jean-Louis Pepin, Johan Verbraecken, Ludger Grote, Jan Hedner, Maria R. Bonsignore, ESADA study group. Chronic kidney disease in European patients with obstructive sleep apnea: the ESADA cohort study. *J. Sleep Res.* (2016) doi:10.1111/jsr.12426.

[21] Oreste Marrone, Fabio Cibella, Jean-Louis Pépin, Ludger Grote, Johan Verbraecken, Tarja Saaresranta, John A Kvamme, Ozen K Basoglu, Carolina Lombardi, Walter T. McNicholas, Jan Hedner, Maria R. Bonsignore, ESADA Network. Fixed But Not Autoadjusting Positive Airway Pressure Attenuates the Time-dependent Decline in Glomerular Filtration Rate in Patients With OSA. *Chest* (2018) doi:10.1016/j.chest.2018.04.020.

[22] Lin Dou, Haitao Lan, Daniel J. Reynolds, Tina M. Gunderson, Rahul Kashyap, Ognjen Gajic, Sean Caples, Guangxi Li, Kianoush B. Kashani. Association between Obstructive Sleep Apnea and Acute Kidney Injury in Critically Ill Patients: A Propensity-Matched Study. *Nephron* (2017) doi:10.1159/000453367.

[23] Besedovsky, L. & Born, J. Sleep, Don't Sneeze: Longer Sleep Reduces the Risk of Catching a Cold. *Sleep* (2015) doi:10.5665/sleep.4958.

[24] Beumer M. C., R. M. Koch, D. van Beuningen, A. M. OudeLashof, F. L. van de Veerdonk, E. Kolwijck, J. G. van der Hoeven, D. C. Bergmans, C W E Hoedemaekers. Influenza virus and factors that are associated with ICU admission, pulmonary co-infections and ICU mortality. *J. Crit. Care* (2019) doi:10.1016/j.jcrc.2018.11.013.

[25] Chung, F., Liao, P., Elsaid, H., Shapiro, C. M. & Kang, W. Factors associated with postoperative exacerbation of sleep-disordered breathing. *Anesthesiology* (2014) doi:10.1097/ALN.0000000000000041.

[26] Azadeh Yadollahi, Joseph M. Gabriel, Laura H. White, Luigi Taranto Montemurro, Takatoshi Kasai, T. Douglas Bradley. A randomized, double crossover study to investigate the influence of saline infusion on sleep apnea severity in men. *Sleep* (2014) doi:10.5665/sleep.4084.

[27] Glaser, J. B. & El-Haddad, H. Exploring novel medicare readmission risk variables in chronic obstructive pulmonary disease patients at high risk of readmission within 30 days of hospital discharge. *Ann. Am. Thorac. Soc.* (2015) doi:10.1513/Annals ATS.201504-228OC.

[28] Gupta, R. M., Parvizi, J., Hanssen, A. D. & Gay, P. C. Postoperative complications in patients with obstructive sleep apnea syndrome undergoing hip or knee replacement: A case-control study. *Mayo Clin. Proc.* (2001) doi:10.4065/76.9.897.

[29] Lavie, L. & Lavie, P. Ischemic preconditioning as a possible explanation for the age decline relative mortality in sleep apnea. *Med. Hypotheses* (2006) doi:10.1016/j. mehy.2005.10.033.

[30] Berger, S., Aronson, D., Lavie, P. & Lavie, L. Endothelial progenitor cells in acute myocardial infarction and sleep-disordered breathing. *Am. J. Respir. Crit. Care Med.* (2013) doi:10.1164/rccm.201206-1144OC.

[31] Steiner, S., Schueller, P. O., Schulze, V. & Strauer, B. E. Occurrence of coronary collateral vessels in patients with sleep apnea and total coronary occlusion. *Chest* (2010) doi:10.1378/chest.09-1136.

[32] Lavie, L. & Lavie, P. Coronary collateral circulation in sleep apnea: A cardioprotective mechanism? *Chest* (2010) doi:10.1378/chest.09-2657.

[33] de Kruif, M. D., Voncken, S. F. J., Laven, S. A. J. S., Feron, T. M. H. & Kolfoort-Otte, A. A. B. Obstructive sleep apnea and risk of COVID-19 infection, hospitalization and respiratory failure. *Sleep and Breathing* (2021) doi:10.1007/s11325-020-02271-2.

[34] Maas, M. B., Kim, M., Malkani, R. G., Abbott, S. M. & Zee, P. C. Obstructive Sleep Apnea and Risk of COVID-19 Infection, Hospitalization and Respiratory Failure. *Sleep Breath.* (2021) doi:10.1007/s11325-020-02203-0.

[35] Voncken S. F. J., T. M. H. Feron, S. A. J. S. Laven, U. Karaca, K. Beerhorst, P. Klarenbeek, J. M. J. A. A. Straetmans, G. J. de Vries, A. A. B. Kolfoort-Otte, M D de Kruif· Impact of obstructive sleep apnea on clinical outcomes in patients hospitalized with COVID-19. *Sleep Breath.* (2022) doi:10.1007/s11325-021-02476-z.

[36] Cade, B. E., Dashti, H. S., Hassan, S. M., Redline, S. & Karlson, E. W. Sleep apnea and COVID-19 mortality and hospitalization. *American Journal of Respiratory and Critical Care Medicine* (2020) doi:10.1164/rccm.202006-2252LE.

[37] Vincent Yi-Fong Su, Chia-Jen Liu, Hsin-Kai Wang, Li-An Wu, Shi-Chuan Chang, Diahn-Warng Perng, Wei-Juin Su, Yuh-Min Chen, Elizabeth Ya-Hsuan Lin, Tzeng-Ji Chen, Kun-Ta Chou. Sleep apnea and risk of pneumonia: A nationwide population-based study. *C. Can. Med. Assoc. J.* (2014) doi:10.1503/cmaj.131547.

[38] Eusebi Chiner, Mónica Llombart, Joan Valls, Esther Pastor, José N. Sancho-Chust, Ada Luz Andreu, Manuel Sánchez-de-la-Torre, Ferran Barbé. Association between obstructive sleep apnea and community-acquired pneumonia. *PLoS One* (2016) doi:10.1371/journal.pone.0152749.

[39] Michael Beal, Andrew Chesson, Thomas Garcia, Gloria Caldito, Fred Stucker, Cherie-Ann Nathan. A pilot study of quantitative aspiration in patients with symptoms of obstructive sleep apnea: Comparison to a historic control group. *Laryngoscope* (2004) doi:10.1097/00005537-200406000-00002.

[40] Mahesh Nagappa, David T Wong, Crispiana Cozowicz, Satya Krishna Ramachandran, Stavros G Memtsoudis, Frances Chung. Is obstructive sleep apnea associated with difficult airway? Evidence from a systematic review and meta-analysis of prospective and retrospective cohort studies. *PLoS One* (2018) doi:10.1371/journal.pone.0204904.

[41] Sefer Elezkurtaj, Selina Greuel, Jana Ihlow, Edward Georg Michaelis, Philip Bischoff, Catarina Alisa Kunze, Bruno Valentin Sinn, Manuela Gerhold, Kathrin Hauptmann, Barbara Ingold-Heppner, Florian Miller, Hermann Herbst, Victor Max Corman, Hubert Martin, Helena Radbruch, Frank L Heppner, David Horst. Causes of death and comorbidities in hospitalized patients with COVID-19. *Sci. Rep.* (2021) doi:10.1038/s41598-021-82862-5.

Chapter 2

Comorbidities: Key Practical Recommendations

Jamal Al-Aghbari[1,*], MD and Mohammed Al-Abri[2], MD, PhD

[1]Department of Medicine, Sultan Qaboos University Hospital, Muscat, Oman
[2]Department of Clinical Physiology, College of Medicine and Health Sciences, Sultan Qaboos University, Muscat, Oman

Abstract

Obstructive sleep apnea (OSA) is a common sleep-disordered breathing associated with repetitive apneas, hypopneas, or respiratory effort-related arousals. OSA is associated with increased prevalence of many comorbidities including cardiovascular diseases like arrhythmias particularly atrial fibrillation, heart failure, stroke, pulmonary hypertension, and metabolic disturbance including diabetes mellitus and dyslipidemia. Depression and mood changes are also common in OSA. Furthermore, there are overlaps in the clinical presentations of some of these comorbidities and OSA symptoms making the possibility of underdiagnoses of OSA or its comorbidities. Some of these comorbidities are a physiological sequela of OSA. Though some comorbidities could be linked to obesity, there is growing evidence of OSA as an independent risk factor. Continuous positive airway pressure (CPAP) has been proven to alleviate some of these comorbidities or their severity while additional detailed studies are required to further characterize benefits in some others.

---

* Corresponding Author's Email: jamaln@squ.edu.om

In: Obstructive Sleep Apnea in Pulmonary Critical Care
Editors: Antonio M. Esquinas and Takatoshi Kasai
ISBN: 979-8-88697-858-2

Keywords: obstructive sleep apnea, comorbidities, cardiovascular diseases, continuous positive airway pressure, sleep-disordered breathing

Introduction

The incidence of cardiovascular diseases and cardiovascular events has increased in OSA patients. Similarly, there is a proportional relationship between all-cause mortality and the severity of OSA [1]. The current available data suggests that CPAP therapy is ineffective as a secondary prevention of cardiovascular diseases or cardiovascular events [2], however, there are many limitations in the current available evidence urging further randomized controlled trials. Many other cardiovascular diseases are associated with OSA including systemic hypertension, ischemic heart disease, arrhythmias particularly atrial fibrillation, heart failure, stroke, and pulmonary hypertension. Depression and metabolic disturbance including diabetes mellitus are also associated with OSA. While CPAP can be effective on reducing some of these comorbidities, still there is a gap in the knowledge of CPAP efficacy on others. Further studies targeting OSA phenotypes might be the key to answer many questions.

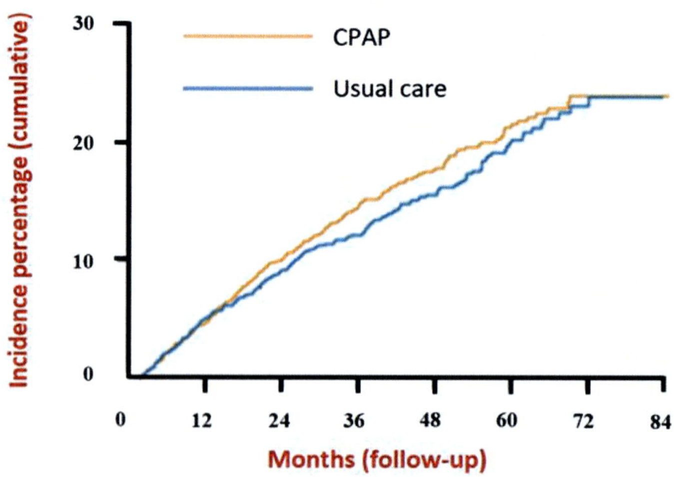

Figure 1. Cumulative incidence of the primary endpoint comparing CPAP group (CPAP plus usual care) and usual care group (usual care alone). N Engl J Med 2016; 375:919-93.

OSA and Cardiovascular Diseases

Cardiovascular Events

Observational studies have shown that OSA is associated with increased cardiovascular disease and increased morbidity and mortality. Sleep-disordered breathing increases all-cause mortality in proportion to the severity of sleep-disordered breathing as classified by apnea/hypopnea index (AHI) with hazard ratios of 0.93, 1.17, and 1.46 for mild, moderate, and severe OSA respectively [1]. This risk is particularly worse in men aged forty to seventy and coronary artery disease follows the same pattern as all-cause mortality [1].

The Sleep Apnea Cardiovascular Endpoints (SAVE) study which was one of the largest randomized controlled trials to investigate the benefit of CPAP in preventing cardiovascular events revealed that CPAP did not prevent cardiovascular events in those with moderate to severe OSA and existing cardiovascular diseases or coronary artery disease (Figure 1). These cardiovascular events include cardiovascular deaths, stroke, myocardial infarction, hospitalizations for unstable angina, transient ischemic attack, or heart failure [2]. However, there are many limitations in this study which include the exclusion of the sleepy population with an Epworth sleepiness score (ESS) of 15 (range of 0-24), or severely hypoxic patients (oxygen saturation <80% for more than 10% of recorded time) and those who are at elevated risk of road traffic accident. Furthermore, the study was conducted on patients with already established cardiovascular disease (i.e., not primary prevention). In addition, the diagnosis of OSA in the studied population was made by Apnea Link (automated oximetry) rather than full polysomnography and the adherence to CPAP was poor (mean of 3.3 hours per night). All these limitations constrain the generalization of these results. Several meta-analyses of RCT showed comparable results [3] with different OSA severity and duration of treatment. Further RCTs are required to indicate CPAP benefit on OSA patients according to patient characteristics or phenotypes (e.g., sleep vs non-sleepy patients).

Coronary Artery Disease

There is convincing evidence that untreated men with severe OSA (mean AHI of 45 events/hour) are associated with increased non-fatal cardiovascular events including stroke, myocardial infarction, and acute coronary syndrome, as well as fatal cardiovascular events irrespective of confounding factors including obesity when it is compared with patient with mild to moderate OSA [4]. This reflects the importance of CPAP treatment. Further RCTs are needed to prove the CPAP effect on cardiovascular outcomes.

Hypertension

There is a well-known association between OSA and hypertension with close to fifty percent of OSA patients being hypertensive. Furthermore, there is an increased prevalence of OSA in patients with resistant hypertension. OSA is also linked to non-dipping nocturnal blood pressure, particularly in those who have cardiovascular risk and moderate to severe OSA [5]. A prospective population-based study for patients with OSA found that after four years of follow-up, there was a proportional relationship between the severity of OSA and the presence of hypertension with an odds ratio of 2.03 and 2.89 for mild and moderate-severe OSA respectively after adjustment for other risk factors [6]. One meta-analysis has shown that using CPAP is associated with a small reduction in systolic blood pressure (mean of 2.6 mmHg) [7]. This little reduction is clinically important as it can lessen cardiovascular risk. Additional studies are required to further characterized benefits in certain groups of OSA patients like sleepy patients and to investigate benefits according to the severity of OSA. Moreover, more evidence is required to examine the effect of withdrawal of CPAP on blood pressure control, the effect on diastolic blood pressure, the effect of CPAP when it is compared to antihypertensive agents, duration of CPAP usage to see the effect and alternative treatment to CPAP and their effect on blood pressure.

Atrial Fibrillation and Other Arrhythmias

Arrhythmias in general and particularly atrial fibrillation are associated with OSA. These arrhythmias were attributed to several physiological changes in OSA which include hypoxia and it is associated with delayed depolarization, fluctuated autonomic system, and respiratory acidosis. The prevalence of atrial fibrillation (AF) in OSA patients is variable from 2% to 5% independent of other risk factors and it is three to four folds higher than the general population. Outcomes of sleep disorders in older men (MrOS) study revealed that the prevalence of atrial fibrillation and complex ventricular ectopy (CVE) are proportionally correlated to the severity of sleep-disordered breathing (SDB) measured by respiratory disturbance index (RDI) in older men. Though this study also showed that CVE is more prevalent in obstructive sleep apnea as compared with AF which was more common in central sleep apnea [8].

Patients with OSA have an elevated risk of recurrent AF after ablation compared with non-OSA patients close to 31%. This risk can increase to 57% if CPAP therapy is not used. Furthermore, CPAP can reduce AF recurrence at a rate close to the non-OSA patient [9].

Other arrhythmias like conduction delay including sinus pause, asystole, and atrioventricular block were reported in old literature but have never been proven in large studies. Ventricular arrhythmia, on the other hand, has been linked to OSA as well [10], yet large RCTs are still required to determine the utility of CPAP or alternative therapy to prevent or reduce the recurrent rate.

Stroke

There is growing evidence of an increased incidence of stroke in OSA patients. Several hypotheses have been proposed as mechanisms for increasing stroke risk. Firstly, OSA is associated with an increase in other cardiovascular risks including diabetes mellitus and insulin resistance, hypertension, heart diseases, and atrial fibrillation. Furthermore, there might be a reduction in cerebral flow velocity secondary to increased intrathoracic pressure because of the obstructive events. Moreover, intermittent hypoxia can attenuate the cerebral vasodilatory response. Similarly, endothelial dysfunction secondary to oxidant stress and an increase in sympathetic drive all can play a role in the pathogenesis of stroke. Likewise, OSA can result in pulmonary hypertension which could lead to right to left shunt in patients with patent foramen ovale (PFO) and therefore possible paradoxical embolism and stroke. The hazard ratio (HR) is 2.89 in one observational study irrespective of confounding factors like diabetes mellitus, hypertension, previous stroke, atrial fibrillation, smoking history, body mass index, age, or gender. This risk corresponds proportionally to the severity of OSA with hazard ratios of 2.44 and 3.56 in patients with AHI (5-15) and >15 events per hour respectively [11]. Using CPAP may alleviate some of the proposed risk factors for stroke like improving blood pressure. Though some RCTs have shown no proven effect on the rate of stroke after CPAP therapy [2]. However large detailed RCTs to investigate the benefit of CPAP in reducing stroke incidence are lacking.

Heart Failure

The prevalence of heart failure in OSA patients is variable in the literature between 50% to 75%. Many physiological changes could explain this correlation which includes reduced preload and increased afterload because of increased negative intrathoracic pressure during obstructive respiratory events. Similarly, increasing sympathetic drive could increase heart failure recurrence. In addition, some of the OSA's symptoms can be confused with heart failure symptoms like paroxysmal nocturnal dyspnea and nocturia due to diuresis which can lead to under recognition of OSA. On other hand, heart failure is proposed as a risk to worsen OSA, particularly in supine positions due to neck edema.

The risk to develop heart failure is worse in men and those with severe OSA. The risk is approximately 59% compared with subjects with no OSA [12]. CPAP therapy reduces the incidence of heart failure in those more than 60 years of age [13].

Pulmonary Hypertension

Pulmonary hypertension due to OSA belongs to group 3 according to the clinical classification of pulmonary hypertension (i.e., pulmonary hypertension due to lung disease and/or hypoxia). The severity of pulmonary hypertension in OSA patients is usually mild if there is no coexisting other potential etiology for pulmonary hypertension. Pulmonary hypertension can also be a prognostic factor in OSA patients. CPAP therapy has been proven to improve systolic pulmonary arterial pressure and pulmonary vascular resistance after a few months of treatment.

OSA and Metabolic Disturbance

Diabetes and insulin resistance are proven in cross-sectional studies to be associated with OSA. Similarly, increasing OSA severity is associated with increasing type 2 diabetes incidence independent of possible confounding factors like body mass index, age, race, gender, and baseline fasting glucose. This risk is less in those who use CPAP [14]. OSA not only leads to an increased risk of diabetes, but it is associated with other metabolic disturbances which can lead to metabolic syndrome. This is attributed to the intermittent hypoxia and its effect on accelerating metabolic derangement in patients with obesity, fatty liver disease, and insulin resistance. This is reflected in increased triglyceride levels and visceral fat in OSA patients [15].

OSA and Depression

There is a major association between depression and OSA. Furthermore, there are some overlapping symptoms that can lead to under detection of either OSA or depression. These symptoms include depressive symptoms, low energy, anxiety, fatigue, poor concentration, and sleep problems. The prevalence of depression is higher in OSA patients than in the general population. Similarly, the prevalence of OSA in major depression disorder (MDD) is 18%. Depression itself carries a risk of coronary artery disease [16].

Conclusion

OSA is associated with increased cardiovascular events and there is dose-response relationship between the severity of OSA and all-cause mortality. Current available data suggests that CPAP therapy is ineffective as a secondary prevention of cardiovascular diseases or cardiovascular events, however more structured studies needed to prove this fact and as well as to investigate the benefits of CPAP as a primary prevention. Many other cardiovascular diseases are associated with OSA including systemic hypertension, ischemic heart disease, arrhythmias particularly atrial fibrillation, heart failure, stroke, and pulmonary hypertension. CPAP therapy has been proven as effective in alleviating some of these comorbidities even if the effect is minimal, as the case for systemic hypertension which can have significant clinical impact. OSA is also associated with metabolic disturbance reflected in insulin resistance, diabetes mellitus, dyslipidemia and fatty liver. This metabolic disturbance can exert additional cardiovascular risk. Depression and OSA are linked comorbidities and their clinical manifestation can be confused with each other. This can lead to underdiagnosis of OSA or depression. The efficacy of CPAP or other OSA treatment modalities in many comorbidities are ambiguous urging further studies targeting different OSA phenotypes.

References

[1] Punjabi N. M., Caffo B. S., Goodwin J. L., Gottlieb D. J., Newman A. B., O'Connor G. T., Rapoport D. M., Redline S., Resnick H. E., Robbins J. A., Shahar E., Unruh M. L. and Samet J. M. Sleep-disordered breathing and mortality: a prospective cohort study. *PLoS Med.* 2009 Aug;6(8): e1000132.

[2] McEvoy R. D., Antic N. A., Heeley E., Luo Y., Ou Q., Zhang X., Mediano O., Chen R., Drager L. F., Liu Z., Chen G., Du B., McArdle N., Mukherjee S., Tripathi M., Billot L., Li Q., Biostat M., Lorenzi-Filho G., Barbe F., Redline S., Wang J., Arima H., Neal B., White D. P., Grunstein R. R., Zhong N. and Anderson C. S. CPAP for Prevention of Cardiovascular Events in Obstructive Sleep Apnea. *N Engl J Med.* 2016 Sep 8;375(10):919–31.

[3] Yu J., Zhou Z., McEvoy R. D., Anderson C. S., Rodgers A., Perkovic V. and Neal B. Association of Positive Airway Pressure with Cardiovascular Events and Death in Adults with Sleep Apnea: A Systematic Review and Meta-analysis. *JAMA.* 2017 jul 11;318(2):156–66.

[4] Marin J. M., Carrizo S. J., Vicente E. and Agusti A. G. N. Long-term cardiovascular outcomes in men with obstructive sleep apnoea-hypopnoea with or without treatment with continuous positive airway pressure: an observational study. *Lancet.* 2005 Mar 19;365(9464):1046–53.

[5] Seif F., Patel S. R., Walia H. K., Rueschman M., Bhatt D. L., Blumenthal R. S., Quan S. F., Gottlieb D. J., Lewis E. F., Patil S. P., Punjabi N. M., Babineau D. C., Redline S. and Mehra R. Obstructive sleep apnea and diurnal nondipping hemodynamic indices in patients at increased cardiovascular risk. *J Hypertens.* 2014 Feb;32(2):267–75.

[6] Peppard P. E., Young T., Palta M. and Skatrud J. Prospective study of the association between sleep-disordered breathing and hypertension. *N Engl J Med.* 2000 May 11;342(19):1378–84.

[7] Fava C., Dorigoni S., Dalle Vedove F., Danese E., Montagnana M., Guidi G. C., Narkiewicz K. and Minuz P. Effect of CPAP on blood pressure in patients with OSA/hypopnea a systematic review and meta-analysis. *Chest.* 2014 Apr;145(4):762–71.

[8] Mehra R., Stone K. L., Varosy P. D., Hoffman A. R., Marcus G. M., Blackwell T., Ibrahim O. A., Salem R. and Redline S. Nocturnal Arrhythmias across a spectrum of obstructive and central sleep-disordered breathing in older men: outcomes of sleep disorders in older men (MrOS sleep) study. *Arch Intern Med.* 2009 Jun 22;169(12):1147–55.

[9] Li L., Wang Z. Wu, Li J., Ge X., Guo L. zhu, Wang Y., Guo W. Hua, Jiang C. Xi and Ma C. Sheng. Efficacy of catheter ablation of atrial fibrillation in patients with obstructive sleep apnoea with and without continuous positive airway pressure treatment: a meta-analysis of observational studies. *Europace.* 2014 Sep;16(9):1309–14.

[10] Raghuram A., Clay R., Kumbam A., Tereshchenko L. G. and Khan A. A Systematic Review of the Association between Obstructive Sleep Apnea and Ventricular Arrhythmias. *J Clin Sleep Med.* 2014 Oct 15;10(10):1155–60.

[11] Valham F., Mooe T., Rabben T., Stenlund H., Wiklund U. and Franklin K. A. Increased risk of stroke in patients with coronary artery disease and sleep apnea: a 10-year follow-up. *Circulation.* 2008 Aug 26;118(9):955–60.

[12] Gottlieb D. J., Yenokyan G., Newman A. B., O'Connor G. T., Punjabi N. M., Quan S. F., Redline S., Resnick H. E., Tong E. K., Diener-West M. and Shahar E. Prospective study of obstructive sleep apnea and incident coronary heart disease and heart failure: the sleep heart health study. *Circulation.* 2010 Jul 27;122(4):352–60.

[13] Holt A., Bjerre J., Zareini B., Koch H., Tønnesen P., Gislason G. H., Nielsen O. W., Schou M. and Lamberts M. Sleep Apnea, the Risk of Developing Heart Failure, and Potential Benefits of Continuous Positive Airway Pressure (CPAP) Therapy. *J Am Heart Assoc.* 2018 Jun 22;7(13):e008684.

[14] Botros N., Concato J., Mohsenin V., Selim B., Doctor K. and Yaggi K. Obstructive Sleep Apnea as a Risk Factor for Type II Diabetes. *Am J Med.* 2009 Dec;122(12):1122–7.

[15] Drager L. F., Togeiro S. M., Polotsky V. Y. and Lorenzi-Filho G. Obstructive Sleep Apnea: A Cardiometabolic Risk in Obesity and the Metabolic Syndrome. *J Am Coll Cardiol.* 2013 Aug 13;62(7):569–76.

[16] Jehan S., Auguste E., Pandi-Perumal S. R., Kalinowski J., Myers A. K., Zizi F., Rajanna M. G., Jean-Louis G. and McFarlane S. I. Depression, Obstructive Sleep Apnea and Psychosocial Health. *Sleep Med Disord.* 2017;1(3):00012.

Chapter 3

Pharmacological Treatment

Diogo Canhoto*, **MD**
Pulmonology Department, Coimbra Hospital and University Centre, Portugal

Abstract

Obstructive sleep apnea (OSA) is managed through a combination of measures aimed at improving upper airway patency, including positive airway pressure treatment and oral appliances. Historically, pharmacotherapy of OSA has been met with relative unsuccess, and lacks sufficient evidence for safe recommendation. This is attributed to suboptimal efficacy and low tolerability, which are often compounded in the intensive care setting.

Keywords: comorbidity, high dependency unit, obstructive sleep apnea, pharmacologic treatment, sedation

Introduction

Obstructive sleep apnea (OSA) is traditionally managed with a combination of interventions aimed at improving upper airway patency and sleep architecture and ventilatory drive. These range from lifestyle adjustments to anatomical interventions on the sleeping patient's upper airway anatomy (oral devices, surgery), to positive airway pressure (PAP) treatment [1].

Pharmacological treatment of OSA takes up a marginal fraction of management efforts, related to its relative lack of efficacy and unwanted side

* Corresponding Author's Email: diogo.mcanhoto@gmail.com.

In: Obstructive Sleep Apnea in Pulmonary Critical Care
Editors: Antonio M. Esquinas and Takatoshi Kasai
ISBN: 979-8-88697-858-2

effects. In the high dependency unit (HDU) setting, control of symptoms and comorbidities, improvement of ventilatory dynamics, and reduction of cardiovascular and metabolic stress may be the most desired benefits of OSA treatment. However, pharmacotherapeutic options have been limited [2, 3]. This derives from the fact that many interventions directed at OSA treatment are most appropriately performed electively and represent an additional burden on an already strained organism suffering from acute illness, and from the fact that they may be rendered futile by the patient's setting (e.g., measures aimed at prevention of airway collapse in an intubated patient).

Comorbidity Management

Comorbidity management, not only important, may also be useful in ameliorating OSA severity and symptoms.

The HDU is an environment prone to disrupt sleep, as 24-h intensive monitorization is in place, the patient's typical zeitgebers may be absent, and interventions to the patient or others admitted may be required in the patient's traditional resting hours, leading to insufficient sleep and sleep fragmentation [4]. These represent fertile grounds for the development of sleep-wake rhythm disorders. Ideally, the unit should be illuminated in a schedule respecting the physiological sleep-wake rhythm, if possible, with natural light. Exercise activities and stimulation such as rehabilitation should also be performed in the beginning of the day. Procedures that may disrupt patient's nightly rest and need not be undertaken urgently may be postponed to the following day [5]. Specific intervention for insomnia or restless legs syndrome may need to be undertaken.

Central sleep apnea (CSA) may derive from neurological (e.g., cerebral vascular accidents) or cardiac (e.g., decompensated heart failure) insults, as well as be secondary to the patient's medication (e.g., opioid analgesia). CSA may co-exist initially with OSA, further contributing to the instability of the patient's ventilatory control or emerge following its treatment. Moreover, it may contribute to the overestimation of OSA severity itself, as obstructive hypopnea scoring in adults is easily overestimated by current scoring methods [6].

Hypervolemia from a myriad of causes may promote upper airway collapse, by accumulation of fluid in the cephalad regions of the body [7].

Psychiatric disturbances, such as mood disorders have been shown to be prevalent in HDU-admitted patients and are frequent comorbidities in OSA patients [8, 9].

Increased sympathetic tone from OSA may promote the development of dysrhythmia (which may be refractory), arterial hypertension (particularly in a non-dipping pattern during the night period), as well as dysglycemia [10].

Obstructive airway disease (including asthma and chronic obstructive pulmonary disease) may be difficult to compensate in OSA patients. In these overlap patients, desaturations may be more pronounced, hypoventilation may occur, and ventilatory management may become more challenging.

General Interventions

In HDU, body positioning is essential to promote venous return, prevent the development of stress ulcers and improve ventilatory dynamics. However, during this process, positions favoring airway collapsibility occur. For instance, patients placed in Trendelenburg position as a response to hypovolemic hypotension may experience worsening of their upper airway collapsibility.

For some patients, owing to trauma or post-operative states, the fraction of time in the supine position is far greater, which contributes to worsening of their apnea-hypopnea index (AHI). A common example are patients with cervical collar immobilization devices.

Catabolism and weight loss are common during acute illness, and even more so in critical patients, where they occur faster and are more pronounced. Although this may have some protective effect on the severity (or even existence) of OSA, nutritional management should be individualized for each patient considering factors that relate not only to dynamic upper airway obstruction during the patient's sleep. For the patients who exhibit significant weight loss, particularly from thoracoabdominal and cervical fat stores, a reduction of respiratory disturbance index and positive pressure requirements may be observed [11].

Musculoskeletal strength and aerobic reconditioning exercises, which may be performed during rehabilitation, may improve sleep efficiency and macrostructure [12].

Nasal patency could be improved by use of nasal corticosteroids or anticholinergics, antihistamine drugs, leukotriene receptor antagonists, as well as short courses of topical sympathomimetics, depending on the etiology of the patient's rhinitis. Although their direct effect on OSA itself is modest at best, improvement of non-invasive interface tolerance could justify their use.

Restriction of Worsening Medication

In the HDU, arousability and muscle tone are often decreased as a product of the underlying pathology (e.g., an intoxication), comorbidities (e.g., myopathy), or iatrogenic intervention (e.g., sedation, neuromuscular blockade). This results in an impairment of the physiological response to obstructive events, leading to prolonged and more severe hypoxemic events.

Notably, some common sedative agents suspected to aggravate OSA are frequently administered in the HDU, often in prolonged infusions. This is the case of benzodiazepines, opioids, as well as barbiturates. These promote a decrease in the state of consciousness as well as a reduction in muscle tone, therefore predisposing to upper airway collapse. Some studies suggest an association not only with OSA, but also with CSA, in some cases in a dose-dependent manner (e.g., opioids). However, these findings are becoming somewhat controversial following a Cochrane systematic review suggesting that the effects of these drugs may have been overestimated [13].

Use of these medications should be limited to the minimum necessary. When benzodiazepines are used for hypnotic purposes, replacement with a Z-drug may have a lesser impact on the AHI (e.g., zolpidem, zopiclone). Lastly, careful down-titration of these drugs needs often be performed progressively as to prevent withdrawal symptoms.

Analogously, treatments aimed at antagonizing or clearing substances that may hinder patient's arousal (e.g., ethanol or opioid detoxication) should be undertaken.

Pharmacologic Treatment

As mentioned previously, the role of pharmacological treatment in OSA is quite limited, as more effective treatment options exist.

Attention should be devoted to the effect of drugs on sleep macrostructure disruption, namely their effect on slow wave sleep (SWS) and rapid eye movement (REM) sleep, as well as the possible promotion of insomnia and restless legs syndrome. Typical examples are the REM suppression provoked by tricyclic antidepressants, or the triggering of restless legs syndrome by selective serotonin reuptake inhibitors. Moreover, should these drugs be withdrawn, rebound of sleep stages may occur. In the case of REM, a possible worsening of OSA may develop, secondary to loss of upper airway tonicity in a greater fraction of the night.

Nocturnal oxygen use is markedly controversial in OSA and has been mainly adjuvant to other (namely PAP) treatments. Caution should be exerted due to its inhibitory effect of respiratory drive, which may promote longer obstructive events, and thus more prolonged hypoxemia. Furthermore, this may occur in the face of an improvement of oxygen saturation, which may cover the more detrimental aspects of its use [14].

Carbonic anhydrase inhibitors (e.g., acetazolamide) may reduce ventilatory instability by reduction of loop gain. Nonetheless, side effects frequently limit their use and are poorly tolerated (electrolyte disturbances, dysgeusia, paresthesia of extremities). Moreover, their efficacy on symptomatic improvement is reduced.

Methylxanthines such as theophylline act by increasing respiratory drive but have narrow therapeutic intervals and modest efficacy. Moreover, their stimulating effect may promote insomnia and their diuretic effect can contribute to the nycturia already observed in OSA.

Experimentation with other drugs has occurred along the history of OSA treatment, which, in one way or another, relate to a relative reduction in REM percentage, improvement of upper airway tonicity, or improvement of arousal. These include progesterone, atomoxetine, oxybutinin, desipramine, fluoxetine, protriptyline, and donepezil. Their efficacy has been mostly negligible to justify their use, and safety concerns frequently arise due to their potential cardiovascular effects [15]. The same concern exists with some stimulants (e.g., modafinil) which are less commonly used to treat residual sleepiness in OSA patients, and whose side effects may be even more relevant in the HDU setting.

Conclusion

Pharmacological treatment of obstructive sleep apnea is multimodal and in the intensive care setting is limited by relative lack of efficacy and side effects. It is necessary to take into account that the spectrum of comorbidities of OSA is broad and these should be aggressively managed, measures such as positioning, and rehabilitation may improve OSA patient's sleep and withdrawal of iatrogenic drugs and treatment of intoxications are paramount for the treatment of sleep apnoea.

References

[1] Pvwoski P, Shelgikar AV. 2017. Treatment options for obstructive sleep apnea. *Neurol. Clin. Pract.* 7(1): 77-85.

[2] Curado TF, Berger S, Polotsky VY. 2019. Pharmacotherapy of Obstructive Sleep Apnea: Is Salvation Just Around a Corner? *Am. J. Respir. Crit. Care Med.* 15;199(10):1186-7.

[3] Vasu TS, Grewal R, Doghramji K. 2012. Obstructive Sleep Apnea Syndrome and Perioperative Complications: A Systematic Review of the Literature. *J. Clin. Sleep Med.* 8(2):199-207.

[4] Chan M, Spieth P M, Quinn K, Matteo P, Zhang H, Slutski A S. 2014. Circadian rhythms: From basic mechanisms to the intensive care unit. *Crit. Care Med.* 40(1):246-53.

[5] Telias I, Wilcox M E. 2019. Sleep and Circadian Rhythm in Critical Illness. *Critical Care.* 23(1): 82.

[6] Zhang J, Wang L, Guo G, Wang Y, Cao J, Chen B. 2020. Treatment-emergent central sleep apnea: a unique sleep-disordered breathing. *Chin. Med. J. (Engl).* 133(22):2721-30.

[7] Bradley T D, Floras J S. 2003. Sleep Apnea and Heart Failure. Part I: Obstructive Sleep Apnea. *Circulation.* 107:1671-8.

[8] Lu M, Tan H, Tsai I, Huang L, Liao X, Lin S. 2017. Sleep apnea is associated with an increased risk of mood disorders: a population-based cohort study. *Sleep Breath.* 21(2):243-53.

[9] Marwale A V, Phadke S S, Kocher A S. 2022. Psychiatric management of patients in intensive care units. *Indian J. Psychiatry.* 64(Suppl 2):S292-307.

[10] Rossi V A, Stradling J R, Kohler M. 2013. Effects of obstructive sleep apnoea on heart rhythm. *Eur. Resp. J.* 41:1439-51.

[11] Corral A, Caples S M, Lopez-Jimenez F, Somers VK. 2010. Interactions Between Obesity and Obstructive Sleep Apnea. *Chest.* 137(3):711-9.

[12] Nobeschi L, Zangirolami-Raimundo J, Cordoni P K, Squassoni S D, Fiss E, Pérez-Riera A R, Abreu LC, Raimundo R D. 2020. Evaluation of sleep quality and daytime somnolence in patients with chronic obstructive pulmonary disease in pulmonary rehabilitation. *BMC Pulm. Med.* 20(1):14.

[13] Mason M, Cates C J, Smith I. 2015. Effects of opioid, hypnotic and sedating medications on sleep-disordered breathing in adults with obstructive sleep apnoea. *Cochrane Database Syst. Rev.* (7):CD011090.

[14] Mehta V, Vasu T S, Phillips B, Chung F. 2013. Obstructive Sleep Apnea and Oxygen Therapy: A Systematic Review of the Literature and Meta-Analysis. *J. Clin. Sleep Med.* 9(3):271-9.

[15] Arredondo E, DeLeon M, Masozera I, Panahi L, Udeani G, Tran N, Nguyen C K, Atphaisit C, de la Sota B, Gonzalez Jr. G, Liou E, Mayo Z, Nwosu J, Shiver TL. 2022. Overview of the Role of Pharmacological Management of Obstructive Sleep Apnea. *Medicina (Kaunas)*. 58(2):225.

Chapter 4

High-Flow Nasal Oxygen Sleep-Disordered Breathing

Stefano Oldani[1,*], MD
Massimo Terenzoni[2], MD
Chiara Martone[3], MD
Emanuele Checcoli[3], MD
Martina Venturi[4], MD
and Andrea De Vito[3], MD

[1]Department Thoracic Diseases, Pulmonary Operative Unit, Forlì Hospital, Health Local Agency of Romagna, Italy
[2]Department of General Surgery, Anaesthesia and Critical Care Unit, Ravenna Hospital, Health Local Agency of Romagna, Italy
[3]Head and Neck Department, ENT Unit, Ravenna - Lugo Hospitals, Health Local Agency of Romagna, Italy
[4]Department ENT & Audiology, University of Ferrara, Ferrara, Italy

Abstract

High Flow Nasal Oxygen (HFNO) is a way to administer oxygen therapy with a reliable and stable Fraction of inspire O2 (FiO2), through a heated and humidified flow of gases, that is usually comfortable enough to be bearable even 24 hours a day for numerous days in a row. HFNO helps patients both in the inspiratory and in the expiratory phase of the breathing cycle, and could gain a potential role in the treatment of sleep disordered breathing, especially in obstructive sleep apnea and/or

* Corresponding Author's Email: stefano.oldani111289@gmail.com.

In: Obstructive Sleep Apnea in Pulmonary Critical Care
Editors: Antonio M. Esquinas and Takatoshi Kasai
ISBN: 979-8-88697-858-2

hypoventilation. In fact, HFNO might help to restore airway patency and to overcome flow limitation of the upper airway.

However, the sample size few studies reported in current literature are too small to adequately evaluate the responses, and with the application of HFNO just for one night. Moreover, there are no published data about the use of HFNO for more than one consecutive nights in the adult population affected by OSA. Furthermore, a retrospective study conducted on a small population of children with OSA showed that home HFNO was feasible and effective in reducing AHI, although 42% of the patients discontinued the treatment due to intolerance issue within 12 months. To summarize, there is no evidence about the effectiveness of HFNO application in patients affected by OSA.

Keywords: high flow nasal oxygen, obstructive sleep apnea, continuous positive airway pressure, flow limitation

Introduction

High flow nasal oxygen (HFNO) has gained popularity in recent years, especially in the management of acute respiratory failure, as filler of the gap in the respiratory support escalation between standard oxygen therapy and noninvasive or invasive mechanical ventilation [1]. The main components of a HFNO system are four:

1) A flow generator, usually a turbine, that can convey 20 to 70 L/min of fresh air
2) An active humidification system, to regulate the temperature and the humidity of the gases provided
3) A source of oxygen, to deliver oxygen to be mixed with the airflow generated by the turbine. All HFNO systems must have a way to monitor and manage the Fraction of inspire O2 (FiO2) provided to the patient. FiO2 can therefore range from 21% (no oxygen added to the air flow) to 100%.
4) An interface. HFNO is usually provided with a peculiar nasal cannula, available in different calibers in order to adapt to the patient's nostrils. In tracheostomized patients, specific connections to the tracheal cannula are usable as well.

Thus, HFNO is a way to administer oxygen therapy with a reliable and stable FiO2, through a heated and humidified flow of gases, that is usually comfortable enough to be bearable even 24 hours a day for numerous days in a row.

Effects of the High Flow Nasal Oxygen on Respiratory Physiology

There are several desirable effects of HFNO on respiratory physiology. In fact, HFNO helps patients both in the inspiratory and in the expiratory phase of the breathing cycle.

During inspiration, high flow sustains the patient's inspiratory effort, reducing it significantly when a flow of at least 20-45 L/min is provided. Moreover, as flow increases, respiratory rate, and minute ventilation decrease, without any resultant hypercapnia, thanks to the ability of high flow to obtain a washout of the physiological dead space of the respiratory airways. In fact, the high flow of air guarantees the replacement of the end expiratory CO2-rich air in the dead space with oxygenated air, contributing to both a better oxygenation and a reduction of the amount of rebreathed CO2 [2].

As aforementioned, HFNO also plays an important role during the expiratory phase. It can oppose the expiratory flow of the patient, hence generating a positive end expiratory pressure (PEEP) that can increase the airway pressure and the end expiratory lung volume (EELV). Groves and Tobin demonstrated that HFNO could generate positive airway pressure, providing approximately 1 cmH2O for every 10L/min of increased flow [3]. Moreover, a linear relationship has been reported between flow provided and EELV, resulting in a 0.7% increase of EELV with each liter of increased flow [4]. HFNO can therefore enhance and maintain alveolar recruitment, improve lung compliance (thus reducing work of breathing), and ameliorate blood oxygenation [5].

All these features have made HFNO a cornerstone of respiratory assistance in the ICU, in respiratory units and in emergency departments. As a matter of fact, HFNO has been shown to be superior to standard oxygen therapy in the management of type 1 respiratory failure, reducing intubation rate. It has also been reported to be useful during the pre-oxygenation procedure before intubation and in the post-extubation phase, to reduce the risk of reintubation. Moreover, there is also some evidence of its potential role during type 2 respiratory failure as a complementary therapy during breaks off NIV, or as an alternative to NIV in mild respiratory acidosis [1]. However, taken into consideration the mechanisms of HFNO, it is compelling to explore the potential role of HFNO in the treatment of sleep breathing disorders, especially in obstructive sleep apnea and/or hypoventilation. In fact, HFNO might help to restore airway patency and to overcome flow limitation of the upper airway.

High Flow Nasal Oxygen as Treatment of OSA

As well known, CPAP represents the main treatment of OSA, especially in cases of severe and symptomatic OSA. However, CPAP has his own limitations. For instance, bulbar dysfunction and poor consciousness are contraindications to CPAP, and long-term decreasing of compliance is significantly reported in the literature [6]. Therefore, in the late '00, an alternative treatment, termed nasal cannula system or trans-nasal insufflation (TNI) was developed. This tool used an air compressor to deliver 20L/min of air through a nasal cannula. TNI was proved to slightly reduced respiratory events and arousals in OSA patients, thanks to his capability to increase peak inspiratory flow and moderately increase pharyngeal pressure as well [7]. Unfortunately, this technique has not been widely used, and evidence is limited to proof of concept studies. More recently, HFNO was created, and it is now provided all over the world specially to treat type 1 respiratory failure.

Theoretically, HFNO can be figured as an evolution of TNI, since it can provide 60L/min via nasal cannula, thus generating a maximum of 6cmH2O of airway pressure. However, studies exploring the role of HFNO as the treatment of OSA are few and often consider a small number of patients. Yan et al. enrolled 56 OSA patients (9 mild, 30 moderate and 17 affected by severe OSA) and performed a polysomnographic recording with and without HFNO. AHI decreased significantly (from 26.9 ± 14.7 to 21.5 ± 17.0 events/h, $p < 0.001$) after HFNC treatment. Moreover, when HFNC was administered, breathing pattern and oxygen saturation stabilized, because of the resolution of flow limitation. However, HFNO flow was titrated only up to 30L/min, since with higher flow, sleep efficacy decreased, AHI and arousal index increased and SpO2 did not changed significantly. Of the patients with mild to moderate severity, 76% achieved any AHI reduction and 24% of patients achieved at least 50% reduction in AHI [8]. Instead, Yu et al. conducted a prospective crossover trial trying to compare the efficacy of HFNO and CPAP on OSA. All the 28 enrolled participants were randomly divided into two groups.

The first group underwent CPAP the first night and HFNO the second night. Conversely, the second group received HFNO the first night and CPAP the second night. Polysomnographic recordings were performed in a sleep laboratory and HFNO were titrated up to 60L/min to maintain sleep and the best AHI at the same time. HFNO was shown to reduce AHI from 34.9 (18.68–56.13) to 14.85 (6.85–27.3), while the median optimal flow rate of HFNC was 60 (40–60) L/min. Thus, AHI was reduced by approximately 69%. However, sleep quality was not improved. When CPAP was compared directly with HFNC, CPAP achieved a lower AHI (CPAP vs. HFNC, 5.0 [2.0–7.0] vs. 10.8 [5.5–20.6] events/h) than HFNC. Furthermore, CPAP resulted in better indices for desaturations and snoring and maintained higher mean and minimal SpO2 values. AHI differences were more pronounced in favor of CPAP while the patients lay in supine position, whereas in non-supine position AHI differences were not significant. Moreover, quality of sleep was better with CPAP. Interestingly, more central apnea events occurred in HFNC, allegedly due to the high flow that exaggerate the ventilatory overshoot and the insufflation of air into the nose and thus wash out the anatomic dead space. This may reduce CO2 rebreathing, thereby contributing to central apnea. Regarding side effects, the most common issues reported with HFNC included loud noise (35.71%), airflow too strong (17.86%), frequent awakenings (17.86%), airflow too hot (17.86%) and nasal stuffiness (21.43%). In contrast, mask discomfort (21.43%) was the main concern with CPAP therapy. Thus, CPAP was perceived to be more comfortable by the patients than HFNO [9].

Evidence available to justify the use of HFNO in the treatment of OSA are scant. In fact, the sample size of these studies may be too small to evaluate the responses. Then, in both studies HFNO was provided just for one night, hence it is possible that the polysomnographic recordings collected during HFNO may show a "first-night-effect" as CPAP that may interfere with the results [10]. Moreover, there are no published data about the use of HFNO for more than one consecutive nights in the adult population affected by OSA. However, a retrospective study conducted on a small population of children with OSA showed that home HFNO was feasible and effective in reducing AHI, although 42% of the patients discontinued the treatment due to intolerance issue within 12 months [11].

Finally, there is no evidence about the effectiveness of HFNO on cardiovascular and other comorbidities typical of OSA, where it is well established that CPAP can help to keep them under control.

Conclusion

Despite being inferior to CPAP in the treatment of OSA, HFNO may be useful for patients with mild to moderate OSA severity and may represent an alternative for those patients who are intolerant to CPAP. However, further trials are needed to establish the role of HFNO in the management of OSA patients.

References

[1] Jean-Damien Ricard, Oriol Roca, Virginie Lemiale, Amanda Corley, Jens Braunlich, Peter Jones, Byung Ju Kang, François Lellouche, Stefano Nava, Nuttapol Rittayamai, Giulia Spoletini, Samir Jaber, Gonzalo Hernandez . Use of nasal high flow oxygen during acute respiratory failure. *Intensive Care Med.* 46, 2238–2247 (2020).

[2] Tommaso Mauri, Laura Alban, Cecilia Turrini, Barbara Cambiaghi, Eleonora Carlesso, Paolo Taccone, Nicola Bottino, Alfredo Lissoni, Savino Spadaro, Carlo Alberto Volta, Luciano Gattinoni, Antonio Pesenti, Giacomo Grasselli. Optimum support by high-flow nasal cannula in acute hypoxemic respiratory failure: effects of increasing flow rates. *Intensive Care Med.* 43, 1453–1463 (2017).

[3] Groves, N. & Tobin, A. High flow nasal oxygen generates positive airway pressure in adult volunteers. *Aust. Crit. Care* 20, 126–131 (2007).

[4] Corley, A., Caruana, L. R., Barnett, A. G., Tronstad, O. & Fraser, J. F. Oxygen delivery through high-flow nasal cannulae increase end-expiratory lung volume and reduce respiratory rate in post-cardiac surgical patients. *Br. J. Anaesth.* 107, 998–1004 (2011).

[5] Delorme, M., Bouchard, P.-A., Simon, M., Simard, S. & Lellouche, F. Effects of High-Flow Nasal Cannula on the Work of Breathing in Patients Recovering From Acute Respiratory Failure*. *Crit. Care Med.* 45, 1981–1988 (2017).

[6] Rotenberg, B. W., Murariu, D. & Pang, K. P. Trends in CPAP adherence over twenty years of data collection: a flattened curve. *J. Otolaryngol. - Head Neck Surg.* 45, 43 (2016).

[7] McGinley, B. M., Patil, S. P., Kirkness, J. P., Smith, P. L., Schwartz, A. R. & Schneider, H. A Nasal Cannula Can Be Used to Treat Obstructive Sleep Apnea. *Am. J. Respir. Crit. Care Med.* 176, 194–200 (2007).

[8] Hu Yan, Li Qinghua, Pi Mengyuan, Chen Yaoyu, Zhao Long, Li Mengjie, Dong Xiaosong, Han Fang High flow nasal cannula therapy for obstructive sleep apnea in adults. *Sleep Breath.* (2021) doi:10.1007/s11325-021-02453-6.

[9] Yu, C.-C., Huang, C.-Y., Hua, C.-C. & Wu, H.-P. High-flow nasal cannula compared with continuous positive airway pressure in the treatment of obstructive sleep apnea. *Sleep Breath.* (2021) doi:10.1007/s11325-021-02413-0.

[10] Gouveris, H., Selivanova, O., Bausmer, U., Goepel, B. & Mann, W. First-night-effect on polysomnographic respiratory sleep parameters in patients with sleep-disordered breathing and upper airway pathology. *Eur. Arch. Oto-Rhino-Laryngology* 267, 1449–1453 (2010).

[11] Ignatiuk, D., Schaer, B. & McGinley, B. High flow nasal cannula treatment for obstructive sleep apnea in infants and young children. *Pediatr. Pulmonol.* 55, 2791–2798 (2020).

Chapter 5

Invasive Mechanical Ventilation

Faruk Seçkin Yücesoy*, MD
St. Bartholomew's Hospital, Barts NHS, London, UK

Abstract

It has been recognised that obstructive sleep apnea (OSA) can accompany core respiratory diseases or manifest severely by itself in respiratory critical care settings. Lots of patients who need invasive mechanical ventilation in respiratory critical care have OSA related physiological derangements like obesity, heart failure, pulmonary hypertension, and diabetes. Clinicians should get prepared to manage sensitive respiratory dynamics of OSA patients. This chapter summarizes the important highlights of induction, maintenance and weaning of invasive mechanical ventilation of OSA patients which still lays in the shadow of limited studies.

Keywords: obstructive sleep apnea, mechanical ventilation, respiratory failure, critical care

Introduction

Obstructive sleep apnoea is an underrated disease seen in many patients with different comorbidities or alone in respiratory critical care [1]. Invasive mechanical ventilation is a non-frequent form of treatment when it comes to ventilatory assistance for patients with obstructive sleep apnoea (OSA). But

---

* Corresponding Author's Email: faruk.seckin@yahoo.com.

In: Obstructive Sleep Apnea in Pulmonary Critical Care
Editors: Antonio M. Esquinas and Takatoshi Kasai
ISBN: 979-8-88697-858-2

patients with OSA may also need invasive mechanical ventilation where oral appliances or non-invasive ventilation is not sufficient for the respiratory failure or procedure [2]. This may be a post-surgery or an extrapulmonary reason like sepsis, trauma as well as a pulmonary disease leading to severe respiratory failure helpless with NIV. Pulmonary critical care units are frequently occupied by patients in need for invasive mechanical ventilation with a long list of diagnosis like Chronic obstructive pulmonary disease (COPD), pneumonia, sepsis, heart failure, thoracic malignancies. These patients may be diagnosed with OSA as well.

Invasive mechanical ventilatory settings in the presence of OSA may show some difference throughout the process; intubation, mechanical ventilation and weaning because of many comorbidities coming with OSA and the disease itself.

Airway Management and Intubation

Considering OSA patients, even the initial step to mask ventilation has its hardships. It is expected that an OSA patient may have a fat, short neck, a swelling face, decreased mouth and jaw movement, a large tongue, and large breasts.

Assisted two hand mask ventilation with an airway may smoothen the airway path for the clinician.

Sedative medications and anaesthetics may increase airway obstruction, so it is important to apply general anaesthetics cautiously. It is also a better option to awake intubate an OSA patient with fibre optics. On the other side, it may not be feasible in the critical care settings to awake intubate OSA patients because of agitation, hypoxia, tachypnea, and lack of cooperation. OSA patients has a high incidence of diabetes and atlanto-occipital joint movement may be limited.

Palm print or prayer sign may be used to evaluate glycosylation of inter-phalangeal joints which is related with duration and severity of the disease [1].

Moderate to severe OSA is independently associated with difficult intubation. A long neck circumference, usually seen in obese patients, is associated with difficult face mask ventilation [2]. OSA patients often have abnormalities like short, thick neck, restricted neck extension, decreased jaw movement which lie behind difficult airway or failed intubation and commonly contribute to airway complications. These airway complications may be irreversible or may lead to death [3, 4]. OSA is a major determinant for difficult airway [3].

Indeed, it has been shown to increase the risk of difficult intubation or mask ventilation compared to non-OSA patients [5].

Mechanical Ventilation

Mechanically ventilated patients may have numerous reasons besides OSA to be treated in pulmonary critical care. A few examples of commonly accompanying diseases are COPD and pneumonia. OSA patients hospitalised with pneumonia are shown to have a higher risk of clinical deterioration but a lower in hospital mortality [6]. It is known that high tidal volumes are detrimental for pulmonary tissue both for healthy and non-healthy lungs [7,8]. Tidal volumes (TV) dosed 6-8 ml/kg is expected to be associated with fewer pulmonary complications postoperatively [9, 10]. Tidal volumes to invasive mechanically ventilate should be calculated based on height and sex, excluding weight [11]. Weight should not be included into pulmonary tidal calculations. Otherwise, obese OSA patients may be exposed to high TV based on actual body weight [11]. PEEP set by clinicians has been shown to be less than what is needed to be in order to make transpulmonary pressure positive at end expiratory phase. Safe range of driving pressure, beach chair position and adequate PEEP may also be implemented in OSA as it has been shown to be important in obese surgery patients [12].

Higher driving pressures are needed to overcome the mobilization of chest wall and lungs in obese OSA patients. But still a limit of 15 cmH2O (which is already higher compared to lean patients) is suggested to be the limit of driving pressure to avoid lung injury [13]. For a better distribution of the flow in the alveoli, there are teams recommending pressure support ventilation (PSV) over volume control. PSV has also been shown to increase oxygenation and decrease inflammation in obese piglets [14]. Neurally-adjusted ventilatory assist (NAVA) may be a choice when it technologically evolves. Decrease in FRC leads to intrinsic PEEP and alters expiratory flow.

Next step is gas trapping and dynamic hyperinflation coming with patient-ventilator asynchrony [15], 10 cmH2O PEEP has been shown to be more successful in obese mechanically ventilated patients, decreasing elastance and improving respiratory mechanics [16]. Lower PEEP is known to increase work of breath and has negative impact on pulmonary health leading to hypoxia and atelectasis.

Recruitment may be beneficial in OSA patients in order to open atelectatic lung and increase oxygenation. 40 seconds expiratory pause with a PEEP level of 40 cm H2O is a reference method. It should only be tried in hemodynamically stabile patients though [17].

Chronic obstructive pulmonary disease (COPD) patients are shown to be less intubated and longer non invasive ventilated if they concomitantly had OSA [18].

Mechanical Ventilation in OSA with Obesity

Overweight and obesity are the most common aetiologies of OSA. Relaxation of the soft tissue throughout the mouth and throat result the collapse or obstruction of airway. Obesity means atelectasis and alters chest wall mechanics and eventually hypoxia and hardship of respiration. Obesity also results in decreased Functional Residual Capacity (FRC) and leads to hypoxia which is well defined during mask ventilation. Increased abdominal pressure pushes diaphragm and increases its workload and oxygen demand [19, 20]. High abdominal pressure also elevates diaphragm and produces intrinsic PEEP, collapsing small airways in dependant lung [21, 22]. The optimum position for oxygenation in OSA patients is beach chair position, pulling diaphragm down and increasing end expiratory lung capacity [23].

FiO2 should be initially set as low as possible to avoid harmful effects of hyperoxia. Tidal volume should start from 4-6 ml/predicted weight kg in patients with deranged pulmonary tissue or ARDS. Still, it is mostly advised to start with a PEEP level of 5-8cmH2O with obese patients without pulmonary issues. While setting higher PEEP values, hemodynamic stability should be considered as recruitment manoeuvres and high PEEP comes at the cost of hemodynamic derangement [24].

In OSA patients, decrease in FRC can be expressed with an alteration in partial arterial oxygen pressure. It increases FRC and decreases work of breath (WOB). It may be of favour to put patients to sitting position especially while weaning and after extubation if not all along mechanical ventilation. Increased thoracic fat alters respiratory muscle function and pulmonary perfusion as well as ventilation/perfusion ratio [25]. Increased body weight also means an increase in demand of total oxygen consumption which comes at the cost of tachypnoea and increased minute ventilation on obese patients. A study with oesophageal balloon technique has shown obese patients' chest wall compliances to be two-fold lower than in lean patients undergoing surgery [3,26]. Supine positioning as in the critical care settings also leads to decrease of expiratory reserve volume which means lower end expiratory lung volume in intubated and PEEP receiving patients. Closing volume overpasses End expiratory Lung Volume (EELV) which lets lungs collapse between each breath [27]. It increases work of breath and makes patients feel more perception of dyspnoea [28]. Ventilation Perfusion mismatch is another problem in obese patients while ventilation is dense at the apex of the lung but perfusion at the basal zones which is another reason for obese to be prone to hypoxia [29]. See Table 1.

Table 1. Highlights of Mechanical Ventilation in OSA Patients

- Risk of difficult intubation and difficult face mask ventilation
- Consider video laryngoscopy
- Consider awake intubation
- Beach chair position favoured during mechanical ventilation (MV)
- Low volume ventilation
- IBM (kg) = height (cm) – 100 for a man and (cm) – 110 for a woman.
- High frequency
- Moderate PEEP with cautious titration
- Recruitment manuever
- Full awake extubation
- Steroid and Cuff leak test before extubation
- Protective HFNC of NIV after extubation
• Consider early extubation if possible

Mechanical Ventilation in OSA with Heart Failure

We know from a large retrospective study that OSA patients are to be male, married, young, obese, and diagnosed more with heart failure than non-OSA patients. [6]. A study on rats showed highly increased sympatho-excitation and increased renal perfusion on hypoxia exposed rats [30]. How OSA leads to atherosclerosis in patients also depends heavily on increased endothelial dysfunction and oxidative stress [31] We also know that a high apnea-hypopnea index (AHI) during REM sleep is associated with cardiac remodelling and ventricular diastolic dysfunction, aortic root size, E/A ratio, left ventricular, and stroke volume [31].

Atherosclerosis, hypertension, and arrhythmia are other problems to be seen in OSA. Inspiration against obstructed pharynx cause severe intrathoracic pressure to decrease in OSA patients which increases left ventricular transmural pressure and afterload [32]. OSA decreases left ventricular preload and increases left ventricular afterload and shorten cardiac output [33].

Intubated OSA patients in critical care settings are no longer expected to create reduced intrathoracic pressures with intracardiac pressure alterations. OSA causes many deteriorations in non-REM sleep and increases atherosclerosis and promotes coronary artery disease. PEEP is a useful booster in heart failure patients. It decreases venous return, right atrial pressure and left ventricle end diastolic pressure by increasing intrathoracic pressure. Use of PEEP increases pleural pressure, reducing transmural pressure and left ventricle afterload. [34]. An early study showed that 8 to 10 cmH2O pressure of PEEP did not decrease cardiac output in heart failure patients [35]. There is no clear data about the PEEP level in OSA related intubated heart failure patients, but we know that a moderate PEEP level is safe in left heart failure (36). Both in patients with heart failure and obesity PEEP is a valuable parameter for homeostasis in intubated patients. Considering OSA patients as one with heart failure and obesity; titrating PEEP has shown to increase cardiac output in heart failure patients and, 5 cm H2O is recommended for start and to increase 2-3 cmH2O in every 15-20 minutes cautiously.

There is also recommendation of applying 10 cmH2O PEEP to obese patients from the beginning as PEEP only prevents decruitment of the lung. It can improve oxygenation and compliance in many obese patients while clinicians should avoid negative effects of high PEEP and consider airway pressures, oxygenation, and cardiac output as it should be individually titrated [17]. Chronic hypoventilation of OSA patients leads to hypercarbia and bicarbonate retention [36].

Weaning OSA Patients from Mechanical Ventilation

Sedation and opiates are certain drug to worsen respiratory muscle relaxation and increase obstruction in OSA patients. Positioning is a major help for obese OSA patients to decrease work of breath, increase FRC and oxygenation. Sitting position means release of abdominal pressure and decrease in alveolar pressure as well as let go of intrinsic PEEP [37]. Completely reversing neuromuscular block in postoperative patients and full awake extubation are helpful facts to care about. Obesity Induced airway hyperreactivity may be another fact to be considered about OSA patients [36]. Especially in times of respiratory tract infection, hypersensitivity of airway may lead to dyspnoea and wheezing. It is also important to determine negative inspiratory force in obese patients to interpret post-extubation clinic. It has also become a standard treatment to apply HFNC or NIV just after extubation prophylactically [38]. NIV after extubation decreases mortality in hypercarbic obese patients. Respiratory physiotherapy and incentive spirometry education should be given to all patients before treatment or surgery.

Patients with OSA who require invasive mechanical ventilation because of pneumonia have a decreased in hospital mortality unknown whether it is the treatment differences compared to non-OSA pneumonia patients [39]. OSA was also associated with decreased non-routine discharge. Another retrospective cohort study was also able to say that no differences in means of ventilator duration and hospital length of stay was shown, but invasive mechanically ventilated OSA patients had significant lower in hospital mortality [40].

Fluid retention due to heart failure or renal failure may be risk factor in developing OSA. OSA patients with heart failure have been proven to better tolerate semirecumbent sleeping position and their apnoea-hypopnea index have been shown to significantly decrease. [41, 42]. Semi recumbent position is already favoured in critical care units to avoid respiratory complications and ventilator associated pneumonia (VAP) which may also be advantageous during follow-up of intubated OSA patients and during weaning [32].

It is known that obese patients have an increased oxygen consumption, respiratory rate, and work of breath. Before induction for intubation, high flow nasal cannula oxygen can be used to pre-oxygenate patients while it is also recognised to give low levels of PEEP [17]. Post extubation stridor is common and can be prevented by steroids beforehand. A cuff leak test is also recommended to investigate laryngeal oedema [43].

Conclusion

We consider that in OSA patient use of invasive mechanical ventilation need to take into account the following key aspects: a) Airways: obese with a short neck, swelling face, decreased mouth and jaw movement, a large tongue and breasts, b) OSA patients are prone to be male, married and young with heart failure, c) Moderate to severe OSA is independently associated with difficult intubation, d) Tidal volumes to invasive mechanically ventilate should be calculated based on height and sex and low tidal volumes is expected to be associated with fewer pulmonary complications in OSA patients. For mechanical ventilation setting a) Lower PEEP is known to increase work of breath and has negative impact on pulmonary health, b) The optimum position for oxygenation in OSA patients is beach chair position, c) Fio2 should be initially set as low as possible to avoid harmful effects of hyperoxia, d) OSA decreases left ventricular preload and increases left ventricular afterload and shorten cardiac output, e) 8 to 10 cmH2O pressure of PEEP did not decrease cardiac output in heart failure patients, f) Full awake extubation in sitting position and a cuff leak test is recommended to investigate laryngeal oedema.

References

[1] Hashim KV, Thomas M. Sensitivity of palm print sign in prediction of difficult laryngoscopy in diabetes: A comparison with other airway indices. *Indian J Anaesth*, 2014; 58(3):298-302.

[2] Seet E, Chung F, Wang CY, Tam S, Kumar CM, Ubeynarayana CU, Yim CC, Chew EFF, Lam CKM, Cheng BCP, Chan MTV. Association of Obstructive Sleep Apnea with Difficult Intubation: Prospective Multicenter Observational Cohort Study. *Anesth Analg*, 2021 Jul 1; 133(1):196-204.

[3] Akoumianaki E, Maggiore SM, Valenza F, Bellani G, Jubran A, Loring SH, Pelosi P, Talmor D, Grasso S, Chiumello D, Guérin C, Patroniti N, Ranieri VM, Gattinoni L, Nava S, Terragni PP, Pesenti A, Tobin M, Mancebo J, Brochard L, PLUG Working Group (Acute Respiratory Failure Section of the European Society of Intensive Care Medicine). The application of esophageal pressure measurement in patients with respiratory failure. *Am J Respir Crit Care Med,* 2014 Mar 1; 189(5):520-31.

[4] Behazin N, Jones SB, Cohen RI, Loring SH. Respiratory restriction and elevated pleural and esophageal pressures in morbid obesity. *J Appl Physiol,* 2010 Jan; 108(1):212-8.

[5] Nagappa M, Wong DT, Cozowicz C, Ramachandran SK, Memtsoudis SG, Chung F. Is obstructive sleep apnea associated with difficult airway? Evidence from a

systematic review and meta-analysis of prospective and retrospective cohort studies. *PLoS One,* 2018 Oct 1; 13(10):e0204904.

[6] Lindenauer PK, Stefan MS, Johnson KG, Priya A, Pekow PS, Rothberg MB. Prevalence, Treatment, and Outcomes Associated with OSA among Patients Hospitalized with Pneumonia. *Chest.,* 2014 May 1; 145(5):1032-8.

[7] Rouby JJ, Constantin JM, Girardi CRDA, Zhang M, Lu Q. Mechanical Ventilation in Patients with Acute Respiratory Distress Syndrome. *Anesthesiology,* 2004 Jul 1; 101(1):228-34.

[8] Amato MBP, Barbas CSV, Medeiros DM, Magaldi RB, Schettino GP, Lorenzi-Filho G, Kairalla RA, Deheinzelin D, Munoz C, Oliveira R, Takagaki TY, Carvalho CR. Effect of a protective-ventilation strategy on mortality in the acute respiratory distress syndrome. *N Engl J Med,* 1998 Feb 5; 338(6):347-54.

[9] Futier E, Constantin J-M, Paugam-Burtz C, Pascal J, Eurin M, Neuschwander A, Marret E, Beaussier M, Gutton C, Lefrant JY, Allaouchiche B, Verzilli D, Leone M, De Jong A, Bazin JE, Pereira B, Jaber S; IMPROVE Study Group. A Trial of Intraoperative Low-Tidal-Volume Ventilation in Abdominal Surgery. *N Engl J Med,* 2013 Aug; 369(5):428-37.

[10] Chaney MA, Nikolov MP, Blakeman BP, Bakhos M. Protective ventilation attenuates postoperative pulmonary dysfunction in patients undergoing cardiopulmonary bypass. *J Cardiothorac Vasc Anesth*, 2000; 14(5):514-8.

[11] Fernandez-Bustamante A, Wood CL, Tran Z V., Moine P. Intraoperative ventilation: Incidence and risk factors for receiving large tidal volumes during general anesthesia. *BMC Anesthesiol*, 2011 Nov. 21;11.

[12] Pirrone M, Fisher D, Chipman D, Imber DAE, Corona J, Mietto C, Kacmarek RM, Berra L. Recruitment Maneuvers and Positive End-Expiratory Pressure Titration in Morbidly Obese ICU Patients. *Crit Care Med*, 2016 Feb 1; 44(2):300-7.

[13] Amato MBP, Meade MO, Slutsky AS, Brochard L, Costa ELV, Schoenfeld DA, Stewart TE, Briel M, Talmor D, Mercat A, Richard JC, Carvalho CR, Brower RG. Driving Pressure and Survival in the Acute Respiratory Distress Syndrome. *N Engl J Med*, 2015 Feb 19; 372(8):747-55.

[14] Aldenkortt M, Lysakowski C, Elia N, Brochard L, Tramèr MR. Ventilation strategies in obese patients undergoing surgery: A quantitative systematic review and meta-analysis. *Br J Anaesth,* 2012; 109(4):493-502.

[15] Dhand R. Ventilator graphics and respiratory mechanics in the patient with obstructive lung disease. *Respir Care*, 2005; 50(2): 246-61.

[16] Pelosi P, Ravagnan I, Gíuratí G, Panigada M, Bottino N, Tredici S, Eccher G, Gattinoni L. Positive end-expiratory pressure improves respiratory function in obese but not in normal subjects during anesthesia and paralysis. *Anesthesiology,* 1999 Nov; 91(5):1221-31.

[17] De Jong A, Chanques G, Jaber S. *Mechanical ventilation in obese ICU patients: From intubation to extubation*. 2017.

[18] Liu W, Guo H, Ding F, Cui Z, Zhang J, Wang J, Yuan Y. Comparison of invasive intubation and noninvasive mechanical ventilation in patients with chronic obstructive pulmonary disease and obstructive sleep apnoea syndrome. *J Int Med Res,* 2021 Dec 1; 49(12).

[19] Brazzale DJ, Pretto JJ, Schachter LM. Optimizing respiratory function assessments to elucidate the impact of obesity on respiratory health. *Respirology,* 2015 Jul 1; 20(5):715-21.

[20] Littleton SW. Impact of obesity on respiratory function. *Respirology,* 2012 Jan; 17(1):43-9.

[21] Arena R, Cahalin LP. Evaluation of cardiorespiratory fitness and respiratory muscle function in the obese population. *Prog Cardiovasc Dis,* 2014 Jan; 56(4):457-64.

[22] Chlif M, Keochkerian D, Choquet D, Vaidie A, Ahmaidi S. Effects of obesity on breathing pattern, ventilatory neural drive and mechanics. *Respir Physiol Neurobiol,* 2009 Sep 30; 168(3):198-202.

[23] Valenza F, Vagginelli F, Tiby A, Francesconi S, Ronzoni G, Guglielmi M, Zappa M, Lattuada E, Gattinoni L. Effects of the beach chair position, positive end-expiratory pressure, and pneumoperitoneum on respiratory function in morbidly obese patients during anesthesia and paralysis. *Anesthesiology,* 2007; 107(5): 725-32.

[24] Ball L, Pelosi P. How I ventilate an obese patient. *Crit Care*, 2019 May 16; 23(1): 1-3.

[25] Sebastian JC. Respiratory physiology and pulmonary complications in obesity. *Best Pract Res Clin Endocrinol Metab*, 2013 Apr; 27(2):157-61.

[26] Mauri T, Yoshida T, Bellani G, Goligher EC, Carteaux G, Rittayamai N, Mojoli F, Chiumello D, Piquilloud L, Grasso S, Jubran A, Laghi F, Magder S, Pesenti A, Loring S, Gattinoni L, Talmor D, Blanch L, Amato M, Chen L, Brochard L, Mancebo J, PLeUral pressure working Group (PLUG—Acute Respiratory Failure section of the European Society of Intensive Care Medicine). Esophageal and transpulmonary pressure in the clinical setting: Meaning, usefulness and perspectives. *Intensive Care Med,* 2016 Sep 1; 42(9):1360-73.

[27] Milic-Emili J, Torchio R, D'Angelo E. Closing volume: A reappraisal (1967-2007). *Eur J Appl Physiol*, 2007 Apr; 99(6):567-83.

[28] Sin DD, Jones RL, Paul Man SF. Obesity is a risk factor for dyspnea but not for airflow obstruction. *Arch Intern Med*, 2002 Jul 8; 162(13):1477-81.

[29] Holley HS, Milic-Emili J, Becklake MR, Bates DV. Regional distribution of pulmonary ventilation and perfusion in obesity. *J Clin Invest,* 1967; 46(4):475-81.

[30] Huang J, Lusina S, Xie T, Ji E, Xiang S, Liu Y, Weiss JW. Sympathetic response to chemostimulation in conscious rats exposed to chronic intermittent hypoxia. *Respir Physiol Neurobiol*, 2009 Apr 30; 166(2):102-6.

[31] Dursunoglu N, Dursunoglu D. [Obstructive sleep apnea syndrome, endothelial dysfunction and coronary atherosclerosis]. *Tuberk Toraks*, 2005 Jan 1; 53(3):299-306.

[32] Van Nieuwenhoven CA, Vandenbroucke-Grauls C, Van Tiel FH, Joore HCA, Strack Van Schijndel RJM, Van Der Tweel I, Ramsay G, Bonten M. Feasibility and effects of the semirecumbent position to prevent ventilator-associated pneumonia: A randomized study. *Crit Care Med*, 2006; 34(2):396-402.

[33] Tolle FA, Judy WV, Yu PL, Markand ON. Reduced stroke volume related to pleural pressure in obstructive sleep apnea. *J Appl Physiol Respir Environ Exerc Physiol,* 1983; 55(6):1718-24.

[34] Luecke T, Pelosi P. Clinical review: Positive end-expiratory pressure and cardiac output. *Crit Care,* 2005 Dec 18; 9(6):607-21.

[35] Schuster S, Erbel R, Weilemann LS, Lu W, Henkel B, Wellek S, Schinzel H, Meyer J. Hemodynamics During PEEP Ventilation in Patients with Severe Left Ventricular Failure Studied by Transesophageal Echocardiography. *Chest,* 1990 May 1; 97(5):1181-9.

[36] Chau EHL, Mokhlesi B, Chung F. Obesity Hypoventilation Syndrome and Anesthesia. *Sleep Med Clin,* 2013 Mar; 8(1):135.

[37] Wiesen J, Ornstein M, Tonelli AR, Menon V, Ashton RW. State of the evidence: mechanical ventilation with PEEP in patients with cardiogenic shock. *Heart,* 2013 Dec 15; 99(24):1812-7.

[38] Mahul M, Jung B, Galia F, Molinari N, de Jong A, Coisel Y, Vaschetto R, Matecki S, Chanques G, Brochard L, Jaber S. Spontaneous breathing trial and post-extubation work of breathing in morbidly obese critically ill patients. *Crit Care,* 2016 Oct 27; 20(1).

[39] Jean RE, Gibson CD, Jean RA, Ochieng P. Obstructive sleep apnea and acute respiratory failure: An analysis of mortality risk in patients with pneumonia requiring invasive mechanical ventilation. *J Crit Care,* 2015 Aug 1; 30(4):778-83.

[40] Taweesedt P, Djurdjevic N, Pattharanitima P, Ali F, Kim JW. Mortality in patients with or without osa who required invasive mechanical ventilation: A propensity score-matched analysis. *Chest,* 2020 Oct 1; 158(4):A2339.

[41] Yumino D, Ruttanaumpawan P, Yau B, Su MC, Lam J, Bradley TD. Relationship between overnight rostral fluid shift and Obstructive Sleep Apnea in nonobese men. *Am J Respir Crit Care Med,* 2009 Feb 1; 179(3):241-6.

[42] Asoglu OK, Keskin B, Tasbakan MS, Gurgun C. Effect of Semirecumbent Sleep Position on Severity of Obstructive Sleep Apnea in Patients with Heart Failure. *J Card Fail,* 2015 Oct 1; 21(10):842-7.

[43] Jaber S, Chanques G, Matecki S, Ramonatxo M, Vergne C, Souche B, Perrigault PF, Eledjam JJ. Post-extubation stridor in intensive care unit patients: Risk factors evaluation and importance of the cuff-leak test. *Intensive Care Med,* 2003 Jan 1; 29(1):69-74.

Chapter 6

Monitoring in Critical Care

Seda Kurtbeyoğlu*, MD
Department of Anaesthesia and Critical Care, Health Sciences University, Ankara City Hospital, Ankara, Turkey

Abstract

Correct monitoring is essential for patient follow-up in the intensive care unit (ICU). All obstructive sleep apnea syndrome patients need the support of mechanical and pharmacological treatments according to the information conveyed by the technical equipment. The main purposes of monitoring are diagnosis, follow-up, and titration of treatment. The patient should be informed about the procedures and treatment to be applied to himself, so that the level of anxiety decreases. Clinical observation is particularly important. Vital values should be monitored. Neurological evaluation should be performed at regular intervals. The standard ones in monitoring are oxygen saturation monitoring with pulse oximetry, heart rate and arterial blood pressure monitoring. In addition, although it is invasive, arterial blood gas monitoring should be performed when necessary. According to the results, it is evaluated whether he needs non-invasive or invasive mechanical ventilation support. Correct monitoring is essential for OSA patient follow-up in ICU. The monitoring options should be evaluated depending on the disease severity.

Keywords: obstructive sleep apnea, intensive care unit, monitoring

---

* Corresponding Author's Email: kurtbeyogluseda@gmail.com.

In: Obstructive Sleep Apnea in Pulmonary Critical Care
Editors: Antonio M. Esquinas and Takatoshi Kasai
ISBN: 979-8-88697-858-2

Introduction

Correct monitoring is essential for patient follow-up in intensive care unit (ICU). Many OSA patients in intensive care unit are hospitalized only for monitoring purposes. All of these patients need the support of mechanical and pharmacological treatments according to the information conveyed by the technical equipments [1].

The main purposes of monitoring are: diagnosis, follow-up and titration of treatment. For this purpose, non-invasive and invasive monitoring methods can be used. Many numerical and subjective data such as vital signs, urine flow, mechanical ventilation, blood gases, hematological and biochemical parameters, coagulation, fluid input and output, physical examination findings can be monitored. The systems used in monitoring should be easily interpretable, specific, sensitive enough to detect small changes, easily reproducible, easy to use, not pose a risk to the patient, and have an acceptable cost-benefit balance [2].

In this chapter, we will go through the main parameters that should be considered in the monitoring of OSA patients, followed in ICU.

Practical Recommendations

First of all, clinical observation is very important. Patients may be worried about both health problems and treatments. The introduction of all procedures to be applied to the patient reduces the anxiety and increases the comfort during ICU. In particular, when the invasive/noninvasive mechanical ventilation needs, patients should be informed and motivated by the clinician and coordination with ventilator should be provided [3]. Since respiratory distress may decrease, the level of consciousness of the patients should be closely monitored.Neurological assessment of the patient should be done routinely. The Glasgow Coma Scale (GCS) can be used to the monitorization of consciousness level. GCS evaluation should be performed more frequently especially in patients who need mechanical ventilation support.The application of improved GCS score in 2 hours intervals have been shown to improve the therapeutic effect. Other than GCS, the level of consciousness can be evaluated directly using the Kelly–Matthay score and a score of > 3 may raise the alarm for depressed consciousness and high risk of NIV failure.

Neurological examination and delirium follow -up is also important, especially in patients with alert and NIV support, the incidence of delirium is around 50%. Delirium is associated with increased mortality and morbidity. Delirium in NIMV reduces the success. Evaluation of delirium with Confusion Assessment Method for the intensive care unit (ICU) every morning from initiation to the termination of NIMV has shown that delirium is independently associated with NIMV failure. The level of conciosness can be evaluated with Richmond-Agitation- Sedation Scale (RASS). Pharmacological treatment may be required [4]. In addition, frequent neurological follow -up is important in early diagnosis due to increased risk of strokes in OSAS patients [5]. Furthermore, maintaining the correct position of the patient is important in the comfort of the patient and in the efficacy of treatment.

Especially in patients with high intra-abdominal pressure or obese patients, supine and semi-sitting positions should be preferred. In the presence of dyspnea, the seating position is generally preferred. If NIV is to be used, the suitability of the interface mask should be followed and it should be observed whether there is a leak or not.

Respiratory Rate and Breathing Pattern

Respiratory rate (RR) should be monitored. Increased RR is an earliest finding of oxygen requirement and respiratory deficiency, and parallel to clinical seriousness. The use of auxiliary respiratory muscles, nasal wing respiration, intercostal and supraklavicular withdrawal and abdominal paradox respiratory, respiratory deficiency are important physical examination findings. Normally, RR increases as a result of an increase in PACO2 and this effect is more pronounced in the presence of hypoxemia [6]. RR should be monitored continuously like a heart rate (HR). While applying NİV, decrease in RR and HR within one hour is a sign of success, but this may not always be seen. However, in successful application, the ventilator is synchronized with respiratory and accessory respiratory muscles decreases. The lack of symptoms of improvement shows bad response and necessary measures should be taken [7-9]. Current clinically available monitoring devices for respiration in suspected or confirmed OSA patients include continuous pulse oximetry (PO), capnography monitor, respiratory volume monitor (RVM), and photoplethysmography (PPG) in addition to clinical observation. PO is a routine oxygenation monitoring method that measures the percentage of oxygenated hemoglobin. By detecting hypoxemic episode, it is the primary objective indicator of respiratory distress in clinical use. PO is recommended as a strategy to reduce the complications of OSA patients such as short term hypoxemia, transfer to intensive care unit and death [10]. In order to understand mild hypoxemia without clinical findings, oxygen saturation should be monitored by continuously monitoring with PO. Although the most common measurement is made from the finger, the ear probes respond faster and are minimized by vasoconstriction [11]. According to the literature, PO is still the most widely used device with its high sensitivity. It is also cost effective and easy to use, but its specificity is low and does not reflect ventilation [12]. Also provides real time, continuous and noninvasive information about arterial oxygenation. In critically ill patients with 90% or higher SaO2 values, the mean difference between SPO2 and SAO2 measured by a reference standard is less than 2%; The standard deviation of the differences between the two measurements is less than 3%. However, the bias and accuracy of PO readings deteriorate when the SAO2 is less than 90%. Although PO is correct in reflecting the single value measurements of SAO2, it does not reliably the changes in SAO2 in patients with intensive care unit (ICU).

Although PO measurements are quite reliable, it is necessary to pay attention to some points to control this reliability. Peripheral pulse or ECG rhythm and the PO wave are similar, suggesting that the measurement is reliable. Hypoxia detection with PO shows the need for nasal CPAP or NIPPV application [13]. PO is beneficial in OSAS patient follow up in intensive care, but does not eliminate the requirement of AKG if NIV is required. PO has advantages such as simplicity, short installation and response time, as well as disadvantages like affected by movement and perfusion. It is also not safe for the detection of hypoventilation in patients with oxygen supplements [14]. PO cannot detect reduced RR, apnea or carbon dioxide levels that indicate ventilation disorder before the SPO2 decrease is displayed. In addition, additional oxygen can sometimes mask existing respiratory depression and cause urgent events [15]. In the meantime, sound wrong alarms caused by signal error during SPO2 monitoring may often occur and mislead the treatment or cause maintenance providers to neglect to determine real emergencies.

Capnography

Capnography is the most widely used device for detecting hypoventilation, but it may not provide reliable data for extubated patients. Even normal baking value cannot exclude the presence of hypoxia. Capnography detects end-tied carbon dioxide (ETCO2), which can provide information about metabolic, circulatory and respiratory activities. ETCO2 measurement is performed by placing a nasal cannula to obtain and analyze breathing gas samples. ETCO2 can detect apnea attacks and respiratory depression indicated by respiratory rate per minute. For earlier detection of apnea, the pulse is considered superior to the oximeter. The difference between ETCO2 and PACO2 will increase with fresh oxygen flow, this change is more pronounced in OSA patients [16, 17]. OSA patients have high nasal airway resistance and mouth breathers. Therefore, it can be difficult to obtain correct ETCO2 measurements through nasal cannula. The difference between EtCO2 and PaCO2 will increase with fresh oxygen flow, a change more obvious in OSA patients. For this reason, Kasuya et al. alternatively used mainstream and a nasal cannula that included an oral guide to reduce the inconsistency between EtCO2 and PaCO2, and it performed better than sidestream capnography for OSA patients [18].

To date, there is no report that the number of respiratorys reflected by the capnography is wrong.

However, in many cases there is a problem of easily removed by patients. ETCO2 is technically reliable in intubated patients. For this reason, capnography should always be interpreted extensively with other physiological parameters and clinical evaluation. Partial obstruction of the airway and mixing of exhaled air with ambient air may also display a normal EtCO2 value, whereas PaCO2 detectable by blood gas analysis is high. Arterial blood gases are the basis for starting NİV treatment and at the same time determining whether the need continues [19]. Thus, the need for intubation can be evaluated. In clinical studies, the frequency of arterial blood gas varies in great differences depending on the patient's condition and clinician's niv experience [20]. ACG is also important in PAO2 and PACO2 measurement in respiratory failure and response to treatment [21].

Clinical findings, laboratory changes and monitoring findings secondary to cell metabolism, which are impaired as a result of inadequate tissue perfusion in critical patients who are followed in intensive care unit, are vital. In cases where the so -called "microcirculation and mitochondrial dystress syndrome eğitim developing secondary to tissue hypoperfusion causes organ dysfunction, necrotic cell death is not performed early without intervention, irreversible organ damage occurs. The cause of hemodynamic instability in intensive care patients may be due to volume changes, excessive vasodilatation or vasoconstriction, as well as a cardiac -induced insufficiency. In order to maintain adequate perfusion of vital organs in critical patients, it is aimed to monitor the variations in hemodynamic parameters simultaneously and effectively in the management of vasoactive drugs.

Hemodynamic Monitorization

Hemodynamic Monitorization (HDM) may even have intensively indication in intensive care, and multiple methods are generally used and evaluated together to detect the hemodynamic variability of the patients. The results obtained provide information about the violence and prognosis of the disease, but are also beneficial in observing the response to the treatment.

These patients should be monitored continuously by electrocardiography. Noninvasive blood pressure can be measured in stable patients. However, if hemodynamic instability, invasive measurement should be performed. If there are cases such as hypoxemia and respiratory acidosis, it may be necessary for extra ventures such as central catheter and urine prostitution. It should be noted that hemodynamic instability plays a role in NIV failure [22]. In addition, increased cardiac events, cerebrovascular disorder and unexpected postoperative mortality were documented [23]. Early recognition of apnea in non -intubated OSA patients has the most important role in mortality and morbidity. In patients with Cardiac complications such as hypertension, cardiac arrhythmia, left heart failure, coronary artery disease, and right heart failure /pulmonary hypertension, in patients with Cardiac complications, ankynamic monitoring methods may be preferred according to the severity of the disease. Since the risk of diabetes increases in OSA patients, blood sugar monitoring is also important.

If non-invasive or invasive mechanical ventilation is applied to the patient, the patient-supplier compliance should be followed closely, and the airway pressure and leakage amount should be measured objectively. CO2 level is essential for the evaluation of Alveolar ventilation adequacy during NİV and the sampling of arterial blood gas is the gold standard. This method is a process of expertise, painful and complication risk [24]. Since there is an arterial line in the intensive care units, sampling can be easier. Hypoventilation is the most common cause of hypercapnia and can cause vital significant respiratory acidosis [24].

Conclusion

Correct monitoring is essential for OSA patient follow-up in ICU. The monitoring options schould be evaluated depending on the disease severity. The availability of different mnitoring modalities and the experience of the staff are other important determinants of monitoring. Basicly regular evaluation schould include assesment of vital signs; respiratory rate, respiratory muscle effort and level of consciousness, continuous SPO2 and ABG.

References

[1] Elnour S, Shankar- Hari M. The critically ill patient: making referral to intensive care. *Br. J. Hosp. Med.* 2011;72:154-6.

[2] Kesici S, Bayrakçı B. Yoğun Bakımda Monitorizasyonda Yenilikler. *Turkiye Klinikleri J. Pediatr.* 2011;7:43-8.

[3] Bello G, De Pascale G, and Antonelli M. Review. Noninvasive ventilation: practical advice. *Curr. Opin. Crit. Care* 2013;19:1-8.

[4] Ely E W, Shintani A, Truman B, Speroff T, Gordon S M, Harrell F E Jr, Inouye S K, Bernard G R, Dittus R S. Delirium as a predictor of mortality in mechanically ventilated patients in the intensive care unit. *JAMA* 2004; 291:1753-62.

[5] Brown D L, Shafie-Khorassani F, Kim S, Chervin R D, Case E, Morgenstern L B, Yadollahi A, Tower S, Lisabeth LD. Sleep-Disordered Breathing Is Associated With Recurrent Ischemic Stroke. *Stroke* 2019; 50:571.

[6] Karakurt S. Respiratory Monitoring in the Intensive Care Unit. *Yoğun Bakım Dergisi* 2002;2(1):5-15.

[7] Ozyilmaz E, Ugurlu A O and Nava S. Timing of noninvasive ventilation failure: causes, risk factors, and potential remedies. *BMC PulmonaryMedicine* 2014;14:19.

[8] Elliott M W, Confalonieri M, Nava S. Where to perform noninvasive ventilation? *Eur. Respir. J.* 2002;19:1159-66.

[9] Mehta S and Hill N S. Noninvasive Ventilation. *Am. J. Respir. Crit. Care Med.* 2001; 163:540-77.

[10] Kaw R. Perioperative complications in patients with obstructive sleep apnea. *Curr. Anesthesiol. Rep.* (2013) 4(1):37–41.

[11] Jubran A. Pulse oximetry. In: Tobin MJ (ed). *Principles and Practice of Intensive Care Monitoring*. New York: Mc Graw Hill, 1998:261-87.

[12] Zhang X, Kassem M A, Zhou Y, Shabsigh M, Wang Q, Xu X. A Brief Review of Non-invasive Monitoring of Respiratory Condition for Extubated Patients with or at Risk for Obstructive Sleep Apnea after Surgery. *Front. Med.* (Lausanne) 2017; 4: 26.

[13] Gross J B, Bachenberg K L, Benumof J L, Caplan R A, Connis R T, Coté C J, Nickinovich D G, Prachand V, Ward D S, Weaver E M, Ydens L, Yu S; American

Society of Anesthesiologists Task Force on Perioperative Management. Practice guidelines for the perioperative management of patients with obstructive sleep apnea: a report by the American Society of Anesthesiologists Task Force on Perioperative Management of patients with obstructive sleep apnea. *Anesthesiology* (2006) 104(5):1081–93.

[14] Kampelmacher M J. Non-invasive home mechanical ventilation: qualification, initiation, and monitoring. *Pneumonol. Alergol. Pol.* 2012; 80(5): 482-88.

[15] Ayas N, Bergstrom L R, Schwab T R, Narr B J. Unrecognized severe postoperative hypercapnia: a case of apneic oxygenation. *Mayo Clin. Proc.* (1998) 73(1):51–4.

[16] Hillman D R, Platt P R, Eastwood P R. The upper airway during anaesthesia. *Br. J. Anaesth.* (2003) 91(1):31–9.

[17] Hillman D R, Loadsman J A, Platt P R, Eastwood P R. Obstructive sleep apnoea and anaesthesia. *Sleep Med. Rev.* (2004) 8(6):459–71.

[18] Kasuya Y, Akca O, Sessler D I, Ozaki M, Komatsu R. Accuracy of postoperative end-tidal Pco2 measurements with mainstream and sidestream capnography in non-obese patients and in obese patients with and without obstructive sleep apnea. *Anesthesiology* (2009) 111(3):609–15.

[19] Singh G, Pitoyo C W. Non-invasiveVentilation in Acute Respiratory Failure. Acta Medica Indonesiana – *The Indonesian Journal of Internal Medicine* 2014;46:1.

[20] Gay P. Management and monitoring of noninvasive mechanical ventilation. *Eurasian journal of pulmonology*. 2002;4(2);275-77.

[21] Huttmann S E, Windisch W, and Storre J H. Techniques for the Measurement and Monitoring of Carbondioxide in the Blood. *Ann. Am. Thorac. Soc.* 2014;11(4):645-652.

[22] International Consensus Conferences in IntensiveCareMedicine: noninvasive positive pressure ventilation in acute respiratory failure. *Am. J. Respir. Crit. Care Med.* 2001;163:283-91.

[23] Lavie L. Oxidative stress in obstructive sleep apnea and intermittent hypoxia – revisited – the bad ugly and good: implications to the heart and brain. *Sleep Med. Rev.* (2015) 20:27–45.

[24] Kondılı E, Xırouchakı N, Georgopoulos D. Monitoring during acute non-invasiveventilation. Inbook: *Non-invasiveVentilation and Weaning: Principles and Practice*, pp.97-106.

Chapter 7

Hypercapnic OSA and COPD: The Overlap Syndrome

Stefano Oldani[1,*]
Andrea De Vito[2]
and Arianna J. De Grauw[1]
[1]Department of Thoracic Diseases, Pulmonary Operative Unit, Morgagni Pierantoni Hospital, Health Local Agency of Romagna, Forlì, Italy
[2]Head and Neck Department, ENT Unit, Ravenna - Lugo Hospitals, Health Local Agency of Romagna, Italy

Abstract

The coexistence of obstructive sleep apnea (OSA) and chronic obstructive pulmonary disease (COPD) has been labeled as Overlap Syndrome (OS). However, there is no clear evidence whether OS is a specific condition or just the concurrent occurrence of two common disorders by chance. In fact, the interpretation of the studies conducted in this field is challenging, due to their wide methodological differences. Typical of OS are intermittent nocturnal oxygen desaturations from a baseline hypoxemia, the latter resulting from the dynamic hyperinflation showed by COPD patients while sleeping. OS patients show increased oxidative stress and systemic inflammation, along with an increased risk of developing cardiovascular disease and mortality due to cardiovascular events. Physical activity, weight loss, smoking cessation and bronchodilation can help in the treatment of OS. However, continuous positive airway pressure (CPAP) remains the cornerstone of treatment of OS patients with OSA dominancy, while bilevel noninvasive ventilation

* Corresponding Author's Email: stefano.oldani11289@gmail.com.

In: Obstructive Sleep Apnea in Pulmonary Critical Care
Editors: Antonio M. Esquinas and Takatoshi Kasai
ISBN: 979-8-88697-858-2

(NIV) can play a role in case of chronic nocturnal hypoventilation with daytime hypercapnia.

Keywords: obstructive sleep apnea (OSA), chronic obstructive pulmonary disease (COPD), overlap syndrome (OS), cardiovascular comorbidities, positive airway pressure (PAP) therapies

Introduction

Obstructive sleep apnea (OSA) and chronic obstructive pulmonary disease (COPD) are two common breathing disorders, both affecting 10% of the adult population. OSA is caused by the partial or total intermittent upper airways collapse, resulting in hypoxemia and arousal during sleeping. COPD is a slowly progressive disease characterized by persistent airflow obstruction, due to exposure to cigarette smoke. The coexistence of these two diseases has been labeled as Overlap Syndrome (OS), although there is no clear evidence whether OS is a specific condition or just the concurrent occurrence of two common disorders by chance. However, there are considerable data that show close interactions between OSA and COPD, that can influence epidemiology, clinical manifestations, co-morbidities and management of the OS patients [1].

Epidemiology

The hypothesis that OSA may predispose to COPD and vice versa has been explored in many studies, but comparison of the results is challenging due to the significant methodological differences. The first report from the Sleep Heart Health Study found no increased prevalence of sleep breathing disorders (SBD) in patients with mild COPD, although nocturnal oxygen desaturations were more pronounced in patients with OS. However, the examined population was relatively old, and other evidence suggests OSA being less common in elderly affected by COPD [2]. Similar results were reported in a sub-analysis of the WHO-sponsored Monica II project [3]. On the other hand, more recent studies have shown a relatively high prevalence of OSA in patients with moderate to severe COPD, while according to another metanalyses the prevalence of OS ranges from 2.9% and 65.9% in COPD patients [4]. These conflicting results may reflect the different populations in exam, the inconsistent definition of the diseases between studies, and the possibility of survival bias in older patients. However, increased body mass index (BMI) and smoking history positively correlates with the likelihood of OSA in COPD patients.

Pathophisiology

Sleep Breathing Disorders in COPD

SBDs are common in COPD, affecting approximately 40% of the patients. SBDs in COPD can be categorized as [5]:

1. Nocturnal oxygen desaturation (NOD): a fall of PaO2 > 10mmHg or SpO2 < 88% for more than five minutes. The prevalence of NOD increases with COPD severity and can occur even in patients with adequate daytime SpO2.
2. OSA: this diagnosis is confirmed either by a detection of an apnea hypopnea index (AHI) ≥ 15 or by an AHI between 5 -14 plus one or more sleep associated conditions, being:
    a. Sleepiness, nonrestorative sleep, fatigue, or insomnia
    b. Waking up with breath holding, gasping, or choking
    c. Habitual snoring, breathing interruptions, or both, noted by a bed partner or other observer
    d. Hypertension, mood disorder, cognitive dysfunction, coronary artery disease, stroke, congestive heart failure, atrial fibrillation, or type 2 diabetes mellitus
3. Sleep related hypoventilation (SRH): defined as a greater than normal increase in $PaCO_2$ during sleep (PaCO2 of > 50 mmHg or rise of PaCO2 of > 10 mmHg for more than 10 minutes compared to wakefulness). SRH is usually present in chronic hypercapnic COPD patients but can also be recorded in COPD patients without daytime hypercapnia, especially during rapid eye movement (REM) sleep.

The normal sleep-related decline in respiratory drive may exacerbate ventilation-perfusion mismatch and hypoventilation in individuals with COPD, especially during REM sleep. In addition, COPD is characterized by air trapping, due to the premature collapse of small airways during the expiratory phase of breathing. Thus, the increase of the closing volume, along with a reduction of functional residual capacity, can also exacerbate ventilation-perfusion mismatch and hypoxemia.

Moreover, sleep is associated with a loss of drive to upper airway dilator muscles, leading to upper airway narrowing and subsequent inspiratory airflow limitation. In COPD patients, this limitation can further compromise ventilation and increase PaCO2. Lastly, while sleeping, COPD patients also lose specific acquired mechanisms to minimize hyperinflation (by prolonging expiratory time) and to preserve alveolar ventilation (with pursed lip breathing) commonly adopted while awake. All these alterations make COPD patients more prone to dynamic hyperinflation, hence NOD and nocturnal hypoventilation [5].

Interaction between COPD and OS

COPD is not a uniform disease; indeed, it presents with different phenotypes. The two extremities of this spectrum are pulmonary emphysema (pink puffers), patients usually with low BMI, hyperinflation, predominant symptoms of dyspnea and preserved gas exchange, and chronic bronchitis (blue bloater), patients with higher BMI, cor pulmonale, productive cough and hypoxemia.

The predominant emphysema phenotype is linked with a lower likelihood of OSA, due to lower BMI and to hyperinflation itself. In fact, hyperinflation is associated with improvement in upper airway collapsibility, which may explain why COPD patients with emphysema typically do not present with concomitant OSA. On the other hand, patients with chronic bronchitis usually show higher BMI and fluid retention, due to cor pulmonale. This predisposes to a rostral shift of the fluid while sleeping in supine position, hence narrowing the upper airways and increasing the risk of OSA [6].

Actually, most COPD patients are affected by a mixture of emphysema and chronic bronchitis, thus the prevalence of OSA likely reflects a balance of these protective or promoting factors [1].

In addition, COPD patients are often current smokers. Cigarette smoking has been shown to enhance upper airway inflammation and edema, and this may also contribute to increase the risk of OSA.

OSA also appears to exacerbate lower airway inflammation in patients with COPD.

Animal models showed intermittent hypoxia to be linked to progressive lung damage by inducing inflammation and oxidative stress. In fact, patients with OS not treated with CPAP have been shown to have a higher mortality and to be more likely to suffer severe COPD exacerbations leading to hospitalization (RR 1.70) when compared to COPD-only patients [7].

The Burden of Overlap Syndrome on Comorbidities

COPD and OSA are linked to a range of overlapping alterations, such as hypoxia and inflammation, which can contribute to cardiovascular and other comorbidities. Therefore, it is likely that OS is associated with a greater risk of comorbidities than either disease alone. Intermittent hypoxemia stimulates the release of systemic inflammatory mediators like TNF-alfa, IL-6, IL-8, CRP, hence promoting oxidative stress and endothelial dysfunction. As a matter of fact, OSA is associated with a greater risk of systemic hypertension, cardiac arrythmias, coronary artery disease, congestive heart failure and stroke, with a greater overall cardiovascular mortality [8]. On the other hand, COPD has been recognized to be associated with nocturnal desaturations, that can predispose to pulmonary hypertension [9]. Moreover, a report showed that patients with OS have higher sympathetic activity when compared to OSA or COPD alone, providing another potential mechanism for the development of cardiac disease [10].

To summarize, patients affected by OS have been shown to have an increased oxidative stress and systemic inflammation along with an increased risk of developing cardiovascular disease and mortality due to cardiovascular events [6] [11].

Clinical Assessment

It is crucial for clinicians to evaluate patients with OSA or COPD for OS. In fact, OS patients may present with clinical features of either OSA or COPD, depending on the balance between the two conditions. Patients with COPD report poor sleep quality and fatigue, while OSA patients usually complain of excessive snoring, unrefreshing sleep, and excessive daytime sleepiness. In any case, it is likely that signs of chronic hypoxemia, hypercapnia or pulmonary hypertension might be detected. Therefore, typical clinical features can be morning headache due to hypercapnia, cyanosis reflecting hypoxemia and peripheral edema due to cor pulmonale and pulmonary hypertension.

Screening questionnaires such as the Stop-BANG or the NOSAS, have been developed to determine the likelihood of OSA in patients admitted to preoperative and sleep clinics, respectively. These scores are easy and swift to perform, and investigate the presence of clinical features, anthropometric measures (eg. neck circumference, BMI, waist to hip ratio…) and comorbidities typical of patients affected by OSA. These tools can therefore be useful to evaluate the likelihood of OSA in COPD patients as well. However, interpolation of data such as age, sex, BMI and the presence of cardiovascular comorbidities may be superior to traditional symptoms of snoring and daytime sleepiness in predicting the presence of OSA [1].

Polysomnography is still the gold standard to detect sleep disorders, although a sleep study focused on cardiorespiratory parameters may be sufficient to detect OSA in a COPD patient. As previously mentioned, intermittent nocturnal oxygen desaturations from a baseline hypoxemia are the typical feature of OS. These intermittent desaturations have been reported to be greater than desaturations shown in OSA alone. This may be the result of OS patients having a lower baseline saturation during sleep, due to their COPD component [6].

Treatment

The treatment of OS should aim to maintain nocturnal oxygenation, reduce intermittent hypoxemia and hypoventilation, resulting in improvement of sleep quality and mortality as well.

Lifestyle modifications. Exercise programs and pulmonary rehabilitation are known to be beneficial both in OSA and COPD. In fact, OSA patients showed improvement of AHI, daytime sleepiness, and overall sleep quality after an exercise program. Similarly, pulmonary rehabilitation can result in improved quality of life, mood index, dyspnea scores and reduced hospital admissions in COPD patients. However, these measures may not be effective in the management of the disease and must be supplemented with other appropriate treatment options. Along with these behavioral modifications, smoking cessation is strongly recommended to reduce morbidity and mortality associated with OS.

*Supplemental oxygen therapy***.** Supplemental oxygen therapy for at least 18h per day is the cornerstone of treatment of chronic respiratory failure in COPD. However, it has been shown not to be beneficial neither in COPD patients with borderline respiratory failure, nor in COPD patients with nocturnal desaturations and normal daytime saturation. Oxygen alone is also not effective in OSA treatment, since although it can help reduce the episodes of NOD, it does not improve quality of sleep or reduce nighttime arousals. Hence, supplemental oxygen therapy alone is not recommended as treatment for OS [12].

Bronchodilators. Bronchodilation can reduce dynamic hyperinflation in COPD patients, thus reducing NOD and improving sleep quality and REM sleep time. However, little is known regarding possible beneficial effects on OSA of bronchodilation treatment of COPD in OS [6].

Positive airway pressure (PAP) therapies. CPAP is the most effective treatment for OSA and OS, since it can enhance upper airway patency, hence reducing upper airways resistance along with nocturnal hypoventilation. It has also been shown to reduce the release of radical oxidant species (ROS) and improve FEV1, PaO2, PaCO2 and mean pulmonary artery pressure. CPAP can furthermore reduce mortality in OS patients, also reducing episodes of AE-COPD [7]. Therefore, in patients where OSA is predominant, CPAP is the preferred therapeutic option. However, where COPD is the dominant component, especially in patients with chronic hypercapnia, bilevel NIV may be more appropriate to reduce hypercapnia, improve quality of life, and, according to some reports, also prolong survival [13].

Conclusion

OSA and COPD are two common breathing disorders, both affecting nearly 10% of the adult population. The coexistence of these two diseases has been labeled as Overlap Syndrome (OS), although there is no clear evidence whether OS is a specific condition or just the concurrent occurrence of two common disorders by chance. In summary we consider that: a) Patients affected by OS have been shown to have increased oxidative stress and systemic inflammation along with an increased risk of development of cardiovascular disease and mortality due to cardiovascular events, b) Most of COPD patients are affected by a mixture of emphysema and chronic bronchitis, and thus the prevalence of OSA likely reflects a balance of protective factors (hyperinflation) or promoting factors (high BMI, upper airway edema), c) Intermittent nocturnal oxygen desaturations from a baseline hypoxemia are the typical feature of OS. These intermittent desaturations have been generally reported to be greater than desaturation shown in OSA alone. This may be the result of OS patients having a lower baseline saturation during sleep, due to their COPD component and d) Physical activity, weight loss, smoking cessation and bronchodilation can help in the treatment of OS. However, CPAP remains the cornerstone of treatment of OS patients with OSA dominancy, while bilevel NIV can play a role in case of chronic nocturnal hypoventilation with daytime hypercapnia.

References

[1] McNicholas, W. T. COPD-OSA Overlap Syndrome. *Chest* 2017, **152**, 1318–1326.

[2] Sanders, M. H., Newman, A. B., Haggerty, C. L., Redline, S., Lebowitz, M., Samet, J., O'Connor, G. T., Punjabi, N. M. & Shahar, E. Sleep and Sleep-disordered Breathing in Adults with Predominantly Mild Obstructive Airway Disease. *Am. J. Respir. Crit. Care Med.* 2003, 167, 7–14.

[3] Bednarek, M., Plywaczewski, R., Jonczak, L. & Zielinski, J. There Is No Relationship between Chronic Obstructive Pulmonary Disease and Obstructive Sleep Apnea Syndrome: A Population Study. *Respiration* 2005, 72, 142–149.

[4] Shawon, M. S. R., Perret, J. L., Senaratna, C. V., Lodge, C., Hamilton, G. S. & Dharmage, S. C. Current evidence on prevalence and clinical outcomes of co-morbid obstructive sleep apnea and chronic obstructive pulmonary disease: A systematic review. *Sleep Med. Rev.* 2017, 32, 58–68.

[5] Budhiraja, R., Siddiqi, T. A. & Quan, S. F. Sleep Disorders in Chronic Obstructive Pulmonary Disease: Etiology, Impact, and Management. *J. Clin. Sleep Med.* 2015, 11, 259–270.

[6] Singh, S., Kaur, H., Singh, S. & Khawaja, I. The Overlap Syndrome. *Cureus* 2018, doi:10.7759/cureus.3453.

[7] Marin, J. M., Soriano, J. B., Carrizo, S. J., Boldova, A. & Celli, B. R. Outcomes in Patients with Chronic Obstructive Pulmonary Disease and Obstructive Sleep Apnea. *Am. J. Respir. Crit. Care Med.* 2010, 182, 325–331.

[8] Young, T., Finn, L., Peppard, P. E., Szklo-Coxe, M., Austin, D., Nieto, F. J., Stubbs, R. & Hla, K. M. Sleep disordered breathing and mortality: eighteen-year follow-up of the Wisconsin sleep cohort. *Sleep* 2008, 31, 1071–8.

[9] Fletcher, E. C., Luckett, R. A., Miller, T., Costarangos, C., Kutka, N. & Fletcher, J. G. Pulmonary Vascular Hemodynamics in Chronic Lung Disease Patients with and without Oxyhemoglobin Desaturation During Sleep. *Chest* 1989, 95, 757–764.

[10] Taranto-Montemurro, L., Messineo, L., Perger, E., Salameh, M., Pini, L., Corda, L., Ferliga, M. & Tantucci, C. Cardiac Sympathetic Hyperactivity in Patients with Chronic Obstructive Pulmonary Disease and Obstructive Sleep Apnea. *COPD J. Chronic Obstr. Pulm. Dis.* 2016, 13, 706–711.

[11] Singh, G., Agarwal, A., Zhang, W., Kuo, Y.-F., Sultana, R. & Sharma, G. Impact of PAP therapy on hospitalization rates in Medicare beneficiaries with COPD and coexisting OSA. *Sleep Breath.* 2019, 23, 193–200.

[12] Lacasse, Y., Sériès, F., Corbeil, F., Baltzan, M., Paradis, B., Simão, P., Abad Fernández, A., Esteban, C., Guimarães, M., Bourbeau, J., Aaron, S. D., Bernard, S. & Maltais, F. Randomized Trial of Nocturnal Oxygen in Chronic Obstructive Pulmonary Disease. *N. Engl. J. Med.* 2020, 383, 1129–1138.

[13] Köhnlein, T., Windisch, W., Köhler, D., Drabik, A., Geiseler, J., Hartl, S., Karg, O., Laier-Groeneveld, G., Nava, S., Schönhofer, B., Schucher, B., Wegscheider, K., Criée, C. P. & Welte, T. Non-invasive positive pressure ventilation for the treatment of severe stable chronic obstructive pulmonary disease: a prospective, multicentre, randomised, controlled clinical trial. *Lancet Respir. Med.* 2014, 2, 698–705.

Chapter 8

Asthma Overlap Syndrome: Concept and Ventilatory Modes

Nursel Dikmen*, MD
Hatay Mustafa Kemal University, Faculty of Medicine,
Department of Chest Diseases, Hatay, Turkey

Abstract

Obstructive sleep apnea syndrome (OSAS) is a syndrome characterized by recurrent episodes of upper airway obstruction during sleep and often progresses with a decrease in blood oxygen saturation. OSAS patients have high mortality and morbidity rates. Asthma, on the other hand, is a heterogeneous disease, usually characterized by chronic airway inflammation, causing bronchial obstruction and secondary respiratory symptoms such as cough, shortness of breath, and wheezing, especially in the form of nocturnal attacks. The co-occurrence of obstructive sleep apnea-hypopnea syndrome (OSAS) and lung diseases such as chronic obstructive pulmonary disease (COPD), asthma, interstitial lung disease (ILD), and cystic fibrosis is called overlap syndrome. In this section, the co-existence of OSAS and asthma was considered an overlap syndrome. Recent data have shown that the presence of OSAS in asthma patients makes it difficult for patients to control their symptoms. Again, some studies have found an increased prevalence of OSAS in asthma patients. This section summarizes OSAS asthma overlap syndrome and treatment modalities considering the current literature.

Keywords: asthma, overlap syndrome, obstructive sleep apnea syndrome, chronic inflammation, continuous positive airway pressure (CPAP)

* Corresponding Author's Email: nurselkayadikmen@gmail.com.

In: Obstructive Sleep Apnea in Pulmonary Critical Care
Editors: Antonio M. Esquinas and Takatoshi Kasai
ISBN: 979-8-88697-858-2

Introduction

Asthma and sleep breathing disorders (especially obstructive sleep apnea syndrome, the most common in this group) are among the most common respiratory system diseases in recent years. Studies have better characterized the underlying pathophysiology of both diseases, but more detailed studies are needed to address the comorbidities associated with both diseases and the close association of the two diseases. Although the main pathophysiology of OSAS is an obstruction in the upper airways, it has been shown in recent years that inflammation in the airways and increased bronchial hyperactivity are independent risk factors for asthma attacks in these patients and that it makes it difficult to control the symptoms of asthma patients [1]. Similarly, the prevalence of asthma has been increasing in recent years. The most important reasons for this increase are thought to be increased air pollution, increased environmental exposure, and increased incidence of obesity. Symptoms in asthma patients are usually shortness of breath and cough, especially more common at night. These symptoms occurring at night cause fragmented sleep and consequently excessive daytime sleepiness in patients and are common in both diseases, suggesting that the relationship between asthma and OSAS should be examined in more detail. In addition, both diseases are closely associated with allergic rhinitis, gastroesophageal reflux (GER), and obesity. And in both diseases, it can cause similar comorbidities (cardiac arrhythmia, HT, heart failure) due to hypoxia and ventilation disorder [2]. Therefore, in this section, whether asthma and OSAS are two similar diseases that coexist and whether they are pathophysiological related will be summarized considering the current literature.

Obstructive Sleep Apnea Syndrome

Clinical manifestations that lead to increased morbidity and mortality caused by pathological changes in the breathing pattern during sleep are called "sleep breathing disorders" (SBD). Obstructive sleep apnea syndrome is the most common sleep breathing disorder. Obstructive sleep apnea syndrome (OSAS) is characterized by episodes of complete or partial upper airway obstruction during sleep. Inadequate ventilation due to obstruction results in intermittent hypoxia and hypercapnia [3]. Cardiac rhythm disturbances, fluctuations in blood pressure, and intrathoracic pressure are seen as an acute result of ventilation disorder that occurs at night, and as the process becomes chronic, the systemic inflammation causes endothelial dysfunction, metabolic disorders, hypertension, and cardiovascular diseases in the long term. In addition, obesity, increased insulin resistance, deterioration in cognitive functions, deterioration in the quality of life, and increased mortality are observed in patients [4].

Although it is seen in all age groups, it is more common, especially in middle-aged men. It is seen in 2-4% of the adult population [5]. Obesity, age (middle age), gender (more common in male gender – smoking status, fat accumulation in different regions, hormonal effects), smoking and alcohol use, comorbidities (hypothyroidism, collagen tissue diseases) are among the risk factors.

The most common complaints of patients were identified as snoring, witnessed apnea, and excessive daytime sleepiness, and decreased quality of life, decreased neurocognitive activities, and susceptibility to anxiety and depression due to insufficient sleep. All-night polysomnography (PSG), in which more than one physiological signal is monitored simultaneously, is the gold standard in the diagnosis of OSAS. In the presence of OSAS symptoms, an apnea-hypopnea index (AHI) of 5 or higher on PSG makes the diagnosis of OSAS [4].

Continuous positive airway pressure (CPAP) therapy is the first choice in the treatment of adult OSAS patients if AHI > 30/h or AHI between 5 and 30, accompanied by symptoms and comorbidities. Other adjunctive therapy modalities are mandibular advancement devices, surgery, or upper airway stimulation therapy. As additional precautions, patients should be advised to lose weight if overweight, avoid sedative treatments and alcohol before sleep, and positional therapy [2].

Asthma

Asthma is a chronic inflammatory disease of the airways characterized by direct or indirect airway responsiveness. Depending on the degree of airway inflammation, respiratory symptoms such as shortness of breath, cough, chest tightness, and wheezing are detected in patients. The frequency and intensity of symptoms can change over time. However, the symptoms are more common, especially at night. Symptoms resolve spontaneously or with treatment. Asthma is thought to affect about 300 million people worldwide. Numerous research results reported from different parts of the world show great variation in prevalence rates. Studies with relatively standardized and comparable methods for children and adults have found that these rates vary between 1-18% in different countries [6].

The presence of atopy, the presence of allergic rhinitis and eczema, and family history are among the important points in the diagnosis. Although the physical examination is usually normal, depending on the degree of airway obstruction, rhonchi, wheezing, decreased breath sounds (silent chest) in a severe asthma attack, tachypnea, and use of accessory respiratory muscles may be observed during auscultation. In all clinical forms of asthma, there is a chronic inflammation of the airways. Airway inflammation is accompanied by thickening of airway smooth muscles and subepithelial lamina reticularis, matrix deposition in the airway wall, increase in micro vessels and neural networks, increased submucosal glands, and mucosal metaplasia [7].

Measurement of respiratory functions provides support for the diagnosis of asthma by showing the severity, reversibility, and variability of airway restriction. However, normal pulmonary function tests do not exclude the diagnosis of asthma.

Asthma medications are divided into two; controller and reliever (symptom reliever). Controller medications are drugs that are used every day and for a long time, which often keep asthma under control thanks to their anti-inflammatory effects. Relievers, on the other hand, are drugs that act quickly to reverse bronchoconstriction, relieve symptoms, and are used when needed [8].

OSAS-Asthma Overlap Syndrome

The term "overlap" is used for clinical conditions that are related to each other and exhibit different characteristics when combined. In sleep disorders, overlap syndrome is a term used for the association of obstructive sleep apnea-hypopnea syndrome (OSAS) with lung diseases such as chronic obstructive pulmonary disease (COPD), asthma, interstitial lung disease (ILD), and cystic fibrosis.

Similar symptoms detected in both asthma and OSAS patients suggested that these two diseases are related to each other. The first study showing the relationship between asthma and OSAS was presented as a case report by Hudgel and Shrucard in 1979 [9]. In the Wisconsin Sleep Cohort study investigating the risk of developing OSAS in asthma patients, the authors evaluated 547 adult asthma patients (52% female, mean age 50 years) by polysomnography every four years since 1988 and found that the relative risk of developing OSAS was high for asthma patients -adjusted for gender, age, and body mass index (BMI)-(RR = 1.39). In the continuation of the same study, they determined that OSAS was not only an independent risk factor for asthma but also helped worsen asthma and increase asthma exacerbations. Additionally, they found that asthma patients had more excessive daytime sleepiness than the normal population [10, 11].

In a study involving 7649 adults, Ekici et al., reported the presence of asthma symptoms in 2713 patients. They found that snoring and witnessed apnea were higher in these patients with a history of asthma compared to the group without a history of asthma (after adjusting for age, gender, BMI, smoking, income, and educational status). They also observed a lower health-related quality of life in these patients [12].

It has been suggested that the presence of OSAS in asthma patients causes worsening of asthma control. The responsible mechanisms for this are thought to be neuromechanical reflex bronchoconstriction, gastroesophageal reflux, inflammation (local and systemic), and deterioration in cardiac functions as a result of its indirect effect on OSAS-induced dyspnea. Also, additional mechanisms such as airway angiogenesis, leptin-related airway changes, and OSAS-induced weight gain are implicated [13].

In OSAS patients, obstruction in the upper airways causes an increase in vagal tone. Studies have shown that this increase in vagal tone causes bronchoconstriction in the airways. Therefore, it is thought that patients with asthma accompanied by OSAS may experience an increase in nocturnal dyspnea, or it may lead to nocturnal asthma [14]. In addition, studies have shown that neural receptors in the larynx and epiglottis as a result of an obstruction in the upper respiratory tract and increased pressure in the pulmonary capillaries due to increased intrathoracic pressure may cause bronchoconstriction [13].

Studies have found that OSAS is accompanied by gastroesophageal reflux in 58-62% of patients. It causes an increase in negative intrathoracic pressure and an increase in transdiaphragmatic pressure secondary to obstruction in the upper airways. These events cause lower esophageal sphincter relaxation and drainage of gastric contents back into the oesophagus. In contrast, the cleansing ability of stomach acid in patients with GERD often decreases at night. This results in pharyngeal spasms and mucosal inflammation, making the airway more prone to collapse during sleep. Besides, laryngitis and edema caused by reflux may worsen the degree of obstruction. Additionally, GERD is one of the most important risk factors that trigger asthma attacks and complicate asthma treatment. Reflex bronchospasm is caused by receptors stimulated in the esophageal mucosa due to reflux [15]. Asthma is a chronic inflammatory disease of the airways. Inflammation in the airways causes extravasation of fluid and mucosal edema, resulting in narrowing of the bronchi. In addition, patients have chronic systemic inflammation. In OSAS patients, along with systemic inflammation, airway inflammation thought to be caused by mechanical trauma of airway obstruction and vibration due to snoring, as well as local oxidative stress, has been detected. In both cases, the resulting inflammation is thought to contribute to airway obstruction and worsen the symptoms. After mechanical trauma in OSAS, edema occurs in the soft palate and uvula due to cytokines released from the mucous membranes [16].

Another mechanism supporting the relationship between asthma and OSAS is vascular endothelial growth factor (VEGF) and airway angiogenesis. VEGF is a hypoxia-sensitive glycoprotein that stimulates vascular growth. Studies have shown that VEGF has an important role in the pathogenesis of asthma. In addition, a correlation has been found between the degree of airway obstruction and increased VEGF levels in patients with asthma [17]. While VEGF levels were increased due to nocturnal hypoxia in OSAS patients, there was a positive correlation between AHI and VEGF levels. Oxygen-free radicals that emerge after recurrent hypoxia cause gene expression of peptides such as endothelin, resulting in an increase in VEGF levels. Some studies have found higher VEGF levels in OSAS patients with airway hyperresponsiveness [18].

Obesity is a significant risk factor for the development of asthma in both adults and children. In obese asthma patients, there is a bidirectional relationship involving more exacerbations, more symptoms, less response to treatment. Many factors have been suggested for the obesity-asthma relationship. These include nutrition, genetic factors, metabolic factors, increased oxidative stress and cytokines, environmental exposures, and mechanical effects such as reduction in functional residual capacity (FRC). In addition, obesity can cause GER, making it difficult to control asthma. Although many sub-phenotypes of asthma are associated with obesity, obesity-associated asthma constitutes a single sub-phenotype [19, 20]. Obesity is one of the most important factors in the development of OSAS. In one of the most important studies showing the effect of obesity on the development of OSAS, Peppard et al., evaluated 690 adults at two different times (at the beginning and 4 years later), and found that individuals with a BMI $\geq$ 30 kg/m2 (n = 268) had an AHI of 7.4 events/hour, those with 30 > BMI $\geq$ 25 kg/m2 (n

= 241) had an AHI of 2.6 events/hour, and those with a BMI < 25 kg/m2 (n = 181) had an AHI of 1.2 events/hour. After 4 years of follow-up, those with more than 10% body weight gain resulted in an approximately 32% increase in AHI, and those with a 10% body weight loss resulted in a 26% reduction in AHI [21]. The increase in adipose tissue in the neck region and consequent pharyngeal narrowing weakens the support of the pharyngeal muscles and causes easier closure. Again, the increase in fat thickness in the abdomen affects the movement of the diaphragm, reducing the compliance of the lungs, and contributing to the closure of the upper airways. In addition, adipose tissues secrete various hormonally active agents such as leptin, TNF-α, IL-6, and inflammatory cytokines contribute to the increase of inflammation in the airways. In OSAS, impaired sleep architecture and intermittent hypoxia lead to neurohormonal abnormalities such as changes in the leptin-ghrelin ratio and subsequently increase oral intake, while reducing daytime activities exacerbates obesity and increases the difficulty in losing weight.

As can be seen from the studies, OSAS and asthma have similar pathogenesis, symptoms, and treatments. This relationship between them indicated that OSAS symptoms should definitely be questioned in asthma patients, and this is more important, especially in asthma that is difficult to control.

Treatment

The first line of treatment in OSAS is continuous positive airway pressure (CPAP) therapy. With CPAP treatment, improvement in clinical findings, reduction in respiratory events, improvement in nocturnal hypoxia, and consequently a decrease in OSAS-associated mortality and morbidity rates are detected. CPAP treatment was determined to have positive effects on asthma in patients with asthma accompanied by OSAS.

Çiftçi et al., evaluated 43 asthma patients who had night-time symptoms despite optimal medication and had a habit of snoring for 6 months according to the Global Initiative for Asthma (GINA) guidelines and detected OSAS in polysomnography in 21 of them (AHI > 5). They applied CPAP treatment to 16 of 19 patients with AHI ≥ 15. They reported a statistically significant improvement in nocturnal asthma after CPAP therapy [22].

Chan et al., detected OSAS in 8 of 9 patients who were receiving maximal asthma treatment and had frequent nocturnal asthma attacks and heavy snoring, and they found a decrease in asthma symptoms and nocturnal bronchodilator use (from 2 to 0 on average per night), and improvement in pulmonary function tests after 2 weeks of nocturnal CPAP treatment in these patients [23].

Many studies have shown that CPAP therapy reduces local and systemic inflammation in OSAS and is also effective in the treatment of asthma accompanying OSAS due to its favourable mechanical and neuromechanical effects on the airways [24].

Conclusion

The presence of OSAS in asthma patients makes it difficult to control the symptoms, increases the frequency of asthma exacerbations, worsens nocturnal symptoms, increases secondary complications, and additionally causes a significant decrease in patients' quality of life. Although asthma and OSAS are evaluated as two different diseases involving the respiratory system, it is not possible to distinguish between the two diseases when considering similar pathophysiological mechanisms, clinical conditions, and symptoms, and accompanying comorbidities. Additional symptoms such as allergic rhinitis and GER, which are frequently seen together in asthma and OSAS, should be treated appropriately. Asthma patients, especially those whose night-time symptoms persist despite maximal therapy, should be questioned for concomitant OSAS. In asthmatic patients with concomitant OSAS, CPAP treatment improved control of asthma symptoms and reduced the need for medical treatment. Studies have shown that CPAP therapy in patients with asthma and comorbid OSAS results in improved asthma control and quality of life, reduction in asthma exacerbations, and reduction in possible comorbid conditions.

References

[1] Ragnoli B, Pochetti P, Raie A, Malerba M. Interrelationship Between Obstructive Sleep Apnea Syndrome and Severe Asthma: From Endo-Phenotype to Clinical Aspects. *Front Med.* (Lausanne). 2021 Jun 30;8:640636. doi: 10.3389/ fmed. 2021.640636.

[2] Prasad B, Nyenhuis S M, Weaver T E. Obstructive sleep apnea and asthma: associations and treatment implications. *Sleep Med. Rev.* 2014 Apr;18(2):165-71. doi: 10.1016/j.smrv.2013.04.004.

[3] American Academy of Sleep Medicine. International classification of sleep disorders. *Diagnostic and coding manual (ICSD-3). 3rd ed*. American Academy of Sleep Medicine: Westchester, IL, 2014.

[4] Heinzer R, Vat S, Marques-Vidal P, Marti-Soler H, Andries D, Tobback N, Mooser V, Preisig M, Malhotra A, Waeber G, Vollenweider P, Tafti M, Haba-Rubio J. Prevalence of sleep-disordered breathing in the general population: the HypnoLaus study. *Lancet Respir. Med.* 2015 Apr;3(4):310-8. doi: 10.1016/S2213-2600(15) 00043-0.

[5] Young T, Peppard P, Palta M, Hla K M, Finn L, Morgan B. Population-based study of sleep-disordered breathing as a risk factor for hypertension. *Arch. Intern. Med.* 1997;157:1746–52.

[6] Global Initiative for Asthma (GINA). *Global strategy for asthma management and prevention (Update 2021).* (Avaliable from:https://ginasthma.org/wp-content/uploads/2021/05/GINA-Main-Report-2021-V2-WMS.pdf).

[7] Mims J W. Asthma: definitions and pathophysiology. *Int. Forum Allergy Rhinol.* 2015 Sep;5 Suppl 1:S2-6. doi: 10.1002/alr.21609.

[8] Chung KF. Precision medicine in asthma: linking phenotypes to targeted treatments. *Curr. Opin. Pulm. Med.* 2018 Jan;24(1):4-10. doi: 10.1097/MCP. 00000000000 00434.

[9] Hudgel D W, Shucard D W. Coexistence of sleep apnea and asthma resulting in severe sleep hypoxemia. *JAMA.* 1979;242(25):2789-90. Doi: 10.1001/ jama.1979. 03300250045031.

[10] Teodorescu M C M, Polomis D A, Hall S V, TeodorescuMC, Gangnon R E, Peterson A G, Xie A, Sorkness C A, Jarjour N N. Association of obstructive sleep apnea risk with asthma control in adults. *Chest.* (2010) 138:543–50. doi: 10.1378/chest.09-3066.

[11] Teodorescu M, Barnet J H, Hagen E W, Palta M, Young T B, Peppard P E. Association between asthma and risk of developing obstructive sleep apnea. *J. Am. Med. Assoc*. (2015) 2014:17822. doi: 10.1001/jama.2014.17822.

[12] Ekici A, Ekici M, Kurtipek E, Keles H, Kara T, Tunckol M, Kocyigit P. Association of asthma-related symptoms with snoring and apnea and effect on health-related quality of life. *Chest.* 2005;128(5):3358-63. Doi: 10.1378/ chest.128.5.3358 PMid:16304284.

[13] Alkhalil M, Schulman E, Getsy J. Obstructive sleep apnea syndrome and asthma: what are the links? *J. Clin. Sleep Med*. 2009 Feb 15;5(1):71-8.

[14] Morrison J F, Pearson S B, Dean H G. Parasympathetic nervous system in nocturnal asthma. *Br. Med. J. (Clin Res Ed).* 1988 May 21;296(6634):1427-9. doi: 10.1136/bmj.296.6634.1427.

[15] Qiao Y X, Xiao Y. Asthma and Obstructive Sleep Apnea. *Chin. Med. J.* (Engl). 2015 Oct 20;128(20):2798-804. doi: 10.4103/0366-6999.167361.

[16] Sekosan M, Zakkar M, Wenig B L, Olopade C O, Rubinstein I. Inflammation in the uvula mucosa of patients with obstructive sleep apnea. *Laryngoscope*. 1996 Aug;106(8):1018-20. doi: 10.1097/00005537-199608000-00021.

[17] Hoshino M, Takahashi M, Aoike N. Expression of vascular endothelial growth factor, basic fibroblast growth factor, and angiogenin immunoreactivity in asthmatic

airways and its relationship to angiogenesis. *J. Allergy Clin. Immunol.* 2001 Feb;107(2):295-301. doi: 10.1067/mai.2001.111928.

[18] Schulz R, Schmidt D, Blum A, Lopes-Ribeiro X, Lücke C, Mayer K, Olschewski H, Seeger W, Grimminger F. Decreased plasma levels of nitric oxide derivatives in obstructive sleep apnoea: response to CPAP therapy. *Thorax.* 2000 Dec;55(12) :1046-51. doi: 10.1136/thorax.55.12.1046.

[19] Sideleva O, Suratt B T, Black K E, Tharp W G, Pratley R E, Forgione P, Dienz O, Irvin C G, Dixon A E . Obesity and asthma: an inflammatory disease of adipose tissue not the airway. *Am. J. Respirat. Crit. Care Med.* (2012) 186:598– 605. doi: 10.1164/rccm.201203-0573OC.

[20] Peters U, Dixon A, Forno E. Obesity and Asthma. *J. Allergy Clin. Immunol.* (2018) 141:1169–79. doi: 10.1016/j.jaci.2018.02.004.

[21] Peppard P E, Young T, Palta M, Dempsey J, Skatrud J. Longitudinal study of moderate weight change and sleep disordered breathing. *JAMA.* 2000;284(23):3015-21. Doi: 10.1001/jama.284.23.3015.

[22] Ciftci T U, Ciftci B, Guven S F, Kokturk O, Turktas H. Effect of nasal continuous positive airway pressure in uncontrolled nocturnal asthmatic patients with obstructive sleep apnea syndrome. *Respir. Med.* 2005 May;99(5):529-34. doi: 10.1016/j.rmed.2004.10.011.

[23] Chan C S, Woolcock A J, Sullivan C E. Nocturnal asthma: role of snoring and obstructive sleep apnea. *Am. Rev. Respir. Dis.* 1988 Jun;137(6):1502-4. doi: 10.1164/ajrccm/137.6.1502.

[24] Alkhalil M, Schulman E S, Getsy J. Obstructive sleep apnea syndrome and asthma: the role of continuous positive airway pressure treatment. *Ann. Allergy Asthma Immunol.* 2008 Oct;101(4):350-7. doi: 10.1016/S1081-1206(10)60309-2.

Chapter 9

Severe Acute Pneumonia

Estefanía Pérez Macho[1,*], MD
Anaura Carrasquel[1], MD
and Alexis Jaspe Codecido[2], MD
[1]Emergency Department, Hospital Universitario Ramón y Cajal, Madrid, Spain
[2]Intensive Care Unit, Hospital General Universitario Gregorio Marañón, Madrid, Spain

Abstract

Obstructive Sleep Apnea (OSA) is a chronic respiratory disease characterized by transitory collapse of the upper airway during sleep due to anatomical variations, resulting in alteration on lung gas exchange with hypoxemia and hypercapnia [1]. Apart from all the effects for cardiovascular diseases (hypertension, diabetes, pulmonary hypertension, heart failure), the association with arrythmias and cerebrovascular events, it has also been described an augment on the risk for respiratory tract infections, such as pneumonia [1, 2]. Several cohort series have shown that OSA is an independent risk factor for pneumonia, with a specific risk from the other comorbidities [2, 3]. Several theories have been proposed to explain these effects. The hypoxemia after a period of airway collapse activates the respiratory center to initiate an inspiration, even against a closed airway, rising the intrathoracic negative pression. The higher gradient increases the amount of the aspiration of oral secretions, compared to the amount aspirated in normal subjects [4]. Many studies have demonstrated the risk for pneumonia due to an uncoordinated deglutition pattern during sleep in patients with OSA [5]. There have also been described negative effects on local immunity with an impaired function of neutrophils and a decreased inflammatory

* Corresponding Author's Email: estefania_7984@hotmail.com.

In: Obstructive Sleep Apnea in Pulmonary Critical Care
Editors: Antonio M. Esquinas and Takatoshi Kasai
ISBN: 979-8-88697-858-2

response to these damages [6]. The main importance to describe and determine these events is because patients with OSA pneumonia may be exposed to more antibiotic intake, hospitalization with possible need of invasive mechanical ventilation and admission to Intensive Care Unit (ICU), with higher resource use, a functional deterioration after discharge and an increased risk of mortality [1]. The treatment with non-invasive mechanical ventilation based on the Continuous Positive Airway Pression (CPAP) can decrease this effect and has already been proven for other comorbidities with favorable results. CPAP improves sleep-related deglutition and the respiratory phase patterns associated [2].

Keywords: hypoxemia, airway tract, respiratory infection, comorbidities, CPAP

Introduction

The American Academy of Sleep Medicine (AASM) proposed a definition of OSA determined by an Apnea Hypopnea Index ≥ 5 [7]. The physiopathology of OSA is characterized by episodes of collapse and obstruction of the upper airway during sleep that causes hypopnea, apnea and oxygen desaturation [1, 5]. Epidemiologic studies suggest a variable prevalence between different ages, countries and gender, with an average of 2-7% in women and 7-14% men [1] and increases with age in both sexes [7].

In a comparative study of a retrospective cohort of patients hospitalized with diagnosis of pneumonia at different hospitals in US, those with OSA were younger, with higher percentages of obesity, chronic obstructive pulmonary disease (COPD), diabetes, heart failure and hypertension than those without OSA. The incidence of serious complications, defined as mechanical ventilation –invasive and non-invasive- and transfer to ICU after the second and third hospital day, was higher in the OSA group. Consequently, this is associated with longer length of stay and higher sanitary costs. In contrast, there was no statistically significant association with more rates of mortality [1].

In a cohort population prospective study that was made from 2000-2010 in Taiwan with two groups of patients with and without diagnosis of OSA, the main outcome was the complication with pneumonia and the stratification risk of severity was defined by the need of using CPAP. During the time of follow-up, the incidence of pneumonia was higher in the group of patients with obstructive sleep apnea, even after a multivariate adjustment. However, in this study, there was no significant increase of mortality associated with pneumonia. Also, the results showed that patients with more severity OSA had more risk of pneumonia [3]. In another case-control study carried out in Spain, the group of individuals hospitalized for community acquired pneumonia (CAP) was associated to higher rates of OSA than the control group with patients hospitalized for other infectious diseases. The OSA severity, defined by Apnea Hypopnea Index (AHI), was related to higher grade of CAP severity [5].

In the context of an acute lower respiratory tract infection the repeated episodes of apnea might result in an increased risk of pulmonary complications. It may be explained because patients with OSA have more risk of hypoxemia associated with the shunt effect caused for the lung occupation in pneumonia. This effect leads to the patients to make a higher effort for breathing to avoid the oxygen desaturation, resulting in muscle fatigue before than other patients and may be a cause for earlier consultation. Patients with OSA pneumonia usually need mechanical ventilation from the time of admission at hospital, being a possible explanation for the lower mortality rates than would be expected. On the other hand, patients without OSA that need mechanical ventilation are associated with acute respiratory distress syndrome (ARDS) and more severity. It has to be mentioned that obesity was not able to be demonstrated as an independent risk factor for mortality, as it would be supposed, maybe due to the metabolic reserve, the hypoxemia and the less time to consultation to hospital [1].

Physiopathology and Risk Factors

The exact mechanisms that are related to development of pneumonia in patients with OSA are not well known yet, and it is supposed to be multifactorial. Some of these mechanisms that may be involved in the pathophysiology are [2, 3]:

1. The hypoxemia secondary to the continuous episodes of apnea-hypopnea may stimulate patients to start an inspiration not following the normal respiratory pattern. In this case, the airway tract could be closed and, as a result, the intrathoracic pressure could become more negative. This effect can cause migration of the content of the upper airway to a higher grade than usual.

2. Patients with OSA usually have a swallowing reflux and a sensation of the upper airway that are deteriorated. This is a risk factor of aspiration of oral and pharyngeal secretions.
3. The sleep of patients with OSA is frequently interrupted coinciding with apnea episodes, in relation with point one, and this is related with local immunity disfunction to control the inflammatory response.
4. The hypercapnia that can be caused by OSA in these patients negatively to the lung neutrophil function.

Deglutition and Respiratory Sleep Pattern Disorders

The clearance of the pharynx by deglutition and the correct coordination with the respiratory phase patterns are fundamental to protect the airway and lung. Deglutition during sleep is uncommon because can display an uncoordinated pattern with respiratory phases. During the act of swallowing in healthy adults, the breath is arrested and is followed by an expiration instead of an inspiration, that reduces the risk of aspiration of oral secretions into the airway tract. In patients with OSA the studies of polysomnography and surface EMG showed more frequently sleep-related deglutition and an uncoordinated respiratory phase pattern, following deglutition by an inspiration. This is related to episodes of aspiration and higher risk of respiratory tract infections [2].

Aspiration of Oral Secretions

There are studies that demonstrate that all healthy people without OSA may have a variant amount of oral secretion aspiration during sleep. Gleason et al. In 1997 carried out a study to quantify it [8]. The results of this study were used years later for Beal et al., to compare patients with symptoms and polysomnography diagnosis of OSA, showing higher volumes in the second group and more risk of pulmonary infections. Other studies have also established that during sleep all individuals aspirate a small quantity of oral secretions but in patients with OSA this amount can be higher than normal, as it has been measured by radioactive 99mTc tracers. Nevertheless, in normal subjects this aspiration of oral content usually does not suppose any infection because it´s controlled by pulmonary defense mechanisms [6]. There must be other factors involved that are not well determined yet and that need more studies to be defined.

Anatomical Variations

In patients with OSA it is important to make an exhaustive physical exploration describing body mass index (BMI) and detecting if there is any anatomical variation (retrognathia, macroglossia, hyoid-jaw distance, neck circumference, tonsillar hypertrophy, alterations on palatine veil). These patients usually have more rates of gastroesophageal reflux (GER) and symptoms of laryngitis. Many studies have shown how treatment of GER may decrease the AHI. In OSA the cough reflex is affected, especially during REEM sleep, and the intrathoracic pressure becomes more negative [5], being a risk for aspiration of oral secretions (as it has been already explained).

Immunity Local Disorders

All these alterations, associated with the airway obstruction, produce intermittent hypoxia and result in metabolic dysregulation. This fact increases the oxidative stress that contributes to chronic systemic inflammation in the airway tract with changes in local microbiota and higher risk of airway infections [5]. There must be other mechanisms that contribute to the development of infections, as it is already hypothesized in the disruption of local immunity [6]. From some studies with mice and rats, it is suggested that hypercapnia, produced because of OSA, may increase the risk of infection by inhibiting expression of IL-6 and TNF of macrophages and increasing bacterial dissemination as a consequence of defective lung neutrophil function [9].

CPAP: For or Against in OSA Pneumonia

CPAP may Reduce Respiratory Tract Infections

There have been published many reports to determine whether the CPAP therapy can be useful in patients with OSA syndrome who may have swallowing disorders during sleep and, in consequence, may precipitate aspiration and pneumonia. Aspiration pneumonia in most cases is related to elderly people with oropharyngeal dysphagia that causes swallowing problems while eating. However, patients with OSA do not have problems of aspiration while awake, they have risk factors that cause silent aspiration during sleep time [2]. In these patients, the amount of deglutition during sleep and uncoordinated with respiratory phase were significantly reduced after the initiation of CPAP therapy. As a result, cases of pneumonia related to aspiration during sleep in patients with OSA are decreased [2]. Other studies have found that colonization of the CPAP machine was not associated with an increase of upper airway infections [10].

In a case- control study carried out in the Mater Dei Hospital in Malta on Jun 2016 patients with formal diagnosis of OSA, using and not using CPAP, were recruited to identify if there are more rates of infections in patients with CPAP machines and to compare the results of the bacterial flora found in the cultures taken in the different groups. They took nasal samples from all the individuals and from masks (nasal and full masks) and humidifiers, if they were using it. The results did not show a statistically significant difference between the two groups about the number of respiratory tract infections, neither about the isolated relevant organisms, the antibiotic treatment administered nor the cases of patients needing hospitalization for pneumonia. There was no difference in the CPAP group with or without humidification dispositive [11].

In case of hospitalized patients, in several prospective studies performed in intensive care units, those with noninvasive ventilation developed less cases of pneumonia compared with patients with endotracheal intubation (Ventilator Associated Pneumonia) [12].

CPAP may Increase the Risk of Respiratory Tract Infections

It is hypothesized that patients with OSA that use CPAP may be exposed to higher risk of airway infections than patients that do not use this dispositive. This is based on the theory that the positive pressure on the airway can translocate the bacteria from the upper tract to the low respiratory tract and may cause pneumonia. Even more during sleep because of the less capacity to block the entrance to the pharynx, especially in these patients. Also, it is hypothesized that the dryness caused by the entrance of the positive pressure with the non-invasive ventilation could cause lesions in the mucosal and favorize bacterial translocation and upper and lower respiratory tract infections. In these patients that may suffer several co-morbidities: cardiovascular risk factors, obesity and others, the infection derived from the use of the device may cause clinical complications and exacerbate other chronic diseases such as heart failure or chronic respiratory pulmonary disease (COPD). In this sense, Sanner et al., conducted a retrospective study taken from 246 patients with formal diagnosis of OSA. They analyze the infectious complications in the group with and without CPAP therapy, including a subgroup with humidifying system. The results showed higher risk of infections in both groups using CPAP [4]. The conclusions of the study made in an extensive cohort population in Taiwan propose that the use of CPAP may reduce quantity of sputum and increase the risk of aspiration of oral and pharyngeal secretions. The use of humidifier is a factor for proliferation for bacteria and contamination of the ventilation systems, pointing at the importance of their correct cleaning and maintenance [3]. However, they weren´t able to demonstrate it in this sample and this cannot be generalized. More studies are required to endorse this hypothesis.

OSA and COVID-19 Pneumonia

COVID-19 is a viral disease caused by SARS-CoV2 with a very variable severity spectrum depending on many factors that have been analyzed during the past two years since the emergence pandemic situation was declared globally. The percentage of patients that normally require hospitalization or Intensive Care Unit admission reported in different series are around 1-6%. The mildest cases course with cough, asthenia, and unspecific symptoms in common with other respiratory viral infections but severe clinical presentation is defined with ARDS and bilateral pneumonia [13].

The risk factors that have been related to severity are age, male sex, obesity, diabetes, cardiovascular disease and affected lung function for other respiratory disorders. OSA has been proposed as an independent risk factor for severe COVID-19 and its role to determine hospitalization and mortality [14]. In a study based on the analysis of databases and epidemiological cohorts in all University Hospitals in Finland, OSA was not a risk of being infected with SARS-CoV2, but patients with OSA resulted in elevated risk for requiring hospitalization for severe COVID-19. The meta-analysis conducted based on the results from this study describes a risk of contracting COVID-19 independently of BMI and other known risk factors for OSA. Other studies also go in line with this, but not all were able to demonstrate the association between OSA and severe COVID-19 with a statistically significant difference after adjusting for BMI. More studies are necessary to evaluate the presence of this association across diverse groups [13].

Conclusion

OSA is a chronic respiratory disease with episodes of apnea- hypopnea and oxygen desaturation that is usually associated to other comorbidities such as hypertension, diabetes, obesity, or heart failure [1]. It has been described a higher risk of respiratory tract infections demonstrated in several studies with different populations, resulting on an increase of the risk of hospitalization, need of mechanical ventilation and death. It is remarkable for primary care doctors to consider sleep disorders in patients with recurrent pneumonias without other risk factors, after a correct screening of the more frequent causes that are described in the general population [3]. In these patients, many series have shown the usefulness of the CPAP therapy; however, there are other studies that have hypothesized a higher risk of infections, not well demonstrated. Additional research is needed to identify the factors that may support these observations.

References

[1] Lindenauer P K, MD, Stefan M S, MD, Johnson K G, MD, Priya A, MA, MSc, Pekow P S, PhD, Rothberg M B, MD-MPH. Prevalence, Treatment and Outcomes Associated With OSA Among Patients Hospitalized With Pneumonia. *CHEST.* 2014; 145 (5): 1032-1038. Accessed December 26, 2013. doi: 10.1378/chest.13-1544.

[2] Sato K, Chitose S, Sato K, Sato F, Ono T. Recurrent aspiration pneumonia precipitated by obstructive sleep apnea. *Auris Nasus Larynx*. 2021; 48: 659-665. doi: 10.1016/j.anl.2020.11.021.

[3] Vincent Yi-Fong Su, Chia-Jen Liu, Hsin-Kai Wang, Li-An Wu, Shi-Chuan Chang, Diahn-Warng Perng, PhD, Wei-Juin Su, Msc, Yuh-Min Chen, PhD, Elizabeth Ya-Hsuan Lin, Bsc, Tzeng-Ji Chen, PhD, and Kun-Ta Chou, MD. Sleep apnea and risk of pneumonia: a nationwide population-based study. *Canadian Medical Association Journal*, 2014, 186 (6). doi: 10.1503/cmaj.131547.

[4] Sanner B M, Fluerenbrock N, Kleiber-Imbeck A, Mueller JB, Zidek W. Effect of continuous positive airway pressure therapy on infectious complications in patients with obstructive sleep apnea syndrome. *Respiration*. 2001; 68 (5): 483-7. doi: 10.1159/000050555.

[5] Chiner E, Llombart M, Valls J, Pastor E, Sancho-Chust J N, Andreu A L, Manuel Sánchez-de-la-Torre M, Barbé F. Association between Obstructive Sleep Apnea and Community-Adquired Pneumonia. *PLoS ONE*. 2016, 11(4): e0152749. doi: 10.1371/journal.pone.0152749.

[6] Beal M, MD, Chesson A, MD, Garcia T, MD, Caldito G, PhD, Stucker F, MD, FACS, Nathan C A, MD, FACS. A pilot stdudy of quantitative aspiration in patients

with symptoms of obstructive sleep apnea: comparition to a historic control group. *Laryngoscope*. 2004, 114 (6): 965-968. doi: 10.1097/00005537-200406000-00002.

[7] Durán J, Esnaola S, Rubio R, Iztueta A. Obstructive sleep apnea-hypopnea and related clinical features in a population-based sample of subjects aged 30 to 70 yr. *Am. J. Respir. Crit. Care Med*, 2001; 163 (3pt 1): 685-689.

[8] Gleeson K, Eggli D F, Maxwell S L. Quantitative aspiration during sleep in normal subjects. *Chest* 1997; 111: 1266-72.

[9] Gates K L, Howell H A, Nair A, Vohwinkel C U, Welch L C, Beitel G J, Hauser A R, Sznajder J I, Sporn P H. Hypercapnia impairs lung neutrophil function and increases mortality in murine Pseudomonas pneumonia. *Am. J. Respir. Cell Mol. Biol.* 2013; 49: 821-8. doi: 10.1165/rcmb.2012-0487OC.

[10] Ferrer M, Esquinas A, Arancibia F, Bauer T T, González G, Carrillo A, Rodriguez-Roisin R, Torres A. Noninvasive ventilation during persistent weaning failure: a randomized controlled trial. *Am. J. Respir. Crit. Care Med.* 2003; 168 (1): 70-76.

[11] Liam Mercieca, Richard Pullicino, Kyra Camilleri, Rodianne Abela, Sean Apap Mangion, Julian Cassar, Matthew Zammit, Christine Gatt, Christopher Deguara, Christopher Barbara, Peter Fsadni, and Stephen Montefort. Continuous Positive Airway Pressure: is it a route for infection in those with Obstructive Sleep Apnea? *Sleep Science*, 2017 Jan-Mar; 10 (1): 28-34. doi: 10.5935/1984-0063.20170005.

[12] Gay P C, MD. Complications of noninvasive ventilation in acute care. *Respir. Care* 2009; 54 (2): 246-257.

[13] Strausz S, Kiiskinen T, Broberg M, Ruotsalainen S, Koskela J, Bachour A, FinnGen, Palotie A, Palotie T, Ripatti S, Ollila HM. Sleep apnea is a risk factor for severe COVID-19. *BMJ Open Resp. Res.* 2021; 8: e000845. doi: 10.1136/bmjresp-2020-00085.

[14] Miller M A, Cappucio F P. A systematic review of COVID-19 and obstructive sleep apnea. *Sleep Medicine Reviews* 55 (2021) 101382. doi: 10.1016/j.smrv.2020.101382.

Chapter 10

Acute Heart Failure

Ryo Naito[1,2,*], MD, PhD

[1]Cardiovascular Respiratory Sleep Medicine, Juntendo University Graduate School of Medicine, Tokyo, Japan

[2]Department of Cardiovascular Biology and Medicine, Juntendo University Graduate School of Medicine, Tokyo, Japan

Abstract

Obstructive sleep apnea (OSA) is a well-recognized risk factor for cardiovascular diseases, including heart failure (HF), which is a leading cause of morbidity and mortality worldwide. However, the relationship between OSA and HF may be bidirectional. OSA can cause HF via multiple pathways, such as hemodynamic changes, oxidative stress, and inflammation owing to repetitive respiratory effort, desaturation, and reoxygenation accompanied by OSA. In contrast, HF may also develop or worsen OSA owing to fluid retention accompanied by decompensated HF and fluid shift from the lower extremity to the upper airway, resulting in pharyngeal edema and upper airway narrowing. OSA is highly prevalent in patients with acute HF. Concomitant OSA is associated with an increased risk of cardiovascular events in patients with HF, suggesting the need for screening and appropriate treatment for OSA in patients with acute HF to improve their prognosis. Treatments for OSA in patients with acute HF include medical therapy for HF and continuous positive airway pressure (CPAP) therapy for OSA. Diuretics may improve OSA by optimizing fluid management that can alleviate pharyngeal edema, resulting in improvement in OSA. CPAP therapy is the standard therapy for OSA, regardless of the presence or absence of concomitant HF. Evidence suggests that CPAP therapy can improve left ventricular

[*] Corresponding Author's Email: rnaitou@juntendo.ac.jp.

In: Obstructive Sleep Apnea in Pulmonary Critical Care
Editors: Antonio M. Esquinas and Takatoshi Kasai
ISBN: 979-8-88697-858-2

ejection fraction (LVEF) in patients with HF with reduced LVEF. However, strong evidence is scarce on the positive prognostic impact of CPAP therapy in patients with HF and OSA. A recent clinical guideline for HF recommends CPAP therapy for patients with HF with reduced LVEF and moderate to severe OSA (apnea–hypopnea index ≥ 15) to improve left ventricular function, while CPAP therapy is less recommended for improving prognosis.

Keywords: obstructive sleep apnea, acute heart failure, prognosis, CPAP

Introduction: Epidemiology

Heart failure (HF) is a leading cause of morbidity and mortality [1]. In developed countries, 1%–2% of the population has HF, with a prevalence rising to ≥ 10% among people aged ≥ 70 years. Despite improvements in both the pharmacological and non-pharmacological management of HF, the prognosis of patients with HF remains unfavorable. The risks of developing HF include traditional atherosclerotic factors such as hypertension, diabetes mellitus, dyslipidemia, and some modern factors such as kidney and pulmonary diseases and sleep apnea. Patients hospitalized with acute decompensated HF have a high prevalence of previously undiagnosed and untreated moderate to severe obstructive sleep apnea (OSA) [2].

OSA is a form of sleep apnea characterized by repetitive desaturation and reoxygenation with respiratory effort during sleep due to upper airway obstruction. Predisposing factors for OSA include obesity, male sex, small lower jaw, and certain other facial configurations. OSA has been recognized as a risk factor for cardiovascular diseases, including hypertension, atrial fibrillation, coronary artery disease and HF.

The prevalence of OSA in patients with acute HF is high [3 4]. OSA is found in 16%–29% of patients with HF with reduced left ventricular ejection fraction (LVEF) under standard medical therapy for HF [5, 6]. Furthermore, undiagnosed OSA is an independent predictor of post-discharge mortality and readmission in patients with HF [7, 8].

The mechanisms underlying the development of HF in patients with OSA can be explained by hemodynamic overload due to transmural pressure against the heart, right ventricular failure via increased pulmonary arterial resistance due to hypoxemic vasoconstriction of the pulmonary arteries, increased venous return, and decreased cardiac output via left ventricular filling disorder due to intraventricular septal shift from the dilated right ventricle [9] (Figure 1). In addition to hemodynamic effects, vascular endothelial dysfunction, oxidative stress, inflammation, enhanced blood coagulation, insulin resistance, and obesity can cause coronary artery disease, myocardial dysfunction, and arrhythmia, all of which consequently lead to HF.

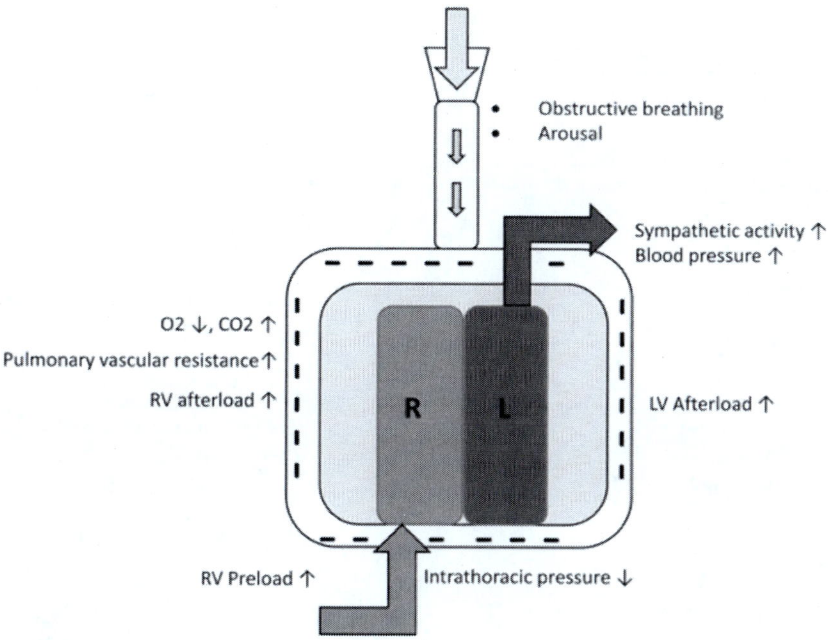

Figure 1. Impacts of obstructive sleep apnea on the cardiovascular system.

Respiratory effort against upper airway obstruction results in negative intrathoracic pressure that increases right ventricular preload and left ventricular afterload. The cessation of airflow results in intermittent hypoxemia and hypercapnia, which can increase pulmonary vascular resistance and right ventricular afterload. An increase in sympathetic nervous activity accompanies an increase in blood pressure [9].

The relationship between OSA and HF may be bidirectional. Patients with HF may develop or worsen OSA due to fluid retention accompanied by decompensated HF and fluid shift from the lower extremity to the upper airway, resulting in pharyngeal edema and upper airway narrowing [9] (Figure 2). A prior observational study investigated association between nocturnal rostral fluid shift and severity of OSA in patients with HF with an LVEF ≤

45% (n = 57). Leg fluid volume and neck circumference were measured, and polysomnography was performed. The overnight change in leg fluid volume was inversely related to both the overnight change in neck circumference ($r = -0.780$, $p < 0.001$) and apnea–hypopnea index (AHI) ($r = -0.881$, $p < 0.001$) in patients with predominant OSA, suggesting that nocturnal rostral fluid shift contributes to the pathogenesis of OSA [11].

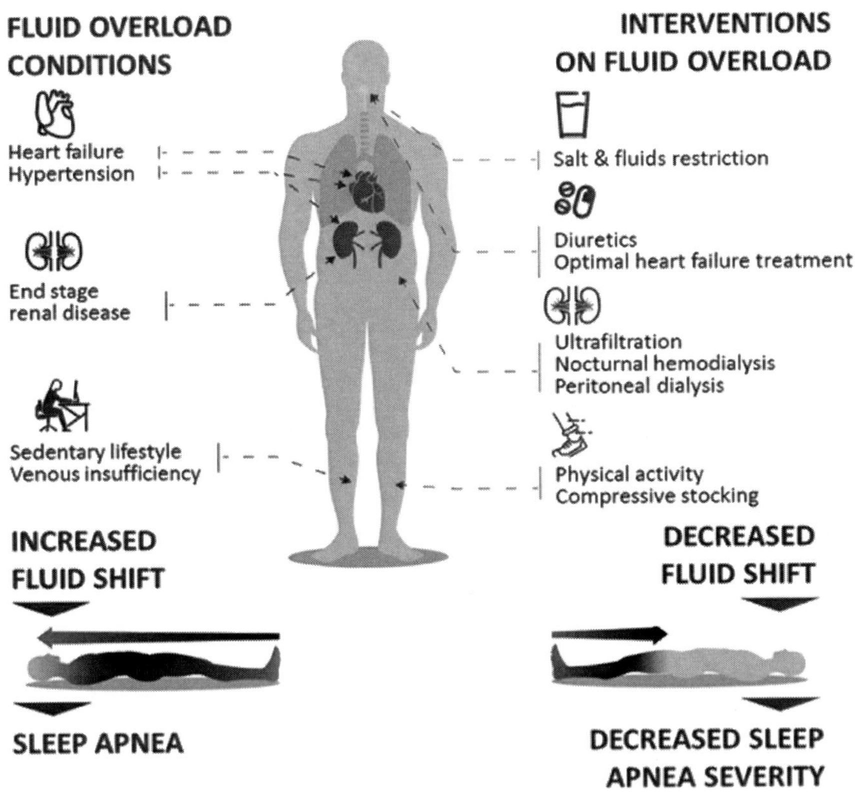

Figure 2. Relationship between fluid shift and obstructive sleep apnea.

Fluid shift from the lower legs to the upper airway may cause obstructive sleep apnea. Pharmacological and non-pharmacological fluid management may reduce severity of obstructive sleep apnea [10].

Based on these data, it is conceivable that the optimization of HF therapy focusing on fluid management remains an important treatment for patients with HF with OSA. However, questions remain regarding how OSA affects the prognosis of patients with acute HF and how it should be treated during the acute phase of HF.

Prognostic Effects in Acute Heart Failure

OSA is associated with clinical events in patients with cardiovascular disease, with higher repeat revascularization in patients with coronary artery disease, higher recurrence rates of atrial fibrillation in patients who underwent pulmonary vein isolation for atrial fibrillation, and higher cardiovascular mortality and readmission rates in patients with HF [7, 8, 12, 13]. The prognostic impact of concomitant OSA in patients with acute HF has been reported in clinical trials. An observational study reported that untreated OSA with an AHI $\geq$ 15 compared with that with an AHI < 15 was associated with an increased risk of death during a mean follow-up of 2.9 years (adjusted hazard ratio [HR], 2.81; 95% confidence interval [CI], 1.11–7.10; $p = 0.029$) in patients with HF with an LVEF $\leq$ 45% [14]. A recent prospective cohort study of hospitalized patients with acute HF reported that 47% of the patients had OSA whose prognoses were worse than those without OSA, with an adjusted HR for mortality of 1.53 (95% CI, 1.1–2.2; $p = 0.02$) for those with OSA during a median follow-up of 3 years post-discharge [3]. In another cohort study, patients with HF complicated with OSA with an AHI $\geq$ 15 and those without were followed up with a mean follow-up of 1 year. OSA was independently associated with the recurrence of acute cardiogenic pulmonary edema (HR, 3.3; 95% CI, 1.2–8.8; $p = 0.01$), incidence of myocardial infarction (HR, 2.3; 95% CI, 1.1–9.5; $p = 0.02$), cardiovascular death (HR, 5.4; 95% CI, 1.4–48.4; $p = 0.004$), and all-cause death (HR, 6.5; 95% CI, 1.2–64.0; $p = 0.005$) [15].

These data indicate that concomitant OSA in acute HF is associated with an increased risk of cardiovascular events in a subset of patients and suggest the need for screening and appropriate treatment for OSA in these patients to improve their prognosis.

Treatment

Treatments for OSA in patients with acute HF should focus on both medical therapy for HF and positive airway pressure (PAP) therapy for OSA. During the acute phase of acute HF, diuretics may improve OSA by optimizing fluid management, which can alleviate pharyngeal edema that can cause upper airway obstruction. In a small single-arm study, 3-day diuretic therapy (intravenous administration of furosemide 20 mg and spironolactone 100 mg daily) significantly decreased the AHI (from 74.89 ± 6.95 to 57.17 ± 5.40, $p < 0.001$) and body weight (from 111.5 ± 3.83 to 109.0 ± 3.63 kg, $p < 0.001$), while the therapy significantly increased the oropharyngeal junction area (from 1.33 ± 0.10 to 1.78 ± 0.16 cm^2, $p < 0.01$) and mean cross-sectional area from the oropharyngeal junction to the glottis (from 2.61 ± 0.18 to 3.27 ± 0.25 cm^2, $p < 0.02$) in hospitalized patients with HF with severe OSA with an AHI ≥ 30, suggesting that diuretic treatment could alleviate pharyngeal edema that may contribute to improvement in OSA in patients with HF [16]. It is recognized that high sodium intake causes fluid retention. An observational study demonstrated that patients with HF with OSA had a higher sodium intake than those without OSA and the AHI was positively correlated with sodium intake [17]. Moreover, a recent randomized trial showed that 1-week sodium restricted diet decreased the AHI (change in the AHI, −10.7 [95% CI, −15.6 to −5.7]) in men with severe OSA (AHI $\geq$ 30) [18]. Physical activity is another potential treatment for OSA. Prior studies have demonstrated that aerobic exercise decreases the AHI in patients with OSA [19,20]. In a meta-analysis including 8 studies and 182 participants with OSA without HF, regular exercise ($\geq$60 min per week) for at least 2 months significantly decreased the AHI (unstandardized mean difference, −0.536; 95% CI, −0.865 to −0.206) in non-HF patients with OSA [21]. Further studies are warranted to investigate the effects of exercise on OSA alleviation in patients with HF.

Optimal therapy for HF leads to a reduction in venous return from the vena cava to the right ventricle, resulting in decreased cervical venous congestion and upper airway edema, thereby improving OSA. Continuous positive airway pressure (CPAP) therapy is an established treatment choice for OSA. A previous guideline stated that CPAP therapy is recommended for OSA in patients with HF, giving it a class IIa recommendation [22]. However, recent guidelines do not specifically recommend CPAP for patients with HF with OSA because the mortality benefits of CPAP in these patients have been shown only in small-scale studies and not in large-scale randomized controlled trials or meta-analyses [23-25]. The potential benefits of PAP in patients with acute HF and OSA are discussed in the following.

Effects of PAP on the Prognosis of Patients with Acute HF with OSA

Effects of CPAP on Cardiac Function

A prior randomized controlled trial demonstrated improvement in LVEF by 9% after 1-month CPAP therapy in patients with HF with severe OSA (26). In a randomized controlled trial, patients with acute HF (n = 49) who had moderate to severe OSA (AHI $\geq$ 15) were treated with either PAP and the standard treatment for HF or the standard treatment alone. The mean differences in changes in the LVEF between the PAP and standard treatment groups showed that the PAP group was superior to the standard treatment group by 4.6% ($p = 0.03$). The prognostic impact of PAP therapy was not demonstrated in this trial [2]. A meta-analysis including six randomized controlled trials reported that LVEF was significantly improved after CPAP treatment in patients with OSA, with a weighted mean difference of 5.18 (95% CI, 3.27–7.08; $p < 0.001$) [27]. The acute effects of PAP therapy were demonstrated in a randomized trial in which patients with acute HF (n = 21) with moderate to severe OSA and pulmonary hypertension with an estimated pulmonary artery systolic pressure $\geq$ 50 mmHg were included. In this trial comparing standard of care with PAP therapy for patients with acute HF and the standard of care alone, 48-h PAP therapy significantly decreased the pulmonary artery systolic pressure with the mean difference of −15.8 ± 3.2 mmHg in the PAP group compared with that in the standard of care alone (−5.2 ± 2.6 mmHg) ($p = 0.025$) [28]. The LVEF was significantly improved by 3.4% ± 1.5% in the PAP plus standard of care group, while that in the standard of care alone group was −0.5% ± 0.5% ($p = 0.01$). PAP therapy improved right ventricular function as assessed by tricuspid annular plane systolic excursion and right ventricular systolic area, while no significant changes were observed in the N-terminal pro-brain natriuretic peptide levels and 6-min walk distance [28]. However, another single center, randomized controlled trial did not follow the positive results of PAP therapy. Hospitalized patients with decompensated HF and OSA (n = 150) were randomized to receive either PAP therapy plus guideline-directed therapy or guideline-directed therapy alone. The primary outcome of changes in the LVEF between baseline and at discharge revealed no significance between those with PAP therapy (25.5% ± 10.4% at baseline and 27.3% ± 11.9% at discharge) and those without (27.3% ± 11.7% at baseline and 28.8% ± 10.5% at discharge) (p

= 0.84) [29]. The on-treatment analysis in the PAP group showed a significant increase in the LVEF in patients who used PAP for 3 h per night (25.4% ± 10.6% at baseline and 29.8% ± 12.5% at discharge) compared with those who used it less (25.3% ± 10.8% at baseline and 24.7% ± 10.7% at discharge) ($p = 0.01$). The readmission rates within 6 months after the intervention were significantly lower in patients with longer PAP use. With the adherence threshold for outpatient CPAP use of 3 h per night, the readmission rates were lower by 67% for those who used CPAP for 3 h or more per night than those who used it less (risk ratio, 0.33; 95% CI, 0.14–0.76; $p = 0.01$). These data emphasize the clinical importance of adherence to CPAP therapy about its beneficial effects on both cardiac function and incident clinical events in patients with decompensated HF and OSA, similar to the results of a previous clinical trial indicating the importance of CPAP adherence in the prevention of cardiovascular events [30].

Effects of CPAP on Clinical Events

A prospective observational study of patients with HF with preserved ejection fraction (HFpEF) and sleep-disordered breathing with an AHI ≥ 15 (n = 109) under optimal medical therapy for HF showed that the all-cause mortality rate in those with CPAP therapy was lower than those without CPAP therapy during a mean-follow-up of 2.5 years (0% vs. 12.8%, log-rank $p = 0.014$). The benefits of 6-month CPAP therapy were also observed for changes in the right ventricular fractional area, % vital capacity of the lungs, and maximal exercise capacity [31]. However, a recently published small observational study showed that even when treated appropriately with CPAP therapy for 36 months, the beneficial effects of CPAP therapy on long-term cardiac function and clinical outcomes were not observed in patients with HFpEF with OSA compared with those without OSA [32].

To date, the prognostic effects of PAP therapy in patients with HF with OSA have not yet been demonstrated in a large-scale clinical trial. The ADVENT-HF trial, which is a multicenter, multinational, randomized, parallel-group, open-label trial, has been conducted to examine the effects of adaptive servo-ventilation that adjusts pressure delivery based on the detection of apnea during breathing in patients with HF with an LVEF < 45% and AHI ≥ 15 (n = 860) [33].

The updated guidelines for HF recommend CPAP therapy for patients with HF with HFpEF and moderate to severe OSA (AHI ≥ 15) to improve left ventricular function (recommendation class IIa, evidence level A) [34]. However, CPAP therapy is less recommended for improving the prognosis (recommendation class IIb, evidence level C).

Conclusion

OSA is a prognostic factor of acute HF. Given the higher prevalence of OSA in patients with acute HF, aggressive screening, and management of OSA are needed to improve their prognosis. The first-line treatment for OSA in patients with acute HF should focus on optimizing fluid management, both pharmacologically and non-pharmacologically. However, evidence of CPAP therapy for improving the prognosis of patients with acute HF and OSA is lacking.

Acknowledgment

This work was supported by AMED under Grant Number JP21ek021 0150s0502.

References

[1] Writing Group Members, Mozaffarian D, Benjamin E J, Go A S, Arnett D K, Blaha M J, Cushman M, Das SR, de Ferranti S, Després J P, Fullerton HJ, Howard V J, Huffman M D, Isasi C R, Jiménez M C, Judd S E, Kissela B M, Lichtman J H, Lisabeth L D, Liu S, Mackey R H, Magid D J, McGuire D K, Mohler E R 3rd, Moy C S, Muntner P, Mussolino M E, Nasir K, Neumar RW, Nichol G, Palaniappan L, Pandey D K, Reeves M J, Rodriguez C J, Rosamond W, Sorlie P D, Stein J, Towfighi A, Turan TN, Virani SS, Woo D, Yeh RW, Turner MB; American Heart Association Statistics Committee; Stroke Statistics Subcommittee. Heart Disease and Stroke Statistics-2016 Update: A Report From the American Heart Association. *Circulation.* 2016 Jan 26;133(4):e38-360.

[2] Khayat R N, Abraham W T, Patt B, Pu M, Jarjoura D. In-hospital treatment of obstructive sleep apnea during decompensation of heart failure. *Chest.* 2009 Oct;136(4):991–7.

[3] Khayat R, Jarjoura D, Porter K, Sow A, Wannemacher J, Dohar R, Pleister A, Abraham WT. Sleep disordered breathing and post-discharge mortality in patients with acute heart failure. *Eur. Heart J.* 2015 Jun 14;36(23):1463–9.

[4] Suda S, Kasai T, Matsumoto H, Shiroshita N, Kato M, Kawana F, Yatsu S, Murata A, Kato T, Hiki M, Chiang S J, Miyazaki S, Daida H. Prevalence and Clinical Correlates of Sleep-Disordered Breathing in Patients Hospitalized with Acute Decompensated Heart Failure. *Can. J. Cardiol.* 2018 Jun;34(6):784–90.

[5] Oldenburg O, Wellmann B, Buchholz A, Bitter T, Fox H, Thiem U, Horstkotte D, Wegscheider K. Nocturnal hypoxaemia is associated with increased mortality in stable heart failure patients. *Eur. Heart J.* 2016 Jun 1;37(21):1695–703.

[6] Arzt M, Oldenburg O, Graml A, Erdmann E, Teschler H, Wegscheider K, Suling A, Woehrle H; SchlaHF Investigators. Phenotyping of Sleep-Disordered Breathing in Patients with Chronic Heart Failure with Reduced Ejection Fraction-the SchlaHF Registry. *J. Am. Heart Assoc.* 2017 Nov 29;6(12):e005899.

[7] Khayat R, Abraham W, Patt B, Brinkman V, Wannemacher J, Porter K, Jarjoura D. Central sleep apnea is a predictor of cardiac readmission in hospitalized patients with systolic heart failure. *J. Card Fail.* 2012 Jul;18(7):534–40.

[8] Ishiwata S, Kasai T, Sato A, Suda S, Matsumoto H, Shitara J, Yatsu S, Murata A, Shimizu M, Kato T, Hiki M, Matsue Y, Naito R, Daida H, Minamino T. Prognostic effect of sleep-disordered breathing on hospitalized patients following acute heart failure. *Clin. Res. Cardiol.* 2022 Jun;111(6):663-672.

[9] Kwon Y, Logan J, Pusalavidyasagar S, Kasai T, Cheong C S, Lee C H. Sleep Apnea and Heart. *Sleep Med. Res.* 2019 Dec;10(2):67–74.

[10] Perger E, Jutant EM, Redolfi S. Targeting volume overload and overnight rostral fluid shift: A new perspective to treat sleep apnea. *Sleep Med. Rev.* 2018 Dec;42:160–70.

[11] Yumino D, Redolfi S, Ruttanaumpawan P, Su MC, Smith S, Newton GE, Mak S, Bradley TD. Nocturnal rostral fluid shift: a unifying concept for the pathogenesis of obstructive and central sleep apnea in men with heart failure. *Circulation.* 2010 Apr 13;121(14):1598–605.

[12] Yatsu S, Naito R, Kasai T, Matsumoto H, Shitara J, Shimizu M, Murata A, Kato T, Suda S, Hiki M, Sai E, Miyauchi K, Daida H. Influence of sleep-disordered breathing assessed by pulse oximetry on long-term clinical outcomes in patients who underwent percutaneous coronary intervention. *Clin. Res. Cardiol.* 2018 Aug;107 (8):711–8.

[13] Ng CY, Liu T, Shehata M, Stevens S, Chugh SS, Wang X. Meta-analysis of obstructive sleep apnea as predictor of atrial fibrillation recurrence after catheter ablation. *Am. J. Cardiol.* 2011 Jul 1;108(1):47–51.

[14] Wang H, Parker J D, Newton G E, Floras J S, Mak S, Chiu KL, Ruttanaumpawan P, Tomlinson G, Bradley T D. Influence of obstructive sleep apnea on mortality in patients with heart failure. *J. Am. Coll. Cardiol.* 2007 Apr 17;49(15):1625–31.

[15] Uchôa C H G, Pedrosa R P, Javaheri S, Geovanini G R, Carvalho M M B, Torquatro A C S, Leite A P D L, Gonzaga C C, Bertolami A, Amodeo C, Petisco A C G P, Barbosa J E M, Macedo TA, Bortolotto LA, Oliveira MT Jr, Lorenzi-Filho G, Drager LF. OSA and Prognosis After Acute Cardiogenic Pulmonary Edema: The OSA-CARE Study. *Chest.* 2017 Dec;152(6):1230–8.

[16] Bucca C B, Brussino L, Battisti A, Mutani R, Rolla G, Mangiardi L, Cicolin A. Diuretics in obstructive sleep apnea with diastolic heart failure. *Chest.* 2007 Aug;132(2):440–6.

[17] Kasai T, Arcand J, Allard J P, Mak S, Azevedo E R, Newton G E, Bradley T D. Relationship between sodium intake and sleep apnea in patients with heart failure. *J. Am. Coll. Cardiol.* 2011 Nov 1;58(19):1970–4.

[18] Fiori C Z, Martinez D, Montanari C C, Lopez P, Camargo R, Sezerá L, Gonçalves SC, Fuchs FD. Diuretic or sodium-restricted diet for obstructive sleep apnea-a randomized trial. *Sleep.* 2018 Apr 1;41(4).

[19] Sengul Y S, Ozalevli S, Oztura I, Itil O, Baklan B. The effect of exercise on obstructive sleep apnea: a randomized and controlled trial. *Sleep Breath.* 2011 Jan;15(1):49–56.

[20] Kline C E, Crowley E P, Ewing G B, Burch J B, Blair S N, Durstine J L, Davis J M, Youngstedt S D. The effect of exercise training on obstructive sleep apnea and sleep quality: a randomized controlled trial. *Sleep.* 2011 Dec 1;34(12):1631–40.

[21] Aiello K D, Caughey W G, Nelluri B, Sharma A, Mookadam F, Mookadam M. Effect of exercise training on sleep apnea: A systematic review and meta-analysis. *Respir. Med.* 2016 Jul;116:85–92.

[22] WRITING COMMITTEE MEMBERS, Yancy C W, Jessup M, Bozkurt B, Butler J, Casey D E Jr, Drazner M H, Fonarow G C, Geraci S A, Horwich T, Januzzi J L, Johnson M R, Kasper E K, Levy W C, Masoudi F A, McBride P E, McMurray J J, Mitchell J E, Peterson P N, Riegel B, Sam F, Stevenson L W, Tang W H, Tsai E J, Wilkoff B L; American College of Cardiology Foundation/American Heart Association Task Force on Practice Guidelines. 2013 ACCF/AHA guideline for the management of heart failure: a report of the American College of Cardiology Foundation/American Heart Association Task Force on practice guidelines. *Circulation.* 2013 Oct 15;128(16):e240-327.

[23] Writing Committee, Maddox T M, Januzzi J L, Allen L A, Breathett K, Butler J, Davis L L, Fonarow G C, Ibrahim N E, Lindenfeld J, Masoudi F A, Motiwala S R, Oliveros E, Patterson J H, Walsh M N, Wasserman A, Yancy C W, Youmans Q R. 2021 Update to the 2017 ACC Expert Consensus Decision Pathway for Optimization of Heart Failure Treatment: Answers to 10 Pivotal Issues About Heart Failure with Reduced Ejection Fraction: A Report of the American College of Cardiology Solution Set Oversight Committee. *J. Am. Coll. Cardiol.* 2021 Feb 16;77(6):772–810.

[24] McDonagh T A, Metra M, Adamo M, Gardner RS, Baumbach A, Böhm M, Burri H, Butler J, Čelutkienė J, Chioncel O, Cleland J G F, Coats A J S, Crespo-Leiro M G, Farmakis D, Gilard M, Heymans S, Hoes A W, Jaarsma T, Jankowska E A, Lainscak M, Lam C S P, Lyon A R, McMurray J J V, Mebazaa A, Mindham R, Munneretto C, Francesco Piepoli M, Price S, Rosano G M C, Ruschitzka F, Kathrine Skibelund A; ESC Scientific Document Group. 2021 ESC Guidelines for the diagnosis and treatment of acute and chronic heart failure. *Eur. Heart J.* 2021 Sep 21;42(36):3599–726.

[25] Patil S P, Ayappa I A, Caples S M, Kimoff R J, Patel S R, Harrod C G. Treatment of Adult Obstructive Sleep Apnea with Positive Airway Pressure: An American

Academy of Sleep Medicine Systematic Review, Meta-Analysis, and GRADE Assessment. *J. Clin. Sleep Med.* 2019 Feb 15;15(2):301–34.

[26] Kaneko Y, Floras J S, Usui K, Plante J, Tkacova R, Kubo T, Ando S, Bradley TD. Cardiovascular effects of continuous positive airway pressure in patients with heart failure and obstructive sleep apnea. *N. Engl. J. Med.* 2003 Mar 27;348(13):1233–41.

[27] Sun H, Shi J, Li M, Chen X. Impact of continuous positive airway pressure treatment on left ventricular ejection fraction in patients with obstructive sleep apnea: a meta-analysis of randomized controlled trials. *PLoS One*. 2013;8(5):e62298.

[28] Sharma S, Fox H, Aguilar F, Mukhtar U, Willes L, Bozorgnia B, Bitter T, Oldenburg O. Auto positive airway pressure therapy reduces pulmonary pressures in adults admitted for acute heart failure with pulmonary hypertension and obstructive sleep apnea. The ASAP-HF Pilot Trial. *Sleep.* 2019 Jul 8;42(7):zsz100.

[29] Khayat R N, Javaheri S, Porter K, Sow A, Holt R, Randerath W, Abraham WT, Jarjoura D. In-Hospital Management of Sleep Apnea During Heart Failure Hospitalization: A Randomized Controlled Trial. *J. Card Fail.* 2020 Aug;26(8):705–12.

[30] Cowie M R, Woehrle H, Wegscheider K, Angermann C, d'Ortho MP, Erdmann E, Levy P, Simonds AK, Somers V K, Zannad F, Teschler H. Adaptive Servo-Ventilation for Central Sleep Apnea in Systolic Heart Failure. *N. Engl. J. Med.* 2015 Sep 17;373(12):1095–105.

[31] Yoshihisa A, Suzuki S, Yamauchi H, Sato T, Oikawa M, Kobayashi A, Yamaki T, Sugimoto K, Kunii H, Nakazato K, Suzuki H, Saitoh S, Takeishi Y. Beneficial Effects of Positive Airway Pressure Therapy for Sleep-Disordered Breathing in Heart Failure Patients with Preserved Left Ventricular Ejection Fraction. *Clin. Cardiol.* 2015 Jul;38(7):413–21.

[32] Arikawa T, Toyoda S, Haruyama A, Amano H, Inami S, Otani N, Sakuma M, Taguchi I, Abe S, Node K, Inoue T. Impact of Obstructive Sleep Apnoea on Heart Failure with Preserved Ejection Fraction. *Heart Lung Circ.* 2016 May;25(5):435–41.

[33] Lyons O D, Floras J S, Logan A G, Beanlands R, Cantolla J D, Fitzpatrick M, Fleetham J, John Kimoff R, Leung R S, Lorenzi Filho G, Mayer P, Mielniczuk L, Morrison D L, Ryan C M, Series F, Tomlinson G A, Woo A, Arzt M, Parthasarathy S, Redolfi S, Kasai T, Parati G, Delgado D H, Bradley T D; ADVENT-HF Investigators. Design of the effect of adaptive servo-ventilation on survival and cardiovascular hospital admissions in patients with heart failure and sleep apnoea: the ADVENT-HF trial. *Eur. J. Heart Fail.* 2017 Apr;19(4):579–87.

[34] Tsutsui H, Isobe M, Ito H, Ito H, Okumura K, Ono M, Kitakaze M, Kinugawa K, Kihara Y, Goto Y, Komuro I, Saiki Y, Saito Y, Sakata Y, Sato N, Sawa Y, Shiose A, Shimizu W, Shimokawa H, Seino Y, Node K, Higo T, Hirayama A, Makaya M, Masuyama T, Murohara T, Momomura SI, Yano M, Yamazaki K, Yamamoto K, Yoshikawa T, Yoshimura M, Akiyama M, Anzai T, Ishihara S, Inomata T, Imamura T, Iwasaki Y K, Ohtani T, Onishi K, Kasai T, Kato M, Kawai M, Kinugasa Y, Kinugawa S, Kuratani T, Kobayashi S, Sakata Y, Tanaka A, Toda K, Noda T, Nochioka K, Hatano M, Hidaka T, Fujino T, Makita S, Yamaguchi O, Ikeda U,

Kimura T, Kohsaka S, Kosuge M, Yamagishi M, Yamashina A; Japanese Circulation Society and the Japanese Heart Failure Society Joint Working Group. JCS 2017/JHFS 2017 Guideline on Diagnosis and Treatment of Acute and Chronic Heart Failure — Digest Version —. *Circulation Journal.* 2019;83(10):2084–184.

Chapter 11

Neurologıcal Dıseases

Ahmet Cemal Pazarlı[1,*], MD
and N. Tibel Tuna[2], MD

[1]Gaziosmanpaşa University Faculty of Medicine,
Department of Pulmonary Diseases, Tokat, Turkey
[2] Ondokuz Mayıs University Faculty of Medicine,
Department of Pulmonary Diseases, Samsun,Turkey

Abstract

Obstructive sleep apnea is a serious, life-threatening condition that causes many comorbidities. It is a common entity among neurological diseases which may worsen the current clinical condition of the patient. Neurological diseases are included among the etiology, differential diagnosis and results of obstructive sleep apnea. Obstructive sleep apnea is a syndrome that includes many neurological symptoms and its relationship with neurological diseases has always attracted attention and led to many studies on this subject. If obstructive sleep apnea is not recognized and treated properly, it can cause many neurological diseases that will potentially exacerbate each other and eventually lead to death.

Keywords: obstructive sleep apnea, neurological diseases, positive airway therapy, epilepsy, Alzheimer's disease

* Corresponding Author's Email: drcemalpazarli@gmail.com.

In: Obstructive Sleep Apnea in Pulmonary Critical Care
Editors: Antonio M. Esquinas and Takatoshi Kasai
ISBN: 979-8-88697-858-2

Introduction

A survey called "Sleep in America" by the American National Sleep Foundation reported that 66% of healthy adults experience at least one sleep disorder symptom on one or more nights a week. In people with health problems, this rate was found as 93% [1]. Sleep apnea is a type of sleep disorder characterized by the interruption of the individual's normal breathing pattern during sleep. This interruption typically occurs repeatedly throughout the night and usually lasts 10 seconds or longer. There are three types of sleep apnea conditions: obstructive sleep apnea (OSA), central sleep apnea (CSA), and a combination of the two. The most common type of sleep apnea is OSA, in which air passage is blocked by relaxation of the soft tissue at the back of the throat. People with sleep apnea often wake up because they have trouble breathing and may not be aware of it in the morning. If left untreated, this condition can cause pulmonary hypertension, psychiatric disorders, myocardial infarction, coronary heart disease, stroke, cognitive impairment, and even death. Typical symptoms known in OSA are witnessed sleep apnea, snoring and excessive daytime sleepiness. It is also a syndrome that includes many neurological symptoms. Typically, OSA may present with headache, amnesia, syncope, cognitive disorders, epileptic seizures, and seizure-like symptoms. Research shows that patients with certain neurological conditions such as myasthenia gravis, parkinsonism, and myotonic dystrophy have a higher risk of suffering from sleep apnea. This is because these conditions can impair the nerves that control the upper airway muscles. Neurological diseases may cause OSA, worsen the prognosis of the existing disease, are included in the differential diagnosis of OSA, or they may occur as a result of OSA. Sleep apnea itself puts a person at risk of suffering from certain neurological conditions, as well as worsening the clinical course of their existing neurological disease. Any neurological condition that causes impaired upper airway muscle tone can contribute to airway obstruction and result in OSA or increase the severity of OSA. Apart from this, some neurological diseases affecting the central nervous system and in some cases affecting the respiratory center may cause sleep apnea related to central apneas. Common neurological and neuromuscular disorders associated with a higher incidence of OSA in adults include congenital myopathies, neuropathies, myotonic dystrophy, Duchenne dystrophy, mitochondrial encephalomyopathy, myasthenia gravis, stroke, epilepsy, Parkinsonism, and Alzheimer's disease [2]. In addition, sleep disturbance is often overlooked, especially in patients with epilepsy, and in case of an existing sleep apnea condition, this may contribute to decreased daytime functionality and increased seizure activity [3]. Epidemiological studies indicate that stroke survivors are at an increased risk for OSA, with an incidence of 50-70% in the first 3 months following stroke [4], whereas in a prospective study conducted with stroke rehabilitation patients with 10-year follow-up, the risk of death in patients with OSA was found as significantly higher than in controls. In neurodegenerative diseases (Parkinson's disease, Alzheimer's dementia), sleep disturbance may become more pronounced as the disease progresses [5, 6]. In this chapter, the relationship between neurological diseases and OSA has been discussed in the light of current literature.

OSA and Epilepsy

Sleep disturbance is often overlooked in patients with epilepsy. However, patients with epilepsy appear to have comorbid OSA more frequently than the general population, leading to hypersomnia, increased seizure frequency and additional health risks. Epilepsy patients with OSA are more often older, heavier, and male patients. Concomitant OSA may worsen seizure control by mediating sleep disturbance and deprivation, increasing the risk of nighttime seizure burden [7]. In their study, Manni et al. found the association of OSA and epilepsy as 10.2% in epilepsy patients (15.4% of men and 5.4% of women) [8]. Epilepsy causes changes in the natural structure and organization of sleep. Antiepileptic drugs also have effects on sleep. Autonomic nervous system activation increases as a result of frequent recurrent apneas and is known to cause nocturnal epilepsy as a result. One third of patients with medically resistant epilepsy have a respiratory disturbance index (RDI) value above 5, and seizures are more common in patients with both epilepsy and OSA than in the general population [9]. Seizures occur most frequently during sleep phase transitions, and reducing sleep fragmentation can reduce the risk of seizures by reducing sleep phase transitions. Patients with obesity and OSA may be at risk for anoxic seizures. CPAP treatment in OSA reduces the frequency of seizures in patients with epilepsy. Vaughn et al. showed that 40% of epilepsy patients treated with OSA became seizure-free, seizures occurring only during sleep were the most responsive to treatment, and factors contributing to treatment response were factors such as decreased sleep fragmentation and improved oxygenation [10]. In addition to the increase in the frequency of OSA in patients with epilepsy, it is assumed that many drugs used to treat existing epilepsy may play a role in the development of OSA.

Valproate, vigabatrin, and gabapentin may promote weight gain and trigger or aggravate pre-existing OSA, as obesity is a clear risk factor for OSA. Benzodiazepines and barbiturates suppress the response to carbon dioxide and hypoxia. In addition, they may cause obstructive apnea or exacerbation by promoting upper airway relaxation. In the light of this information, it is very important that patients with epileptic attacks, especially in multidrug-resistant epilepsy patients, are carefully evaluated for possible OSA and treated with appropriate modalities if detected.

OSA and Cerebrovascular Accident

Obesity, like other risk factors (hypertension, cardiac arrhythmia, etc.), has an important place among the main risk factors of stroke. It is known that OSA not only poses risks through proinflammatory cytokine release, increase in free oxygen radicals, sympathetic nervous system activation and endothelial dysfunction, but also causes disruption of cerebrovascular autoregulatory mechanisms depending on the severity of the disease [11]. The incidence of OSA is higher in patients who have had a stroke or transient ischemic attack than in the general population. Patients presenting with stroke or transient ischemic attack are 3 to 4 times more likely to have OSA than control subjects. Studies conducted on this subject have shown that 60% to 80% of patients with stroke and transient ischemic attack, regardless of gender, have Apnea-Hypoxia Index (AHI) >10.20-22 [12]. In their study, Palomaki *et al.* compared 177 consecutive male patients with brain infarction with controls of the same age, and found that the odds ratio for snoring and brain infarction was 2.13, and if sleep apnea, daytime sleepiness and obesity were also present, the odds ratio increased to 8.0, concluded that snoring may be a risk factor for ischemic stroke, possibly due to the higher prevalence of OSA among snorers [13]. In another study involving 400 patients who had cerebrovascular accident (CVA), it was shown that snoring is an important risk factor for both as a cause of CVA and poor prognosis [14]. In addition, there are many studies in the literature showing the positive effects of CPAP therapy on platelet activation, coagulation factors, and vascular functions in patients with OSA. For this reason, OSA symptoms should be reviewed in patients with CVA and necessary precautions should be taken.

OSA and Parkinson's Disease

Parkinson's disease (PD) is a progressive neurodegenerative disease associated with distinctive motor and non-motor symptoms such as sleep disturbances and cognitive dysfunction. Neuroimaging showed structural and functional changes in OSA patients; and in animal models, it has been shown that OSA causes brain inflammation and oxidative damage, including key areas involved in PD pathophysiology, such as the locus coeruleus. Incresed tone or dyskinesias in the upper respiratory tract due to the effect of the disease itself or the pharmacological drugs may predispose Parkinson's patients to obstructive apnea. It is also seen that coordination disorders in respiratory muscle activation and disorders in respiratory stimuli contribute to nocturnal respiratory problems in PD. It is also associated with autonomic dysfunction, which can impair respiratory control, particularly during non-REM sleep, where breathing is predominantly chemically driven. Although respiratory disorders in PD are generally thought to correlate with the severity of rigidity and tremor, since respiratory disorders typically do not improve with L–dopa administration, the treatment of sleep apnea in Parkinson's must be treated as in the healthy adult population [15].

OSA and Alzheimer's Disease

Alzheimer's disease (AD) and OSA are highly common chronic conditions with intriguing but poorly understood epidemiological overlap. Knowing the prevalence of Alzheimer's disease, as well as the prevalence of OSA in Alzheimer's patients, is important for planning resources and changing treatment for comorbidities. Although studies are far from clear, it has been suggested that there is a causal relationship between untreated OSA and the triggering of neurodegenerative processes underlying AD [16]. The additive effect of progressive changes in sleep quality and structure, changes in cerebral blood flow, and cellular redox status in OSA patients may all be contributing factors to cognitive decline and exacerbate AD progression. Although there is currently no conclusive evidence that OSA therapy in AD will have a major impact on the course of AD, many authors have argued that there is sufficient clinical evidence that CPAP therapy may be at least beneficial in eliminating excessive daytime sleepiness, hypersomnia, and lethargy. In a randomized, double-blind, placebo-controlled study conducted with CPAP therapy used in patients with Alzheimer's disease and OSA coexistence, significant cognitive improvements were observed in patients using CPAP when pre-treatment and post-treatment neuropsychological test scores were compared at the end of the 3rd week [17]. In their meta-analysis, Emamian et al. emphasized that the high rate of OSA in AD patients should alert clinicians regarding the importance of screening AD patients for OSA, and the effects of CPAP therapy were also shown [18].

OSA and Neuromuscular Diseases

OSA and neuromuscular diseases are tightly linked. Malfunctions in the muscles and the neuromuscular junctions can cause serious damage in respiratory functions. Any neuromuscular disease condition that causes weakness of the upper respiratory tract muscle structure creates the basic pathophysiology of OSA and causes the individual to be predisposed to develop OSA. Many neuromuscular diseases affect respiratory muscles such as upper airway dilators, intercostals, or diaphragm. Therefore, it is not surprising that many patients with neuromuscular disease are susceptible to OSA. OSA is an important consideration in neuromuscular disease at any level, such as nerve, neuromuscular junction, or muscle. Common neuromuscular disorders associated with a high incidence of OSA in adults and included in the etiology of OSA are amyotrophic lateral sclerosis, congenital myopathies, myotonic dystrophy, Duchenne muscular dystrophy, mitochondrial encephalomyopathy, myasthenia gravis (MG) disease [2]. OSA is seen in 70% of patients with type 1 myotonic dystrophy, and these patients may also have symptomatic narcolepsy with marked hypersomnia [19]. Patients with neuromuscular disorders, particularly myopathy or motor neuron disease, may develop sleep-related hypoventilation, usually initially during sleep and particularly during the REM phase. It is important to screen these patients with overnight home portable oximetry monitoring, to identify mild early respiratory failure, and to apply appropriate supportive non-invasive positive pressure ventilation during sleep. Early diagnosis and early intervention of OSA in patients with neuromuscular diseases improves quality of life and prolongs survival.

OSA and Multiple Sclerosis

Multiple sclerosis (MS), which causes demyelination of the brain and spinal cord, is one of the leading neurological diseases in young adults. Sleep-related problems in MS have been reported in approximately 50% of patients. Fatigue affects up to 90% of MS patients at some point in the disease course [20]. This extremely debilitating symptom has significant socioeconomic consequences and is a leading cause of reduced quality of life in people with MS. OSA may exacerbate the severity of fatigue in MS. However, despite its impact in the general population, the extent to which OSA contributes to fatigue in people with MS is not fully understood, and the prevalence of OSA in MS remains unclear. Although some researchers argue that the prevalence of OSA is higher in MS patients than in the general population, heterogeneity in study subjects, sample size, and outcome measures have led to highly variable estimates. Although OSA is considered as an important public health problem, its prevalence in people with MS is not known exactly, and there are estimates ranging from 0% to 58% in published studies [21, 22]. In conclusion, there is evidence that sleep disturbances, particularly OSA, can be quite common in patients with MS, but what contributes to fatigue in people with MS is poorly understood. Clinicians should keep the screening threshold of OSA in MS patients low and try to identify underlying nocturnal symptoms that may affect sleep quality and contribute to daytime fatigue.This raises the possibility that a significant portion of MS-related fatigue can be eliminated by diagnosis and successful treatment of OSA in patients with MS.

Conclusion

OSA is the most common cause of mortality and morbidity among sleep respiratory disorders. As a result of the increase in life expectancy worlwide, the prevalence of many chronic diseases increases as well as the prevalence of neurological diseases. Many studies have shown that the incidence of OSA is increasing in patients with neurological disorders, necessitating careful physician evaluation. The diagnosis and effective treatment of the presence of OSA in addition to the neurological disease will contribute to the improvement of the patient's current neurological status. In summary, a) Neurological diseases include disease groups in which patient care management is very important, which are common in the society, and whose frequency increases with age, b) Although OSA is common in the general population, patients with neurological disease should be carefully evaluated for the possible presence of OSA, since sleep-related breathing disorders seen in neurological diseases will impair the patient's current neurological status, c) It should be kept in mind that effective treatment of OSA in many neurological diseases will regress the patient's neurological symptoms, d) Positive airway pressure therapy, which is still considered as the most effective treatment for OSA, should be carefully evaluated in such patients and the appropriate modality should be decided on a patient basis and e) In addition to the association between OSA and many neurological diseases, it should be kept in mind that drugs used in neurological diseases may also cause the development of OSA or increase existing OSA symptoms.

References

[1] National Sleep Foundation. "Sleep in America" Poll. National Sleep Foundation Web site. http ://www.sleepfoundation. org/sites/default/fi les/2002. Sleep In America Poll. pdf. Accessed August 17, 2011.

[2] Kryger M, Roth T, Dement W. Principles and practice of sleep medicine (3rd ed.). Philadelphia: Saunders. Bazil, C. W. Sleep and epilepsy. *Current Opinion in Neurology,* 2000 13 (2), 171-175.

[3] Bazil CW. Sleep and epilepsy. *Current Opinion in Neurology,* 2000 13(2), 171-175.

[4] Johnson KG, Johnson DC. Frequency of sleep apnea in stroke and TIA patients: A meta-analysis. *J Clin Sleep Med,* 2010; 6:131-137.

[5] Sahlin C, Sandberg O, Gustafson Y, Bucht G, Carlberg B, Stenlund H, Franklin KA. Obstructive sleep apnea is a risk factor for death in patients with stroke: A 10-year follow-up. *Arch Intern Med,* 2008; 168:297-301.

[6] Boeve BF, Silber MH, Saper CB, Ferman TJ, Dickson DW, Parisi JE, Benarroch EE, Ahlskog JE, Smith GE, Caselli RC, Tippman-Peikert M, Olson EJ, Lin S-L, Young T, Wszolek Z, Schenck CH, Mahowald MW, Castillo PR, Del TrediciK, Braak H. Pathophysiology of REM sleep behaviour disorder and relevance to neurodegenerative disease. *Brain,* 2007; 130:2770-2788.

[7] Malow BA, Levy K, Maturen K, Bowes R. Obstructive sleep apnea is common in medically refractory epilepsy patients. *Neurology,* 2000; 55(7):1002-1007.

[8] Manni R, Terzaghi M, Arbasino C, Sartori I, Galimberti CA, Tartara A. Obstructive sleep apnea in a clinical series of adult epilepsy patients: Frequency and features of the comorbidity. *Epilepsia,* 2003 44, 836-840.

[9] Sonka K, Juklícková M, Pretl M, Dostálová S, Horínek D, Nevsímalová S. Seizures in sleep apnea patients: Occurrence and time distribution. *Sb Lek,* 2000; 101:229-232.

[10] Vaughn BV, D'Cruz OF, Beach R, Messenheimer JA. Improvement of epileptiseizure control with treatment of obstructive sleep apnoea. *Seizure,* 1996. 5: 73-78.

[11] Cereda C, Lavie L, Bassetti CL. *Sleep disorders in neurology*. New York, NY: Nova Science Publishers, 2012.

[12] Bassetti C, Aldrich MS. Sleep apnea in acute cerebrovascular diseases: Final report on 128 patients. *Sleep,* 1999; 22:217-223.

[13] Palomaki H. Snoring and the risk of ischemic brain infarction. *Stroke,* 1991; 22:1021-1025.

[14] Qureshi AI, Giles WH, Croft JB, Bliwise DL. Habitual sleep patterns and risk for stroke and coronary heart disease: A 10−year follow−up from NHANES I. *Neurology,* 1997; 48: 904-11.

[15] Larsen JP, Tandberg E. "Sleep disorders in patients with Parkinson's disease: Epidemiology and management, *CNS Drugs,* 2001. vol. 15, no. 4, pp. 267-275.

[16] Rosenzweig I, Williams SC, Morrell MJ. The impactof sleep and hypoxia on the brain:Potential mechanisms for the effects of obstructive sleep apnea. *Curr Opin Pulm Med,* 2014 20, 565-571.

[17] Ancoli-Israel S, Palmer BW, Cooke JR, Corey-Bloom J, Fiorentino L, Natarajan L, Liu L, Ayalon L, He F, Loredo JS. Cognitive effects of treating obstructive sleep apnea in Alzheimer's disease: A randomized controlled study. J *Am Geriatr Soc,* 2008; 56 (11): 2076-2081.

[18] Emamian F, Khazaie H, Tahmasian M, Leschziner GD, Morrell MJ, Hsiung GY, Rosenzweig I, Sepehry AA. The Association between Obstructive Sleep Apnea and Alzheimer's Disease: A Meta-Analysis Perspective. *Front Aging Neurosci,* 2016; 8:78.

[19] Laberge L, Bégin P, Montplaisir J, Mathieu J. Sleep Complaints in Patients with Myotonic Dystrophy. J *Sleep Res,* 2004; 13:95-100.

[20] Krupp LB, Alvarez LA, LaRocca NG, Scheinberg LC. Fatigue in multiple sclerosis. *Arch Neurol,* 1988; 45:435-7.

[21] Veauthier C, Radbruch H, Gaede G, Pfueller CF, Dörr J, Bellmann-Strobl J, Wernecke KD, Zipp F, Paul F, Sieb JP. Fatigue in multiple sclerosis is closely related to sleep disorders: A polysomnographic cross-sectional study. *Mult Scler,* 2011; 17:613-22.

[22] Kaminska M, Kimoff RJ, Benedetti A, Robinson A, Bar-Or A, Lapierre Y, Schwartzman K, Trojan DA. Obstructive sleep apnea is associated with fatigue in multiple sclerosis. *Mult Scler,* 2012; 18:1159-69.

Chapter 12

Interstitial Lung Diseases: Pathophysiology and Treatment

Mariana Martins* **MD**
Pulmonology Department,
Centro Hospitalar Universitário, São João, Porto, Portugal

Abstract

Obstructive sleep apnoea (OSA) is a common comorbidity in interstitial lung diseases (ILD), mainly in idiopathic pulmonary fibrosis (IPF). Although, there is a lack of consensus regarding the true prevalence of OSA in ILD, proving this a challenging aspect for pulmonologists across the world to effectively diagnose and manage OSA in this population. Older age and higher body mass index (BMI) are risk factors for OSA in patients with ILD, being the later a variable found to be an independent predictive factor for OSA. Therefore, further emphasis must be placed on the screening patients with ILD who are obese and/or symptomatic (presenting daytime somnolence and severe fatigue) via nocturnal polysomnography to promptly identify cases of OSA. The relationships between ILD and OSA are complex and possibly bidirectional, with multiple mechanisms postulated for the pathogenic and physiologic links. In patients with ILD and OSA, APAP treatment could be sufficient to correct oxygen desaturation. Neither OSA severity nor adherence to CPAP was associated with improved outcomes in ILD patients except those requiring supplemental oxygen. Growing evidence shows that sleep disturbances are associated with worse quality of life in ILD, may also predict more rapid disease progression and increased mortality. Nocturnal oxygen saturation is associated with poorer prognosis in ILD

* Corresponding Author's Email: mariana-martins@campus.ul.pt.

In: Obstructive Sleep Apnea in Pulmonary Critical Care
Editors: Antonio M. Esquinas and Takatoshi Kasai
ISBN: 979-8-88697-858-2

patients and may contribute towards the pathogenesis of pulmonary vascular disease.

Keywords: obstructive sleep apnoea, interstitial lung diseases, continuous positive airway pressure, idiopathic pulmonary fibrosis, severity

Introduction

Interstitial lung diseases (ILD) are a heterogeneous group of diseases with varying degrees of inflammation and fibrosis, which cause damage to the lung parenchyma, resulting in restrictive lung disease and impaired gas exchange [1]. Frequently, these patients have exercise intolerance and hypoxemia that can progress to respiratory failure, pulmonary hypertension, and death [2].

The patients with ILD also exhibit a range of comorbidities that have a substantial impact on the prognostic outcome of the disease and quality of life. Studies have suggested that one of the most common comorbidities existing with ILD is OSA. OSA is characterized by airflow impairment during sleep due to repetitive collapse of the pharyngeal muscles and there is increasing recognition of OSA as a phenotypic heterogeneous syndrome with different predisposing factors and pathophysiological traits, or endotypes, including both anatomical and non-anatomical factors. While OSA has been postulated to contribute to the pathogenesis of ILD through tractional or aspiration-related injury and intermittent hypoxia, it is equally plausible that impaired respiratory mechanics and gas exchange in ILD may also predispose the individual towards developing OSA [3].

It is challenging to accurately define the exact prevalence of OSA in patients with ILD. There is a four-fold difference in the reported prevalence of OSA in ILD patients, ranging from 22% to 90%, with some studies suggesting up to two-thirds of patients have moderate-to-severe OSA. Variations in the reported prevalence are likely affected by differences in the diagnostic criteria for OSA and polysomnographic scoring of hypopnea events used. In addition, differences in ILD diagnoses and demographic structure of studied populations may explain the observed variations, as the prevalence of OSA is higher in patients with IPF than those with other ILDs, with a preponderance of males 3. According to Margaritopoulos et al., the prevalence of OSA is of 60-90% in IPF, 50% in systemic sclerosis associated interstitial lung disease (SSc-ILD) and 65% in sarcoidosis [4].

Importantly, the prevalence of OSA consistently increases with age, which is of significant relevance to patients with ILD who most often have onset age of over 60 years old. Other parameters identified as risk factors for OSA in patients with ILD are higher BMI, diabetes mellitus, FEV1(%), duration of immunosuppressant treatment, the minimum O2 saturation during sleep and the time spent under 90% of O2 saturation (T90) [5, 6]. In a cohort prospective study, BMI was the only variable that remained an independent predictive factor for OSA after a multivariate analysis, thus revealing that excess of weight should be considered in ILD patients and that OSA should at least be screened in overweight patients with those diseases [6].

Pathophysiology

The pathogenic links between OSA and ILD are complex, possibly bidirectional, and not clearly understood until now. Marked alterations have been reported in sleep architecture in patients with ILD, such as decreased sleep efficiency, decreased REM sleep stage and increased stage 1, more arousals and sleep fragmentation. It has been proposed that the decreased lung volumes observed in restrictive pulmonary diseases can reduce the upper airway stability and increase resistance due to reducing traction on the upper airway. These changes can facilitate the upper airway collapse, especially during REM sleep when functional residual capacity is further reduced due to reduced activity of the intercostal muscles [7].

In detail, postulated factors contributing to this unique relationship include recurrent mechanical stretch causing tractional injury, repetitive micro aspiration from gastroesophageal reflux, and oxidative stress related to intermittent hypoxia and, more recently, circadian dysregulation, which is yet under evaluation. Recurrent tractional injury has been raised as a pathogenic mechanism once during apneas and hypopneas, patients with OSA generate swings in pleural pressures, which could result in alveolar injury via local traction [3].

OSA is associated with increased nocturnal gastroesophageal reflux but in the only study that evaluated the link between OSA and gastroesophageal reflux in ILD, there was no association between the presence and severity of OSA with gastroesophageal reflux. However, the diagnostic evaluations of both conditions, polysomnography, and oesophageal pH with or without impedance monitoring, were not conducted simultaneously [8]. Intermittent hypoxia is a common feature of OSA. Recurrent apneas and hypopneas during sleep result in cycles of desaturation and re-oxygenation like a hypoxia-reperfusion injury. This process induces increased levels of oxidative stress which have been demonstrated in lung and blood samples from patients with ILD [9].

Upper airway obstruction is considered the pathophysiological endpoint of several interacting and related processes in OSA, which can be divided into anatomical and non-anatomical traits or endotypes. Anatomical traits include the size, shape, and collapsibility of the upper airway, which are strongly linked with obesity, and reduced lung volumes. Non-anatomical traits include ventilatory control instability (also termed as elevated loop gain), low respiratory arousal threshold, and lower upper airway dilator muscle responsiveness/effectiveness. Typically, OSA patients experience an anatomical narrowing because of increasing BMI and fat deposition in the upper airway. This may not happen in cases of ILD patients who have a normal BMI. In these patients, non-anatomical factors play a more important pathogenic role than the anatomical factors [3].

Due to lung parenchymal infiltration and fibrosis, a key pathophysiological feature of ILD is decreased lung compliance and reduced lung volume resulting in increased pharyngeal collapsibility, which is a vital factor in the anatomical contribution to OSA pathogenesis in patients with ILD. This process occurs particularly during REM sleep, when skeletal muscle atonia leads to further reduction in functional residual capacity [1].

Ventilatory control instability, or elevated loop gain, is an important non-anatomical factor implicated in the development of OSA. The loop gain integrates three tracts: controller gain (the sensitivity of the central chemoreceptors to hypercapnia and hypoxia), feedback gain (the sensitivity of the peripheral chemoreceptors to hypercapnia and hypoxia) and plant gain (the efficiency at which ventilation changes blood gases). Although there are no direct data on the effects of ILD on plant gain, it is reasonable to assume that reduced lung volumes and gas transfer in ILD will result in a concomitant increase in plant gain and, subsequently, loop gain [3].

Increased work of breathing during sleep secondary to respiratory loading may cause patients with chronic lung diseases to reach arousal threshold more often, but more studies are required in this area. Skeletal muscle dysfunction is a well-known phenomenon in ILD. Hence, upper airway dilator muscle dysfunction may contribute to OSA in some patients with ILD, however remains to be evaluated [1].

Diagnosis

The Epworth Sleepiness Scale (ESS), and Pittsburgh Sleep Quality Index (PSQI) scores are higher in ILD patients than in normal controls, indicating poorer quality of sleep. Nevertheless, in ILD patients who underwent polysomnography, the ESS and other tools do not reliably predict severity of sleep-disordered breathing [10]. Zhang et al., suggested different cut-off scores for the STOP-Bang questionnaire, with < 3 points for rule-out and > 6 points for rule-in, could improve its predictive performance in patients with ILD. Overnight oximetry is a potential alternative tool for risk stratifying for OSA, which is widely available and easily used. An oxygen desaturation index cut-off > 9 has superior performance in identifying ILD patients with OSA, compared to the STOP-Bang questionnaire [11].

Level 1 polysomnography is the gold standard for the diagnosis of OSA in patients with ILD. Not to forget that isolated nocturnal hypoxemia without OSA is an important observation in ILD and, in addition, a significant number of patients with ILD receive supplemental oxygen, which obscures oxygen dips and may degrade nasal pressure and thermistor signals. So, respiratory effort and electroencephalogram recordings must be present to accurately score hypopnea events [12].

Idiopathic Pulmonary Fibrosis (IPF)

IPF represents a specific form of ILD of unknown cause, with poor survival that occurs primarily in older adults. Many comorbid conditions are described, and these may influence the prognosis and modify the natural course of the disease. In fact, sleep-related disorders, such as OSA have been recognized as an important, high-prevalence comorbidity in the latest official guidelines for the diagnosis and management of IPF. Although, it is considered too precocious to characterize this as an overlap syndrome and, until now, there are still no common biomarkers in IPF and OSA. Patients with OSA and IPF often present atypical symptoms such as daytime fatigue, sleep onset and maintenance insomnia and nocturnal cough. Furthermore, the presence of OSA has been associated with a more rapid clinical deterioration independent of the severity of IPF [13].

Neither the Epworth Sleepiness Scale nor the Sleep Apnoea Scale of Sleep Disorders Questionnaire, alone or in combination, was a strong screening tool.

So, the optimal tool for OSA screening in patients with IPF has yet to be determined making inevitable the need of an evaluation with overnight polysomnography [7]. Effective CPAP treatment in IPF patients with comorbid moderate-to-severe OSA results in a significant improvement in daily living activities, quality of sleep and life. Treatment of comorbidities such as OSA may also influence mortality in IPF [13].

Treatment Pulmonary Rehabilitation

Pulmonary rehabilitation is recommended for patients with ILD, with the beneficial effects of improved dyspnea, functional exercise capacity, and quality of life. Although the effects of pulmonary rehabilitation on co-morbid OSA in the ILD population are unknown, a recent study demonstrated that pulmonary rehabilitation had beneficial effects on overnight oxygenation status, independent of CPAP administration, in a group of newly diagnosed OSA patients without significant cardiorespiratory disease. Also, both anthropometric parameters and respiratory function significantly improved in the intervention group, compared to the control group. The mechanisms whereby exercise training alleviates the severity of OSA are yet to be determined and are likely multifactorial [3].

ILD Targeted Therapies

A significant proportion of patients with ILD receive corticosteroids during their disease course, and the mechanisms by which steroid administration may influence the development of OSA is through weight gain, fluid retention and nocturnal rostral fluid shifts. No studies have explored the effects of other immunosuppressive agents or anti-fibrotic therapies on OSA in patients with ILD.

Continuous Positive Airway Pressure (CPAP)

The recommended treatment for OSA remains CPAP therapy. In patients with co-morbid ILD and significant OSA, CPAP has the potential to improve sleep quality, reduce daytime sleepiness and improve quality of life. Recently,

Adegunsoye et al., demonstrated that adherence to CPAP therapy is not associated with improved all-cause mortality or PFS in most patients with coexistent ILD and OSA [14]. However, in a secondary analysis of the study, our results suggest that in the subpopulation requiring oxygen supplementation, CPAP therapy is associated with improved PFS and preservation of FVC, findings that would need to be prospectively validated. However, compared to nasal cannula, CPAP can worsen oxygen delivery by not allowing supplied oxygen to blend adequately with the air because of turbulent flow generated by CPAP. As such, caution needs to be exercised when oxygen is added to CPAP and close monitoring is necessary to ensure adequate oxygen delivery during sleep while wearing CPAP. In hypoxemic patients receiving supplemental oxygen, CPAP therapy effectively abolishes the upper airway obstruction during sleep, decreases stress-induced inflammation, and relieves alveolar hypoxia by permitting unrestricted influx of air into the alveoli. CPAP can maintain upper airway patency, relieve intermittent hypoxemia/hypercapnia and microarousal due to obstructive apneas and hypopneas, improve end-expiratory lung volume and make the lungs less prone to alveolar collapse, potentially leading to preservation of lung volumes, better pulmonary function, and improved quality of life [4]. This is of critical importance in LD, given that untreated moderate-to-severe OSA is a modifiable risk factor, which could be significantly improved when treated with CPAP during sleep.

Oxygen Therapy

While a benefit in sleep-related quality was reported following institution of CPAP, it wasn't until 2019 that Troy et al., showed that nocturnal oxygen saturation is associated with poorer prognosis in ILD patients and may contribute towards the pathogenesis of pulmonary vascular disease [15]. Supplemental oxygen reduces the loop gain without altering the other pathophysiological factors that influence OSA. So, if elevated loop gain plays an important role in the development of OSA in ILD populations, treating OSA with oxygen therapy could be an appropriate intervention.

Conclusion

OSA is common in ILD patients, with prevalence estimates ranging from 22% to 90%. Although there is a strong theoretical basis and emerging evidence for adverse pathophysiological impacts of OSA in ILD, the underlying complex interrelationships remain unclear.

The gold standard for the diagnosis of OSA in patients with ILD is level 1 polysomnography. In these patients who underwent polysomnography, the ESS and other tools do not reliably predict severity of sleep-disordered breathing. The optimal tool for OSA screening in patients with IPF has yet to be determined making an evaluation by a sleep physician necessary.

Management of OSA in IPF is very important due to their significant impact in life expectancy and quality of life. OSA and nocturnal hypoxemia may predict worse quality of life and disease outcomes in ILD. CPAP and supplemental oxygen might be therapeutic options, but neither OSA severity nor adherence to CPAP was associated with improved outcomes in ILD patients, except those requiring supplemental oxygen.

References

[1] Myall K J, West A, Kent B D. Sleep, and interstitial lung disease. *Curr. Opin. Pulm. Med.* 2019 Nov;25(6):623–8.

[2] Cardoso A V, Pereira N, Neves I, Santos V, Jesus J M, Melo N, Mota P C, Morais A, Drummond M. Obstructive sleep apnoea in patients with fibrotic diffuse parenchymal lung disease—characterization and treatment compliance assessment. *Can. J. Respir. Ther.* 2018 Jun 28;54(2):35–40.

[3] Khor Y H, Ryerson C J, Landry S A, Howard M E, Churchward T J, Edwards B A, Hamilton GS, Joosten SA. Interstitial lung disease and obstructive sleep apnea. *Sleep. Med. Rev.* 2021 Aug;58:101442.

[4] Margaritopoulos G A, Antoniou KM, Wells AU. Comorbidities in interstitial lung diseases. *Eur. Respir. Rev.* 2017 Mar 31;26(143):160027.

[5] Lee J H, Park C S, Song J W. Obstructive sleep apnea in patients with interstitial lung disease: Prevalence and predictive factors. Adrish M, editor. *PLOS ONE.* 2020 Oct 5;15(10):e0239963.

[6] Pereira N, Cardoso A V, Mota P C, Santos A C, Melo N, Morais A, Drummond M. Predictive factors of obstructive sleep apnoea in patients with fibrotic lung diseases. *Sleep Med.* 2019 Apr;56:123–7.

[7] Schiza S E, Bouloukaki I, Bolaki M, Antoniou K M. Obstructive sleep apnea in pulmonary fibrosis. *Curr. Opin. Pulm. Med.* 2020 Sep;26(5):443–8.

[8] Pillai M, Olson A L, Huie T J, Solomon J J, Fernandez-Perez ER, Brown K K, Hanna P, Lee-Chiong T, Swigris J J. Obstructive sleep apnea does not promote esophageal reflux in fibrosing interstitial lung disease. *Respir. Med.* 2012 Jul;106(7):1033–9.

[9] Canora A, Nicoletta C, Ghinassi G, Bruzzese D, Rea G, Capaccio A, Castaldo S, Coppola A, Polistina G E, Sanduzzi A, Bocchino M. First Description of the Hyperpnea–Hypopnea Periodic Breathing in Patients with Interstitial Lung Disease-Obstructive Sleep Apnea: Treatment Implications in a Real-Life Setting. *Int. J. Environ. Res. Public Health.* 2019 Nov 26;16(23):4712.

[10] Margaritopoulos G A, Kokosi M A, Wells A U. Diagnosing complications and co-morbidities of fibrotic interstitial lung disease. *Expert. Rev. Respir. Med.* 2019 Jul 3;13(7):645–58.

[11] Zhang X L, Dai H P, Zhang H, Gao B, Zhang L, Han T, Wang C. Obstructive Sleep Apnea in Patients with Fibrotic Interstitial Lung Disease and COPD. *J. Clin. Sleep. Med.* 2019 Dec 15;15(12):1807–15.

[12] Cheng Y, Wang Y, Dai L. The prevalence of obstructive sleep apnea in interstitial lung disease: a systematic review and meta-analysis. *Sleep Breath.* 2021 Jan 6 [cited 2021 Aug 16]; Available from: https://link.springer.com/10.1007/s11325-020-02282-z.

[13] Schiza S, Mermigkis C, Margaritopoulos G A, Daniil Z, Harari S, Poletti V, Renzoni EA, Torre O, Visca D, Bouloukaki I, Sourvinos G, Antoniou KM. Idiopathic pulmonary fibrosis, and sleep disorders: no longer strangers in the night. *Eur. Respir. Rev.* 2015 Jun;24(136):327–39.

[14] Adegunsoye A, Neborak J M, Zhu D, Cantrill B, Garcia N, Oldham J M, Noth I, Vij R, Kuzniar T J, Bellam S K, Strek M E, Mokhlesi B. CPAP Adherence, Mortality, and Progression-Free Survival in Interstitial Lung Disease and OSA. *Chest.* 2020 Oct;158(4):1701–12.

[15] Troy L K, Young I H, Lau E M T, Wong K K H, Yee B J, Torzillo P J, Corte T J. Nocturnal hypoxaemia is associated with adverse outcomes in interstitial lung disease. *Respirology.* 2019 Oct;24(10):996–1004.

Chapter 13

COVID-19 Pandemic

Michalis Agrafiotis[1], MD
Athanasios Voulgaris[2], MD
and Paschalis Steiropoulos[2,*], MD, PhD

[1]Department of Respiratory Failure, Aristotle University of Thessaloniki, "Georgios Papanikolaou" General Hospital of Thessaloniki, Thessaloniki, Greece
[2]Department of Pneumonology, Medical School, Democritus University of Thrace, Alexandroupolis, Greece

Abstract

The COVID-19 pandemic is associated with increased morbidity and mortality worldwide and has exerted a significant impact on healthcare systems functionality and medical practice. Although many of the characteristics and comorbidities associated with obstructive sleep apnea (OSA) have been identified as risk factors for severe COVID-19 infection vulnerability (i.e., male gender, obesity, chronic cardiovascular disease, and diabetes), OSA per se has also been linked to adverse outcomes. Diligent management of OSA patients is therefore essential for reducing the risk of transmission and protecting them against potential consequences of COVID-19 infection. Experts concede that during pandemic peaks, sleep studies and positive airway pressure (PAP) titration procedures should be postponed or performed at the home setting. Sleep equipment and PAP devices must be meticulously disinfected and, if possible, the use of disposable items should be preferred. Patients attending sleep clinics should be screened/tested for COVID-19 infection, while healthcare providers must conform to the

---

* Corresponding Author's Email: steiropoulos@yahoo.com.

In: Obstructive Sleep Apnea in Pulmonary Critical Care
Editors: Antonio M. Esquinas and Takatoshi Kasai
ISBN: 979-8-88697-858-2

recommended protective practices. Finally, telemedicine can aid OSA management, while minimizing the risk of transmission.

Keywords: obstructive sleep apnea, sleep-disordered breathing, SARS-COV-2, COVID-19, acute respiratory distress syndrome, sleep study, disinfection

Introduction

In late December 2019, a novel coronavirus strain emerged in Wuhan, Hubei Province, China and quickly spread throughout the world, resulting in a devastating worldwide pandemic [1]. Officially termed "severe acute respiratory distress coronavirus-2" (SARS-CoV-2) on February 12, 2020, this newly discovered pathogen has been established as a novel cause of respiratory tract infections, ranging from mild upper airway symptoms to severe viral pneumonia, although several other systems, including the cardiovascular, nervous and gastrointestinal system are also frequently involved [2, 3]. SARS-CoV-2 is transmitted primarily via airborne droplets and aerosols, however direct contact and fomites are also potential, albeit less significant, sources of dissemination [4]. As of February 3, 2022, the SARS-CoV-2 pandemic (coronavirus disease-19, COVID-19) has claimed 5,680,741 lives worldwide for a total of 380,321,615 confirmed cases [5]. A number of factors including, male gender, obesity, active smoking status, cardiovascular diseases, chronic respiratory and kidney disease, diabetes, and malignancy have been identified as predictors of severe COVID-19 infection and adverse outcome [6–8]. An unprecedented race for effective vaccine development resulted in the emergency authorization of several new vaccines in late 2020, most of them utilizing novel biotechnology strategies, such as the viral vector and the mRNA platform [9]. Although evidence for waning immune response over time and the emergence of new SARS-CoV-2 variants (i.e., Delta and Omicron) have fueled doubts regarding the long-term effectiveness of COVID-19 vaccines, recent data suggest that booster doses of currently available vaccines are still remarkably effective in preventing severe COVID-19 infection [10].

Not surprisingly, the COVID-19 pandemic has imposed a considerable strain on healthcare systems, challenging traditional practices and influencing resource allocation. A systematic review, conducted in the early phases of the pandemic, observed a 32% intensive care unit (ICU)-admission rate for patients with COVID-19 infection with the mortality in those patients reaching 39% [11]. When compared to the wild-type strain, Beta and Delta SARS-CoV-2 variants showed even higher ICU-admission rates and mortalities [12]. Notwithstanding issues pertaining to ICU bed availability and lack of trained personnel, the COVID-19 pandemic has also exerted a negative impact on the management of non-COVID health conditions. A study examining non-COVID admissions in four USA hospitals between March and May 2020 reported a significant decline in admissions for various disease types during the peak COVID-19 period. These diseases included exacerbations of chronic respiratory and cardiovascular diseases, acute medical events, and trauma [13]. Likewise, a UK-based report, assessing data from cancer patients between January 2019 and June 2020, showed a decline in urgent referrals by 40% and in chemotherapy attendances by 71% [14]. Non-COVID related excess deaths, due to deferment of care, contributed to the excess all-cause mortality observed during pandemic peaks and represent the collateral damage associated with the changes in healthcare services configuration and patients' attitudes [15–18]. In fact, 40% of the adult USA patients were reluctant to visit healthcare facilities and seek medical care, because of concerns for exposure to SARS-CoV-2 [19]. Given that several chronic medical conditions also represent risk factors for severe COVID-19 disease, it is not surprising that these patients are more likely to be under-referred and avoid visiting healthcare facilities during surges of COVID-19 pandemic.

Obstructive Sleep Apnea and the COVID-19 Pandemic

Sleep health and its disorders are not spared from the ramifications of the COVID-19 pandemic and its impact on healthcare management policies. Normal, undisturbed sleep is essential for proper mental and physical functioning as it is known that several sleep diseases and disorders have been linked to impaired immune response, poor concentration, and a higher risk for accidents [20]. Fear and uncertainty of the unknown may increase distress levels in the general population and induce or exacerbate mental and sleep disorders [21].

An online survey, questioning participants recruited from the Italian general population during a lockdown period, revealed a high frequency of poor sleep quality, depressive and stress symptoms, while half of the interviewees reported significant somatic and cognitive symptoms related to pre-sleep arousal [22]. Overall, sleep problems are reported to be common during the COVID-19 pandemic, affecting 32% of the general population and 36% of the healthcare personnel, but peaking at 75% in patients with active infection [23]. A more recent meta-analysis showed that 41% of the general population complained of sleep problems during the COVID-19 pandemic, with children, adolescents and COVID-19 patients being the most vulnerable groups [24].

The repercussions of COVID-19 pandemic on the management of patients with sleep-disordered breathing (SDB) are considerable. According to a telephone survey, 38% of OSA patients were concerned about contracting COVID-19 infection and 29% felt that, in the latter case, they would be at a higher risk for complications, because of their underlying OSA [25]. A study that interviewed respiratory patients attending telemedicine appointments during a lockdown period (half of them with probable or previously diagnosed SDB) showed that 70% reported at least one sleep complaint. Confinement at home without working was linked to difficulty falling asleep, early morning waking and frequent awakenings. In addition, patients with probable SDB were more likely to complain of non-restorative sleep, while in those with known SDB, positive airway pressure (PAP) treatment was associated with less likelihood to report any sleep problem [26]. Notably, a large prospective study reported that adherence to continuous positive airway pressure (CPAP) increased in OSA patients during the lockdown period [27].

Interestingly, despite being one of the most common sleep disorders in the general population, obstructive sleep apnea (OSA) was not assessed in early COVID-19 prognostication models [6–8]. Although several risk factors and comorbidities associated with OSA (e.g., male gender, obesity, cardiovascular disease, diabetes) have also been implicated in severe COVID-19 infection, emerging evidence suggests that OSA per se is also linked to worse outcomes. Sleep hypoxemia was associated with a 31% higher rate of hospitalization and mortality in a case-control study that included patients who tested positive for COVID-19 and had previous sleep studies [28]. A recent study, assessing data from the FinnGen database, reported that 38 out of 445 (8.5%) patients with COVID-19 infection had OSA. These patients had a 50% hospitalization rate due to severe COVID-19, while OSA was shown to be an independent risk factor for hospitalization, but not for contracting COVID-19 infection [29]. A multicenter observational study of hospitalized patients with COVID-19 infection reported that, while body mass index (BMI) was the only pre-admission factor independently associated with death or invasive mechanical ventilation within seven days of admission (primary outcome), OSA also predicted a higher risk for death by day 7 (secondary outcome) [30].

By evaluating a database of medical records from ten hospitals in the Chicago metropolitan area, Maas et al. demonstrated that, after adjusting for diabetes, hypertension, and BMI, OSA patients had an 8-fold higher risk for acquiring COVID-19 infection, as well as increased risk for hospitalization and respiratory failure [31]. A prospective observational multicenter study, including hospitalized and home-treated patients with COVID-19 infection, showed that, those at a higher risk for OSA, according to the Berlin Questionnaire, were more likely to manifest clinical worsening and require supplemental oxygen [32]. These conclusions, however, were not supported by other authors. Thus, in a retrospective review of 1,738 patients hospitalized with COVID-19 infection, OSA was not associated with a higher risk for ICU admission, after correcting for age, gender, BMI, and comorbidities [33]. To resolve this controversy, Hariyanto and Kurniawana conducted a meta-analysis of 20 retrospective cohort and one case-control study, including in total 54,276 patients with COVID-19 infection. This analysis showed that presence, as opposed to absence of OSA, is associated with a higher risk for severe COVID-19 disease, ICU admission, requirement for mechanical ventilation and increased mortality [34].

Although the role of OSA as a risk factor for adverse outcome in patients with COVID-19 infection has not yet been unequivocally established, there is strong physiologic rationale to support such a connection. OSA could worsen hypoxemia, which is commonly observed in patients with severe COVID-19 infection [28, 35]. In untreated OSA patients, repetitive episodes of partial or complete interruption of airflow can induce dysregulation of the renin-angiotensin pathway, which is also implicated in the pathogenesis of COVID-19 infection [36]. Sleep deprivation can increase the levels of inflammatory mediators (e.g., IL-1β, IL-6, TNF-α) and augment the cytokine storm, which is responsible for multiorgan failure in patients with COVID-19 infection [35, 37]. Therefore, it is reasonable to assume that effective diagnosis, treatment, and follow-up of OSA patients could offer them an advantage in case they contract COVID-19 infection.

Management of Obstructive Sleep Apnea in the Era of COVID-19 Pandemic

The COVID-19 pandemic has drastically influenced the practice of sleep medicine worldwide. Investigators from the European Sleep Apnea Database

(ESADA), a network of sleep centers from 19 European countries, examined the impact of COVID-19 pandemic on the management of patients with SDB. They reported that, during the pandemic, the proportion of the centers performing in-lab polysomnographies and CPAP titration procedures, decreased from 93% to 20% and from 90% to 18%, respectively. Direct follow-up was also heavily reduced (from 83% to 8%), while distance follow-up (telephone calls, telemonitoring) increased, but only by little. Overall, 80% of OSA management in Europe was shut down as a result of the pandemic [38].

In view of the new circumstances imposed by the COVID-19 pandemic, sleep societies have updated their recommendations regarding the diagnosis and treatment of sleep disorders [39–42]. Most of these recommendations were based on good clinical judgement and expert opinion, considering the limited time available for designing and testing new practice strategies. Preventive measures in sleep labs and outpatient clinics as well as PAP therapy implementation represent the fundamental areas of concern (Table 1) [43].

Table 1. Preventive measures against COVID-19 in sleep medicine

• Postpone diagnostic sleep and PAP titration studies, unless absolutely necessary • Prefer the home setting for diagnostic and PAP titration studies • Use disposable equipment parts • Adhere to the recommended disinfection practices • Screen/test patients for COVID-19 infection • Wear personal protective equipment • Avoid setting-up PAP devices in sleep service facilities • Perform in-lab PAP titrations only in negative pressure rooms • Implement double-limb circuits, filters and non-vented masks and avoid humidification • Advise infected patients to use their PAP device in isolation or, if possible, temporarily discontinue treatment • Apply telemedicine for diagnosis, treatment, and follow-up

Experts agree that, unless considered urgent, sleep studies should be postponed in areas with increased epidemiologic COVID-19 burden. When a sleep study is deemed necessary, type-3 home studies should be favored over in-lab polysomnographies (type-1 studies) [39–42]. The former requires less installation time and fewer sensors, minimizing patient-healthcare provider contact, although in-lab polysomnographies could be the only option for complicated cases, such as neuromuscular disease or chronic heart failure [44]. Some sleep centers have opted to deliver sleep equipment by mail accompanied and written set-up instructions; however, older patients are often unable to comprehend the instructions and require assistance for using the equipment. In any case, sleep equipment should be managed within sealed plastic bags and the users should be instructed to wash their hands before and after setting it up [44].

Additional preventive strategies should also be considered in the setting of sleep service facilities. Patients should have their body temperature measured upon arrival and be questioned about symptoms compatible with COVID-19 infection. Testing for COVID-19 infection should ideally be performed within a reasonable timeframe before the study. Physical distancing, hand hygiene and face masks are minimum protective measures for both healthcare providers and patients [43]. In high-risk situations, healthcare providers should wear a full set of personal protective equipment (PPE) including gloves, gowns, face masks, respirators (N95) and face shields [39–42].

Although in the aftermath of the first stage of the pandemic manufacturers updated their recommendations for sleep equipment disinfection procedures, disposable parts should be preferred, when possible. Non-disposable parts can be reused, but strict adherence to the protocol-guided disinfection procedures is recommended [39–42]. Given the susceptibility of SARS-CoV-2 to ultraviolet (UV) radiation, the use of UV boxes is an alternative, cost-effective and expeditious method of sanitization [45]. Implementing a 72-hour equipment quarantine after use is an additional precaution, although this option may not be feasible in centers with high demand for sleep studies [46].

Serious concerns have also been expressed about the transmissibility of the SARS-CoV-2 virus because of PAP therapy [47]. When in-lab PAP titration is required, it should be conducted in an isolation room under negative pressure. Home titration, using auto-PAP devices, is the recommended method for avoiding potential dispersion within healthcare facilities, while meeting the patients' immediate needs [39–42]. In the latter case, it is preferable to prescribe a PAP device as soon as diagnosis is made rather than using one of the sleep center's devices. Use instructions can be provided to the patient via teleconsultation or during short visits to the sleep center but setting up the PAP device at the sleep center should be avoided, unless necessary. The selection of the appropriate interface is a challenging task and can be based on the healthcare provider's experience and facilitated by the use of fitting templates [44].

If PAP-treated patients contract COVID-19 infection, they should be advised to use their device in isolation from the rest of the household members. Additional preventive measures include the implementation of double-limb circuits, filters, and non-vented masks, while humidification is discouraged. Alternatively, if the potential benefit from avoiding transmission outweighs the risk due to therapy interruption, PAP treatment could be temporarily discontinued [39–42].

Telemedicine has emerged as an important strategy for the management of OSA under the complicated circumstances imposed on sleep medicine practice by the COVID-19 pandemic [48, 49]. Telemedicine can reduce long waiting lists due to the time-consuming procedures of infection control and prevention, minimize clinic visits and facilitate patient follow-up. Thus, synchronous tele-visits can be initially implemented to obtain medical and demographic data and assess OSA risk, while standardized questionnaires can be downloaded from the sleep center's website and self-answered by the patient. Relevant medical documents can be uploaded or sent to the sleep center by email [49]. Raw data from home sleep studies can be transmitted via the web to the sleep center [50]. PAP devices can also be adjusted remotely, and the patient can be contacted by telephone or email and questioned about persistent or emerging symptoms as well as response to therapy and its adjustments. Follow-up can be aided by remote PAP monitoring which allows us to detect several therapy-related problems, including treatment compliance, leaks, and residual respiratory events [51]. However, in-lab assessment might be necessary for more complex cases (e.g., heart failure, obesity hypoventilation syndrome, neuromuscular disease) [44].

Compelling evidence suggests that OSA is an additional risk factor for severe COVID-19 infection. Therefore, early diagnosis, treatment and uninterrupted OSA management are essential protective measures for OSA patients. However, OSA management in the era of the COVID-19 pandemic is not without risks. To minimize the risk of dissemination, sleep studies and PAP titration should be postponed or, preferably, performed at home. Standard personnel protective strategies and diligent equipment sanitization should be meticulously implemented to minimize transmission risk. In addition, telemedicine practices can facilitate patient assessment, treatment, and follow-up.

Conclusion

Strong evidence indicates that OSA is a risk factor for adverse outcome in patients with COVID-19 infection. Patients referred to sleep labs for evaluation should be screened/tested for COVID-19 infection. Sleep lab personnel must conform to the recommended protective practices, including physical distancing, hand washing and use of PPE. Sleep studies and PAP titration procedures should be preferably performed at home in periods with increased epidemiologic burden. PAP implementation increases aerosol generation and should be avoided within healthcare facilities or configured in a manner to minimize dispersion. Sleep equipment must be carefully sanitized before reuse. Disposable parts should be favored, if available. Telemedicine is an alternative option for managing patients with OSA without increasing transmission risk.

References

[1] Zhu N, Zhang D, Wang W, Li X, Yang B, Song J, Zhao X., Huang B, Shi W, Lu R, Niu P, Zhan F, Ma X, Wang D, Xu W, Wu G, Gao GF, & Tan, W. A Novel Coronavirus from Patients with Pneumonia in China, 2019. *N Engl J Med* 2020; 382:727–33.

[2] Gandhi RT, Lynch JB, Del Rio C. Mild or Moderate Covid-19. *N Engl J Med* 2020;383:1757–66.

[3] Berlin DA, Gulick RM, Martinez FJ. Severe Covid-19. *N Engl J Med* 2020;383:2451–60.

[4] Meyerowitz EA, Richterman A, Gandhi RT, Sax PE. Transmission of SARS-CoV-2: A Review of Viral, Host, and Environmental Factors. *Ann Intern Med* 2021;174:69–79.

[5] WHO Coronavirus (COVID-19) Dashboard. https://covid19.who.int (accessed 3 Feb2022).

[6] Izcovich A, Ragusa MA, Tortosa F, Lavena Marzio MA, Agnoletti C, Bengolea A, Ceirano A, Espinosa F, Saavedra E, Sanguine V, Tassara A, Cid C, Catalano HN, Agarwal A, Foroutan F, Rada G. Prognostic factors for severity and mortality in patients infected with COVID-19: A systematic review. *PLoS One* 2020;15:e0241955.

[7] Yang J, Zheng Y, Gou X, Pu K, Chen Z, Guo Q, Ke Pu, Chen Z, Guo Q, Ji R, Wang H, Wang Y, Zhou Y. Prevalence of comorbidities and its effects in patients infected with SARS-CoV-2: a systematic review and meta-analysis. *Int J Infect Dis* 2020; 94:91–5.

[8] Hoong CWS, Hussain I, Aravamudan VM, Phyu EE, Lin JHX, Koh H. Obesity is Associated with Poor Covid-19 Outcomes: A Systematic Review and Meta-Analysis. *Horm Metab Res* 2021;53:85–93.

[9] Hadj Hassine I. Covid-19 vaccines and variants of concern: A review. *Rev Med Virol* 2021;e2313.

[10] Thompson MG, Natarajan K, Irving SA, Rowley EA, Griggs EP, Gaglani M, Nicola P Klein, Shaun J Grannis, Malini B DeSilva, Edward Stenehjem, Sarah E Reese, Monica Dickerson, Allison L Naleway, Jungmi Han, Deepika Konatham, Charlene McEvoy, Suchitra Rao, Brian E Dixon, Kristin Dascomb, Ned Lewis, Matthew E Levy, Palak Patel, I-Chia Liao, Anupam B Kharbanda, Michelle A Barron, William F Fadel, Nancy Grisel, Kristin Goddard, Duck-Hye Yang, Mehiret H Wondimu, Kempapura Murthy, Nimish R Valvi, Julie Arndorfer, Bruce Fireman, Margaret M Dunne, Peter Embi, Eduardo Azziz-Baumgartner, Ousseny Zerbo, Catherine H Bozio, Sue Reynolds, Jill Ferdinands, Jeremiah Williams, Ruth Link-Gelles, Stephanie J Schrag, Jennifer R Verani, Sarah Ball, Toan C Ong. Effectiveness of a Third Dose of mRNA Vaccines Against COVID-19–Associated Emergency Department and Urgent Care Encounters and Hospitalizations Among Adults During Periods of Delta and Omicron Variant Predominance — VISION Network, 10 States, August 2021–January 2022. *MMWR Morb Mortal Wkly Rep* 2022; 71:139–45.

[11] Abate SM, Ahmed Ali S, Mantfardo B, Basu B. Rate of Intensive Care Unit admission and outcomes among patients with coronavirus: A systematic review and Meta-analysis. *PLoS ONE* 2020;15: e0235653.

[12] Lin L, Liu Y, Tang X, He D. The Disease Severity and Clinical Outcomes of the SARS-CoV-2 Variants of Concern. *Front Public Health* 2021; 9:775224.

[13] Blecker S, Jones SA, Petrilli CM, Admon AJ, Weerahandi H, Francois F, Horwitz LI. Hospitalizations for Chronic Disease and Acute Conditions in the Time of COVID-19. *JAMA Intern Med* 2021; 181:269.

[14] Lai AG, Pasea L, Banerjee A, Hall G, Denaxas S, Chang WH, Katsoulis M, Williams B, Pillay D, Noursadeghi M, Linch D, Hughes D, Forster MD, Turnbull C, Fitzpatrick NK, Boyd K, Foster GR, Enver T, Nafilyan V, Humberstone B, Neal RD, Cooper M, Jones M, Pritchard-Jones K, Sullivan R, Davie C, Lawler M, Hemingway H. Estimated impact of the COVID-19 pandemic on cancer services and excess 1-year mortality in people with cancer and multimorbidity: near real-time data on cancer care, cancer deaths and a population-based cohort study. *BMJ Open* 2020;10: e043828.

[15] Kontopantelis E, Mamas MA, Deanfield J, Asaria M, Doran T. Excess mortality in England and Wales during the first wave of the COVID-19 pandemic. *J Epidemiol Community Health* 2021; 75:213–23.

[16] Strongman H, Carreira H, De Stavola BL, Bhaskaran K, Leon DA. Factors associated with excess all-cause mortality in the first wave of the COVID-19 pandemic in the UK: A time series analysis using the Clinical Practice Research Datalink. *PLoS Med* 2022;19: e1003870.

[17] Tiotiu A, Chong Neto H, Bikov A, Kowal K, Steiropoulos P, Labor M, Cherrez-Ojeda I, Badellino H, Emelyanov A, Garcia R, Guidos G. Impact of the COVID-19

pandemic on the management of chronic noninfectious respiratory diseases. *Expert Rev Respir Med* 2021; 15:1035–48.

[18] Kyriakopoulos C, Gogali A, Exarchos K, Potonos D, Tatsis K, Apollonatou V, Loukides S, Papiris S, Sigala I, Katsaounou P, Aggelidis M, Fouka E, Porpodis K, Kontakiotis T, Sampsonas F, Karampitsakos T, Tzouvelekis A, Bibaki E, Karagiannis K, Kostikas, K. Reduction in Hospitalizations for Respiratory Diseases during the First COVID-19 Wave in Greece. *Respiration* 2021; 100:588–93.

[19] Wong L, Hawkins J, Langness S, Murrell K, Iris P, Sammann A. Where Are All the Patients? Addressing Covid-19 Fear to Encourage Sick Patients to Seek Emergency Care. *NEJM Catalyst Innovations in Care Delivery* Published Online First: 14 May 2020. https://catalyst.nejm.org/doi/full/10.1056/CAT.20.0193 (accessed 4 Feb 2022).

[20] Medic G, Wille M, Hemels ME. Short- and long-term health consequences of sleep disruption. *Nat Sci Sleep* 2017; 9:151–61.

[21] Shigemura J, Ursano RJ, Morganstein JC, Kurosawa M, Benedek DM. Public responses to the novel 2019 coronavirus (2019-nCoV) in Japan: Mental health consequences and target populations. *Psychiatry Clin Neurosci* 2020; 74:281–2.

[22] Gorgoni M, Scarpelli S, Mangiaruga A, Alfonsi V, Bonsignore MR, Fanfulla F, Ferini-Strambi L, Nobili L, Plazzi G, De Gennaro L, Arnaldi D, Bonanni E, Bonetti GA, Castronovo C, Maestri M, Garbarino S, Guarnieri B, Manni R, Palagini L, Vicini C. Pre-sleep arousal and sleep quality during the COVID-19 lockdown in Italy. *Sleep Med* 2021; 88:46–57.

[23] Jahrami HA, Alhaj OA, Humood AM, Alenezi AF, Fekih-Romdhane F, AlRasheed MM, Saif ZQ, Bragazzi NL, Pandi-Perumal SR, BaHammam AS, & Vitiello MV. Sleep disturbances during the COVID-19 pandemic: A systematic review, meta-analysis, and meta-regression. *Sleep Med Rev* 2022; 62:101591.

[24] Jahrami H, BaHammam AS, Bragazzi NL, Saif Z, Faris M, Vitiello MV. Sleep problems during the COVID-19 pandemic by population: a systematic review and meta-analysis. *J Clin Sleep Med* 2021; 17:299–313.

[25] Thorpy M, Figuera-Losada M, Ahmed I, Monderer R, Petrisko M, Martin C, Akhtar J, Thorpy J, & Haines C. Management of sleep apnea in New York City during the COVID-19 pandemic. *Sleep Med* 2020; 74:86–90.

[26] Pinto J, van Zeller M, Amorim P, Pimentel A, Dantas P, Eusébio E, Neves A, Pipa J, Santa Clara E, Santiago T, Viana P, & Drummond M. Sleep quality in times of Covid-19 pandemic. *Sleep Med* 2020; 74:81–5.

[27] Attias D, Pepin JL, Pathak A. Impact of COVID-19 lockdown on adherence to continuous positive airway pressure by obstructive sleep apnoea patients. *Eur Respir J* 2020; 56:2001607.

[28] Pena Orbea C, Wang L, Shah V, Jehi L, Milinovich A, Foldvary-Schaefer N, Chung MK, Mashaqi S, Aboussouan L, Seidel K, & Mehra R. Association of Sleep-Related Hypoxia with Risk of COVID-19 Hospitalizations and Mortality in a Large Integrated Health System. *JAMA Netw Open* 2021;4:e2134241.

[29] Strausz S, Kiiskinen T, Broberg M, Ruotsalainen S, Koskela J, Bachour A, FinnGen Palotie A, Palotie T, Ripatti S, & Ollila HM. Sleep apnoea is a risk factor for severe COVID-19. *BMJ Open Respir Res* 2021;8:e000845.

[30] Cariou B, Hadjadj S, Wargny M, Pichelin M, Al-Salameh A, Allix I, for the CORONADO investigators.. Phenotypic characteristics, and prognosis of inpatients with COVID-19 and diabetes: the CORONADO study. *Diabetologia* 2020; 63:1500–15.

[31] Maas MB, Kim M, Malkani RG, Abbott SM, Zee PC. Obstructive Sleep Apnea and Risk of COVID-19 Infection, Hospitalization and Respiratory Failure. *Sleep Breath* 2021; 25:1155–7.

[32] Peker Y, Celik Y, Arbatli S, Isik SR, Balcan B, Karataş F, Fatma Işıl Uzel, OSACOVID-19 Study Collaborators. Effect of High-Risk Obstructive Sleep Apnea on Clinical Outcomes in Adults with Coronavirus Disease 2019: A Multicenter, Prospective, Observational Clinical Trial. *Ann Am Thorac Soc* 2021; 18:1548–59.

[33] Mashaqi S, Lee-Iannotti J, Rangan P, Celaya MP, Gozal D, Quan SF, Parthasarathy S. Obstructive sleep apnea and COVID-19 clinical outcomes during hospitalization: a cohort study. *J Clin Sleep Med* 2021; 17:2197–204.

[34] Haryanto TI, Kurniawan A. Obstructive sleep apnea (OSA) and outcomes from coronavirus disease 2019 (COVID-19) pneumonia: a systematic review and meta-analysis. *Sleep Med* 2021;82:47–53.

[35] McSharry D, Malhotra A. Potential influences of obstructive sleep apnea and obesity on COVID-19 severity. *J Clin Sleep Med* 2020; 16:1645.

[36] Ekiz T, İnönü Köseoğlu H, Pazarlı AC. Obstructive sleep apnea, renin-angiotensin system, and COVID-19: interactions. *J Clin Sleep Med* 2020; 16:1403–4.

[37] Leisman DE, Deutschman CS, Legrand M. Facing COVID-19 in the ICU: vascular dysfunction, thrombosis, and dysregulated inflammation. *Intensive Care Med* 2020; 46:1105–8.

[38] Grote L, McNicholas WT, Hedner J, ESADA collaborators. Sleep apnoea management in Europe during the COVID-19 pandemic: data from the European Sleep Apnoea Database (ESADA). *Eur Respir J* 2020; 55:2001323.

[39] Zhang XL, Xiao Y. Sleep health service in China during the coronavirus disease outbreak. *J Clin Sleep Med* 2020; 16:1221–2.

[40] Summary of CDC recommendations during COVID-19 | Sleep Medicine. American Academy of Sleep Medicine – Association for Sleep Clinicians and Researchers. https://aasm.org/covid-19-resources/covid-19-mitigation-strategies-sleep-clinics-labs/ (accessed 12 Feb2022).

[41] ARTP Guidance - Respiratory Function Testing and Sleep Services During Endemic COVID-19. https://www.artp.org.uk/News/artp-guidance-respiratory-function-testing-and-sleep-services-during-endemic-covid-19 (accessed 12 Feb2022).

[42] COVID-19 resources for respiratory and sleep clinicians. https://www.sleep.org.au/Public/Public/Resource-Centre/COVID.aspx (accessed 12 Feb 2022).

[43] Voulgaris A, Ferini-Strambi L, Steiropoulos P. Sleep medicine and COVID-19. Has a new era begun? *Sleep Med* 2020; 73:170–6.

[44] Spicuzza L, Sanna A. Continuum of care for patients with obstructive sleep apnea after one year from the COVID-19 pandemic onset: no time for further delays: practical issues for a safe and effective management. *Sleep Med* 2021; 84:98–106.

[45] Heßling M, Hönes K, Vatter P, Lingenfelder C. Ultraviolet irradiation doses for coronavirus inactivation - review and analysis of coronavirus photoinactivation studies. *GMS Hyg Infect Control* 2020;15:Doc08.

[46] van Doremalen N, Bushmaker T, Morris DH, Holbrook MG, Gamble A, Williamson BN, Tamin A, Harcourt JL, Thornburg NJ, Gerber SI, Lloyd-Smith JO, de Wit E, & Munster VJ. Aerosol and Surface Stability of SARS-CoV-2 as Compared with SARS-CoV-1. *N Engl J Med* 2020; 382:1564–7.

[47] Wilson NM, Norton A, Young FP, Collins DW. Airborne transmission of severe acute respiratory syndrome coronavirus-2 to healthcare workers: a narrative review. *Anaesthesia* 2020; 75:1086–95.

[48] Shamim-Uzzaman QA, Bae CJ, Ehsan Z, Setty AR, Devine M, Dhankikar S, Donskoy I, Fields B, Hearn H, Hwang D, Jain V, Kelley D, Kirsch DB, Martin W, Troester M, Trotti LM, Won CH, Epstein LJ. The use of telemedicine for the diagnosis and treatment of sleep disorders: an American Academy of Sleep Medicine update. *J Clin Sleep Med* 2021; 17:1103–7.

[49] Voulgaris A, Ferini-Strambi L, Economou NT, Nena E, Steiropoulos P. Sleep Telemedicine Practices: Checkpoint List and Practical Considerations in the COVID-19 Era. *Front Neurol* 2021; 12:664274.

[50] Borsini E, Blanco M, Bosio M, Fernando DT, Ernst G, Salvado A. 'Diagnosis of sleep apnea in network' respiratory polygraphy as a decentralization strategy. *Sleep Sci* 2016; 9:244–8.

[51] Schutte-Rodin S. Telehealth, Telemedicine, and Obstructive Sleep Apnea. *Sleep Med Clin* 2020; 15:359–75.

Chapter 14

Weaning Mechanical Ventilation

Vijay Hadda*, MD
and Rahul Tyagi†, MD
Pulmonary, Critical Care, and Sleep Medicine,
All India Institute of Medical Sciences, New Delhi, India

Abstract

Obstructive sleep apnea (OSA), a frequently undiagnosed disease, is common among patients admitted to ICU with respiratory failure and requiring mechanical ventilation. Patients with OSA present a unique set of problems due to changes in respiratory mechanics. Sleep disordered breathing (SDB) may play a significant role while weaning these patients from mechanical ventilation; OSA can manifest as recurrent hypoxia and hypoventilation causing failure of weaning and prolonged mechanical ventilation. Use of sedatives and neuromuscular blockade may further complicate weaning process due to aggravation of OSA. Hence, it is important to have a high risk of suspicion of OSA, especially in patients who are facing difficulty in weaning. The general principle of weaning of these patients remains same with certain modifications to accommodate the physiological changes due to OSA. Daily assessment for readiness to wean, spontaneous breathing trial (SBT) when deemed fit to wean, and extubation on successful SBT followed by extubation to NIV may be the best strategy.

Keywords: obstructive sleep apnea, OSA, mechanical ventilation, extubation

---

* FCCP (USA), FISCCM, International Fellow of NIV, Additional Professor, Corresponding Author's Email: vijayhadda@yahoo.com.

† Senior Resident.

In: Obstructive Sleep Apnea in Pulmonary Critical Care
Editors: Antonio M. Esquinas and Takatoshi Kasai
ISBN: 979-8-88697-858-2

Introduction

Obstructive sleep apnea (OSA), a disorder characterized by repetitive episodes of nocturnal cessation of breathing and collapse of airways, is a common and frequently undiagnosed and untreated disease [1]. It has been estimated that there are 1 billion people suffering from OSA globally [1]. These estimates are based on observations focused only on the adults between 30 to 69 years of age; hence, the overall burden is likely to be more. Over last few years, OSA is being increasingly recognized as a contributor to poor health outcomes. There are good studies describing the health effects of OSA. Notably, many of OSA (diagnosed or undiagnosed) patients are admitted in intensive care unit (ICU) with respiratory failure requiring mechanical ventilation. OSA patients also have high incidence of coexisting co-morbidities such as obesity, diabetes mellitus, hypertension, heart failure, ischemic heart disease and cerebrovascular diseases [2]. Due to the presence of certain abnormalities in the upper airway, lung mechanics and associated comorbidities, OSA is expected to have significant effect on clinical outcomes, especially weaning, among these patients. In this chapter, we will discuss the extent of problem and relevant pathophysiology of OSA and weaning protocol for these high-risk patients.

Pathophysiology

OSA is characterized by intermittent upper airway obstruction during sleep usually involving retropalatal, retroglossal and hypopharyngeal areas [2]. The upper airway narrowing, snoring and reduced airflow in OSA occur due to the reduced action of upper airway dilator muscles in a sleep-stage dependent manner [2]. Ventilatory inadequacies and consequent intermittent hypoxemia lead to transient arousals and sleep state fragmentation throughout the night and cause over compensatory response of the autonomic nervous system. Systemic effects of OSA are well known and include – cardiovascular (hypertension, stroke, coronary artery disease and arrhythmia), impairment of glucose metabolism and neurocognitive effects [2].

Obesity is a risk factor for OSA and obesity hypoventilation syndrome (OHS). Among the fat distribution patterns, central obesity which is characterized by increased deposition of fat in the chest, abdomen, and visceral organs has more effects on pulmonary mechanics [3]. In obesity, fat deposits in mediastinum and abdominal organs result in reduced compliance of the chest wall, the lungs, and entire respiratory system and reduced outward movement of chest wall and downward movement of diaphragm. These changes cause a reduction in Functional Residual Capacity (FRC) and Expiratory Reserve Volume (ERV), and an increase in respiratory system resistance.

There is a subset of patients who have Chronic Obstructive Pulmonary Disease (COPD) and OSA both, an entity known as "overlap syndrome." These patients are estimated to be between 0.5 to 1% of general population above 40 years of age [4] and face a unique problem of having inspiratory flow limitation due to OSA and expiratory flow limitation due to COPD.

Burden of OSA in ICU

Studies demonstrated that OSA is common among patients admitted to ICU with respiratory failure and requiring mechanical ventilation [5-8]. As reported by Diaz et al., among patients requiring prolonged mechanical ventilation for more than 21 days, 94.7% had OSA proven by polysomnography [8]. It is pertinent to note that majority of patients in this study were obese with a mean BMI of 44 kg/m^2. This clearly indicates the high incidence of prolonged ventilation in patients admitted in ICUs and have underlying OSA. Patients with obesity and OSA present a unique set of airway management related complications as compared to general population [9-10]. Sleep disordered breathing (SDB) may play a significant role while weaning patients from mechanical ventilation as it can cause recurrent hypoxia and hypoventilation causing failure of weaning and prolonged mechanical ventilation [10].

There can be a myriad of indications for which an OSA patient may require mechanical ventilation. The need for mechanical ventilation may solely be related to an acute event like acute respiratory distress syndrome (ARDS), exacerbation of a chronic respiratory illness (COPD, asthma, interstitial lung disease) or an acute illness complicating an underlying undiagnosed OSA. Considering the high prevalence in general population and relatively slow progression of symptoms, OSA remains undiagnosed in vast majority. Various features such as obesity, snoring, observed apneas, non-refreshing sleep, excessive day time sleepiness point toward an underlying sleep disorder, however, these symptoms get less attention during evaluation in the ICU. Various scores like Epworth's Sleepiness Score (ESS) and STOP BANG (**S**noring, **T**iredness, **O**bserved apnea, high Blood **P**ressure, **B**MI, **A**ge, **N**eck circumference, and male **G**ender) score may prove pivotal in screening for the presence of a sleep breathing disorder (Table 1). A polysomnography, the "gold standard" for the diagnosis of OSA, may not be feasible in ICU settings. However, with a careful history, it is not difficult to make a clinical diagnosis of OSA with reasonable certainty.

Table 1. Factors used to assess likelihood of OSA in Critically Ill patient

1.	History (from relative): Snoring, witnessed apneas, recent weight gain, morning headaches, excessive day time sleepiness
2.	Obesity, Neck circumference > 40 cm
3.	STOP BANG > 3 (More than 90% sensitivity and specificity to diagnose moderate to severe OSA).

Weaning from Invasive Mechanical Ventilation

Weaning from mechanical ventilation is defined as a process of reducing the ventilator support of the patient with an aim to achieve spontaneous breathing and extubation [11]. It is recommended that all patients on mechanical ventilation need to be assessed daily for the readiness to undergo weaning [11]. Despite following the best protocol, the weaning process itself may take almost 40 to 50% of total duration of mechanical ventilation [11]. Prolonged mechanical ventilation increases the cost, the risk of developing Ventilator Associated Pneumonia (VAP), and airway trauma [11]. Hence, early weaning is essential to avoid adverse outcomes and reduce the cost of care. On the other hand, premature extubation culminating into the weaning failure and reintubation is associated with prolonged ICU stay, increased duration of hospitalization and increased mortality [9]. A protocolized approach for extubation can minimize both, the unnecessary prolonged intubation as well as the risk of weaning failure and re-intubation.

General Weaning Protocol

The most crucial factor which determines the time spent on mechanical ventilation is the physician's decision that discontinuation of ventilator support is feasible. There are certain features which can be used to assess the feasibility of weaning (Table 2).

The liberation from mechanical ventilation is a 3-step process: assessment of readiness for spontaneous breathing trial (SBT), spontaneous breathing trial (SBT), and extubation.

Table 2. Criteria used to assess the feasibility of discontinuation of ventilator support

1.	Condition which led to requirement of ventilation has reversed
2.	PaO2/FiO2 ratio > 150 on PEEP < 8 cm of H_2O; pH> 7.25
3.	No or minimal requirement of vasopressor
4.	Patient should be breathing spontaneously.

Step 1. Assessment of Readiness for SBT

The process of weaning starts when the physician, considering the overall condition of the patient, feels that weaning may be possible [11]. There are few important questions to be answered in patients being considered for weaning [2]:

1. Has the underlying condition for which patient required ventilation improved?
2. Is the general condition of patient optimal for weaning?
3. Is there a likelihood of any airway related issues?
4. Is patient breathing adequately?

Has the Underlying Condition for which Patient Required Ventilation Improved?

The most important question that needs answer before weaning is – has the underlying condition for which patient required ventilation improved? First, the cause of worsening needs to be identified. The common causes of admission to ICU and requirement of ventilation in patients with OSA could be hypercapnic/hypoxemic respiratory failure, congestive heart failure, stroke, arrhythmia, pulmonary embolism, or infection [12]. Hypercapnic respiratory failure, in a patient with OSA, may occur due to poor compliance to the prescribed CPAP therapy or exacerbation of co-existing COPD. Pneumonia in patients with OSA may lead to hypoxemic respiratory failure. Association of OSA with cardiovascular complications including heart failure, arrhythmias, myocardial infarction, and stroke is well described [13].

It is essential that the underlying condition that precipitated intubation and mechanical ventilation has improved before weaning is considered. The documentation of improvement may require clinical (ventilator parameters, vitals, sensorium, cough reflex), radiological, and laboratory assessment (clinical chemistry and blood gases). Also, a reasonable Glasgow Coma Score, at least to a level where patient will be able to manage his secretions, is must before considering these patients for weaning.

Is the General Condition of Patient Optimal for Weaning?

The several factors which need to be looked at before consideration for weaning include [11]:

1. *Respiratory drive*: To ensure optimal respiratory drive, sedatives and hypnotics need to be stopped. Metabolic/respiratory alkalosis/acidosis, due to any cause need to be corrected.
2. *Neuromuscular weakness*: Correctable causes of neuromuscular weakness like electrolyte abnormalities, thyroid disorders, Guillain-Barré syndrome need to be addressed.
3. *Respiratory mechanics*: Respiratory mechanics need to be optimized with use of bronchodilators, pleural effusion/pneumothorax drainage. The underlying cause of respiratory failure and intubation needs to be addressed for improving the respiratory mechanics.

Is There a Likelihood of Any Airway Related Issues?

Airway related issues may prove as an impediment in weaning a patient from mechanical ventilation. Following airway related factors need consideration while assessing fitness to wean [11].

1. Will the patient be able to maintain his airway after extubation? An appropriate consciousness level along with good upper airway reflexes (adequate cough reflex and minimal secretions) are essential to ensure that patient will not fail extubation.

2. Post extubation laryngeal edema may occur in up to 16% of patients requiring endotracheal tracheal intubation and mechanical ventilation [14]. Due to the presence of supra-glottic edema, patients with OSA are at increased risk of post extubation stridor. In presence of endotracheal (ET) tube, direct visualization of upper airway is difficult; and indirect methods such as cough leak test need to be applied. For cough leak test, ET tube cuff is deflated and the amount of air leak around the cuff is assessed. A cuff leak volume of 130 ml and 12% of inspiratory Tidal Volume (V_T) has a sensitivity and specificity of 85% and 95%, respectively, for identification of patients at risk of post extubation stridor.

Is Patient Breathing Adequately?

Patient must have spontaneous breathing effort before considering him/her for weaning. A spontaneous breathing trial (SBT) is the usual method employed to assess weather patients will be able to sustain breathing on their own once the ventilator is removed. The common methods used for SBT include – a T-piece trial, Continuous Positive Airway Pressure (CPAP), or Pressure Support Ventilation (PSV) [11]. The duration of SBT can vary from 30 min to 120 min.

Step 2. Spontaneous Breathing Trial

Patients fulfilling readiness criteria are subjected to SBT. Different methods have been used by clinicians over the years for SBT, before liberating patients from mechanical ventilation. Brochard et al., [15] compared T-piece, Synchronized Intermittent Mandatory Ventilation (SIMV), and PSV and demonstrated that PSV was better than SIMV or T piece in patients for weaning. Currently, PSV is preferred method of SBT. In patients with OSA also, weaning with PSV may help in improving the respiratory mechanics during period of extubation as it will reduce the respiratory muscle load. During the SBT, patient should be monitored for signs of SBT failure (Table 3). Those who show no sign of SBT failure are considered for extubation; whereas the SBT is terminated for those who developed signs of failure. The patients who failed SBT are switched back to assisted mode with same settings of ventilator which patient was being managed prior to SBT and will be assessed daily for fitness for SBT.

Table 3. Features suggesting SBT failure

1. Clinical criterion: a. Agitation/depressed mental status b. Diaphoresis c. Cyanosis d. Use of accessory muscle of respiration or worsening dyspnea e. RR > 35/min or rise in RR of more than 50% f. HR > 140 or rise of more than 20%.
2. ABG Criterion: a. Fall in Spo2 < 90% or PaO2 < 60 mm Hg on FiO2 of 0.5 b. PaCO2 > 50 mm Hg or rise of more than 8 mm Hg c. pH < 7.32.

Table 4. Features of extubation failure

Signs of respiratory failure • Respiratory rate - >30 breaths/min or <12 breaths/min • Diaphoresis • Use of accessory muscle • Drowsiness
Hypoxemia • Oxygen saturation – less than 90% • PaO2 – less than 64 mmHg • PaO2/FiO2 – 130 or less on a flow of >6 L/min or an FiO2 50% or more
Respiratory acidosis • PaCO2 – Increase of 10% or more • pH – less than 7.35

Step 3. Extubation and Post-Extubation

Those patients who successfully passed SBT are eligible for extubation. However, before extubation, the sensorium and cough reflex must be assessed once again. Patients with acceptable sensorium and cough reflex are extubated and monitored closely. All patients will require oxygen supplementation following extubation. Lately, the use of NIV/CPAP and high-flow oxygen using high-flow nasal cannula (HFNC) immediately after extubation has increased, especially in high risk group (age >65 yrs. with chronic cardiac or pulmonary diseases, hypercapnic respiratory, heart failure, APACHE > 14, prolong intubation, re-intubation etc.). Hence, the protocol has been modified little bit with the use of CPAP/NIV/HFNC for initial 6-24 hrs. following extubation. A close monitoring of patients is required to identify the extubation failure at the earliest (Table 4).

Specific Issues Related to OSA

One of the most important risk factors for OSA is obesity. Almost 40% of obese individuals have OSA and more than 70% of patients with OSA are obese [16]. Obesity complicates respiratory mechanics even without presence of a critical illness [13]. The effects of obesity on ventilator mechanics include ventilatory restriction (due to increased intra-abdominal pressure), and reduced compliance of the chest wall and respiratory system. Association of obesity with obstructive ventilatory pattern is also known [17].

Principal factors which will need consideration while weaning a patient with OSA include [17]:

1. Obstructive sleep apnea might get aggravated due to the effects of narcotic and analgesic drugs used for sedation during mechanical ventilation.
2. Due to co-existence of obesity among patients with OSA, there is an increased intra-abdominal pressure which is risk factor for atelectasis of the dependent regions of the lungs.
3. Obese patients are at greater risk of infections such as catheter related infection, blood stream infection and pneumonia.
4. There may be coexisting Obesity Hypoventilation Syndrome (OHS) and daytime hypercapnia, especially in morbidly obese patients.

How to Wean Critically Ill Patients with Suspected OSA

The general principle of weaning in a patient with OSA remains same with certain modifications to accommodate the physiological differences due to OSA. As soon as the treating physician feels that the underlying condition of patient, which caused the need for intubation is improving the patient must be assessed for fitness to wean on daily basis. Broad criteria used to assess the feasibility of discontinuation of ventilator support are summarized in Table 2 [18].

Avoidance of excessive use of sedation/analgesia may be an important intervention among patients with OSA that can facilitate early weaning. However, many a times, OSA is diagnosed after sedation being administered during or after surgery [19]. The use of sedatives worsens already existing the upper airway muscle dysfunction in these patients and results in worsening of respiratory failure. Awake drive will help patients maintain the upper airway patency and prevents apneas and hypopneas.

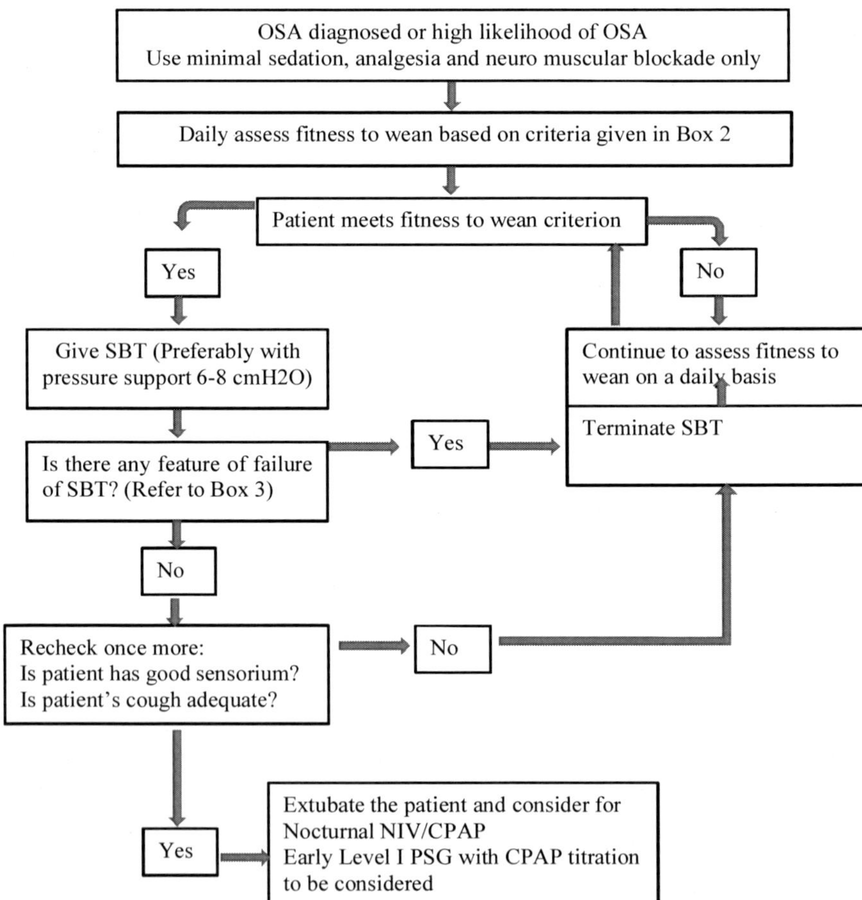

Figure 1. Protocol for weaning among patients with OSA.

Once patient is deemed fit for weaning, SBT should be given, preferably, using pressure-support for a duration of 30-120 min. During this time patients should be closely monitored for various features suggestive of failure of SBT (Table 3) [20]. If none of those criteria are met, the patients are considered for extubation. In patients with suspected OSA, it is desirable to extubate them to NIV/CPAP and continue nocturnal NIV/CPAP for first 6-24 hrs. Once the patient is stable, an in-lab monitored polysomnography and CPAP titration should be conducted. Figure 1 summarizes the protocol for weaning among patients with OSA.

Conclusion

OSA is a frequent problem and may lead to requirement of prolonged mechanical ventilation. It must be suspected in all "difficult to wean" patients. High level of suspicion combined with specific measures to target OSA during and post weaning can help in successful extubation and early weaning of these patients.

References

[1] Benjafield A. V., Ayas N. T., Eastwood P. R., Heinzer R., Ip M. S. M., Morrell M. J., Nunez C. M., Patel S. R., Penzel T., Pépin J. L., Peppard P. E., Sinha S., Tufik S., Valentine K., Malhotra A. Estimation of the global prevalence and burden of obstructive sleep apnoea: a literature-based analysis. *Lancet Respir Med.* 2019 Aug;7(8):687-698. doi: https://doi.org/10.1016/S2213-2600(19)30198-5. Epub 2019 Jul 9. PMID: 31300334; PMCID: PMC7007763.

[2] Dempsey J. A., Veasey S. C., Morgan B. J., O'Donnell C. P. Pathophysiology of sleep apnea. *Physiol Rev.* 2010 Jan;90(1):47-112. doi: https://doi.org/10.1152/physrev.00043.2008. Erratum in: Physiol Rev. 2010 Apr;90(2):797-8. PMID: 20086074; PMCID: PMC3970937.

[3] Dixon A. E., Peters U. The effect of obesity on lung function. *Expert Rev Respir Med.* 2018 Sep;12(9):755-767. doi: https://doi.org/10.1080/17476348.2018.1506331. Epub 2018 Aug 14. PMID: 30056777; PMCID: PMC6311385.

[4] Verbraecken J., McNicholas W. T. Respiratory mechanics and ventilatory control in overlap syndrome and obesity hypoventilation. *Respir Res.* 2013 Nov 20;14(1):132. doi: https://doi.org/10.1186/1465-9921-14-132. PMID: 24256627; PMCID: PMC3871022.

[5] Bailly S., Galerneau L. M., Ruckly S., Terzi N., Schwebel C., Dupuis C., Renaud Tamisier, Bruno Mourvillier, Jean-Louis Pépin, Jean-François Timsit. Impact of

Obstructive sleep apnea on ICU patient's prognosis- insights from a French ICU cohort. *European Respiratory Journal* 2019 54: PA866; doi: https://doi.org/10.1183/13993003.congress-2019.PA866.

[6] Bailly S., Galerneau L. M., Ruckly S., Seiller A., Terzi N., Schwebel C., Dupuis C., Tamisier R., Mourvillier B., Pepin J. L., Timsit J. F. Impact of obstructive sleep apnea on the obesity paradox in critically ill patients. *J Crit Care.* 2020 Apr;56:120-124. doi: https://doi.org/10.1016/j.jcrc.2019.12.016. Epub 2019 Dec 20.

[7] Lin P., Li X., Zhang J., Liang Z. Association Between Obstructive Sleep Apnea and Reduced Mortality in Critically Ill Patients: A Propensity Score-Based Analysis. *Int J Gen Med.* 2021 Aug 21;14:4723-4729. doi: https://doi.org/10.2147/IJGM.S330752. PMID: 34456584; PMCID: PMC8387641.

[8] Johnson D. C., Johnson K. G. Obstructive sleep apnea and prolonged mechanical ventilation. *Respir Care.* 2012 Feb;57(2):326-7. doi: https://doi.org/10.4187/respcare.01723. PMID: 22304801.

[9] Cavallone L. F., Vannucci A. Review article: Extubation of the difficult airway and extubation failure. *Anesth Analg.* 2013 Feb;116(2):368-83. doi: https://doi.org/10.1213/ANE.0b013e31827ab572. Epub 2013 Jan 9. PMID: 23302983.

[10] Diaz-Abad M., Verceles A. C., Brown J. E., Scharf S. M. Sleep-disordered breathing may be under-recognized in patients who wean from prolonged mechanical ventilation. *Respir Care.* 2012 Feb;57(2):229-37. doi: https://doi.org/10.4187/respcare.01260. Epub 2011 Jul 12. PMID: 21762560.

[11] Jeremy Lermitte, B. M. F. R. C. A., Mark J. Garfield, M. B. Ch. B. F. R. C. A., Weaning from mechanical ventilation, *Continuing Education in Anaesthesia Critical Care & Pain*, Volume 5, Issue 4, August 2005, Pages 113–117, https://doi.org/10.1093/bjaceaccp/mki031.

[12] Hang L. W., Chen W., Liang S. J., Lin Y. C., Tu C. Y., Chen H. J., Chiu K. L. Clinical characteristics and outcomes of patients with obstructive sleep apnoea requiring intensive care. *Anaesth Intensive Care.* 2010 May;38(3):506-12. doi: https://doi.org/10.1177/0310057X1003800315. PMID: 20514960.

[13] Lim D. C., Pack A. I. Obstructive Sleep Apnea: Update and Future. *Annu Rev Med.* 2017 Jan 14;68:99-112. doi: https://doi.org/10.1146/annurev-med-042915-102623. Epub 2016 Oct 5. PMID: 27732789.

[14] Jaber S., Chanques G., Matecki S., Ramonatxo M., Vergne C., Souche B., Perrigault P. F., Eledjam J. J. Post-extubation stridor in intensive care unit patients. Risk factors evaluation and importance of the cuff-leak test. *Intensive Care Med.* 2003 Jan;29(1):69-74. doi: https://doi.org/10.1007/s00134-002-1563-4. Epub 2002 Nov 22. PMID: 12528025.

[15] Brochard L., Rauss A., Benito S., Conti G., Mancebo J., Rekik N., Gasparetto A., Lemaire F. Comparison of three methods of gradual withdrawal from ventilatory support during weaning from mechanical ventilation. *Am J Respir Crit Care Med.* 1994 Oct;150(4):896-903. doi: https://doi.org/10.1164/ajrccm.150.4.7921460. PMID: 7921460.

[16] Wolk R., Shamsuzzaman A. S., Somers V. K. Obesity, sleep apnea, and hypertension. *Hypertension.* 2003 Dec;42(6):1067-74. doi: https://doi.org/10.1161/01.HYP.0000101686.98973.A3. Epub 2003 Nov 10. PMID: 14610096.

[17] Miehsler W. Mortality, morbidity, and special issues of obese ICU patients. *Wien Med Wochenschr*. 2010 Mar;160(5-6):124-8. doi: https://doi.org/10.1007/s10354-010-0767-4. PMID: 20364415.

[18] Haas C. F., Loik P. S. Ventilator discontinuation protocols. *Respir Care*. 2012 Oct;57(10):1649-62. doi: https://doi.org/10.4187/respcare.01895. PMID: 23013902.

[19] Kearny M. E. Cadieux R., Kofke W. A., Kales A. The occurrence of Obstructive sleep apnea in a recovery room Patient. *Anesthesiology* 1987;66:232-4.

[20] Boles J. M., Bion J., Connors A., Herridge M., Marsh B., Melot C., Pearl R., Silverman H., Stanchina M., Vieillard-Baron A., Welte T. Weaning from mechanical ventilation. *Eur Respir J*. 2007 May;29(5):1033-56. doi: https://doi.org/10.1183/09031936.00010206. PMID: 17470624.

Chapter 15

Extubation Period: Clinical and Practical Implications

Ferhat Çetinkaya[1], MD
Pelin Duru Çetinkaya[2], MD
and Dilek Özcengiz[1,*], MD
[1]Çukurova University Faculty of Medicine, Department of Intensive Care, Adana, Turkey
[2]Çukurova University Faculty of Medicine, Department of Chest Diseases, Adana, Turkey

Abstract

Obstructive sleep apnea (OSA) is a disease characterized by obstructive apneas, hypopneas and/or excitations related to respiratory effort caused by repetitive collapse of the upper airway during sleep. OSA is the most common sleep-related breathing disorder. Its prevalence is increasing. Extubation is the removal of the endotracheal tube (ETT) used for ventilation support. Meanwhile, extubation means the ending of artificial invasive breathing support. It is the last step in weaning a patient from mechanical ventilation. Extubation is not only a major step in the patient's recovery but also a very important procedure that carries the risk of complications or failure. Successful extubation depends primarily on two factors: the ability to tolerate spontaneous breathing without mechanical ventilation support and the ability to maintain patency of the airway after removal of the endotracheal tube. The mechanism of CPAP involves maintaining positive pharyngeal transmural pressure so that the intraluminal pressure exceeds the ambient pressure. CPAP also stabilizes the upper airway through increased expiratory lung volume. As a result,

* Corresponding Author's Email: dilekozcengiz@gmail.com.

In: Obstructive Sleep Apnea in Pulmonary Critical Care
Editors: Antonio M. Esquinas and Takatoshi Kasai
ISBN: 979-8-88697-858-2

respiratory events due to upper airway collapse (e.g., apneas, hypopneas) are prevented. Routine use of positive airway pressure (PAP) therapy is recommended in the post-operative post-extubation period in compatible patients with a known diagnosis of OSA. Use of PAP is recommended when hypoxemia, airway obstruction, apnea, or hypoventilation occurs for patients with or without a diagnosis of OSA but who are not compatible or intolerant of PAP therapy. There are several studies supporting the routine use of continuous positive airway pressure (CPAP) in postoperative patients with OSA. It has been reported that the use of CPAP for 24-48 hours postoperatively after extubation can reduce the risk of postoperative complications and extubation failure in severely obese OSA patients admitted to the intensive care unit and cause a decrease in mortality in patients with hypercapnia.

Keywords: obstructive sleep apnea, positive airway pressure therapy, extubation, extubation failure

Introduction

Obstructive sleep apnea (OSA) is a disease characterized by obstructive apneas, hypopneas and/or excitations related to respiratory effort caused by repetitive collapse of the upper airway during sleep. OSA is the most common sleep-related breathing disorder. Its prevalence is increasing. This may be related to increased obesity rates or increased OSA diagnosis rates [1-4]. The estimated prevalence of OSA increased from 11% to 14% in adult males and from 4% to 5% in adult females from 1990 to 2010 [5].

Extubation is the removal of the endotracheal tube (ETT) used for ventilation support. Meanwhile, extubation means the ending of artificial invasive breathing support. It is the last step in weaning a patient from mechanical ventilation. Patients should not be extubated unless the condition which causes the intubation is improved and clinical criteria for weaning are met. Extubation is not only a crucial step in the patient's recovery but also a very important procedure that carries the risk of complications or failure. Extubation failure and subsequent reintubation are associated with mechanical ventilation, increased mortality, greater need for tracheostomy, and higher medical costs [6, 7].

Successful extubation depends primarily on two factors: the ability to tolerate spontaneous breathing without mechanical ventilation support and the ability to maintain patency of the airway after removal of the endotracheal tube. Generally, extubation failure is defined as the need for reintubation within 24-72 hours after planned extubation [8, 9]. Extubation failure depends on both patient factors and the reasons for intubation. In general, extubation failure is relatively uncommon after general anesthesia for elective surgery; It is more common in patients who are intubated due to respiratory failure, airway obstruction, and bronchospasm, and in intensive care patients [10, 11]. Extubation criteria and, 11 evaluation criteria for spontaneous breathing for successful extubation are shown in Tables 1 and 2. In general, patients in the ICU should not be extubated unless they have undergone successful weaning.

Table 1. Criteria for a successful extubation

Extubation criteria	
1.	The patient's condition leading to intubation must be stable
2.	Must have successfully completed a weaning process
3.	Cough strength and secretion clearance should be evaluated.
4.	Cough strength: assessed by the gag reflex or assessed indirectly during deep aspiration at the bedside without this assessment.
5.	Secretion clearance: Generally, those who need aspiration every 2-3 hours should not be extubated.
6.	The risk of stridor should be evaluated after extubation (The cuff leak test)
7.	Mental state should be evaluated (Glasgow Coma Scale >8)
8.	The potential difficulty with reintubation should be evaluated.

Table 2. Clinical criteria used to determine readiness for trials of spontaneous breathing (Reference [10])

Required criteria	
1.	The cause of the respiratory failure has improved
2.	$PaO2/FiO2 \geq 150$* or $SpO2 \geq 90$ percent on $FiO2 \leq 40$ percent and positive end-expiratory pressure (PEEP) ≤ 5 cmH_2O
3.	$pH > 7.25$
4.	Hemodynamic stability (no or low dose vasopressor medications)
5.	Able to initiate an inspiratory effort.
Additional criteria (optional criteria)	
1.	Hemoglobin ≥ 7 mg/dL
2.	Core temperature ≤ 38 to 38.5°Centigrade
3.	Mental status awake and alert or easily arousable.

*A threshold of $PaO2/FiO2 \geq 120$ can be used for patients with chronic hypoxemia. Some patients require higher levels of PEEP to avoid atelectasis during mechanical ventilation.

Adequate cough strength, adequate consciousness level, and amount of secretion should also be considered before extubation. The patient's cough strength following extubation and his ability to clear his own secretions should be evaluated before extubation. In general, patients who need aspiration every 2-3 hours should not be extubated. Studies are reporting that successful extubation is directly related to spontaneous cough strength and inversely proportional to the frequency of aspiration [12-16].

Ideally, patients should be extubated, preferably without sedation, while awake and able to follow commands. The importance of the level of consciousness for successful extubation has been shown in observational studies [13, 17].

When starting extubation, the patient is placed in an upright position as concomitant medical or surgical conditions permit. The extubation procedure is explained to the patient before the ETT is removed. Both the oral cavity and the lower airways (inside the endotracheal tube) should be aspirated. The syringe is attached to the cuff, the patient is instructed to take a deep breath and then exhale or cough. During exhalation/cough, the cuff is rapidly deflated and the ETT is removed in a single, smooth motion. The patient typically coughs during removal and any remaining oral secretions are aspirated again to prevent aspiration. Following extubation, supplemental oxygen therapy is administered to achieve the predefined peripheral saturation target. In some cases, non-invasive mechanical ventilation (NIV) is required. NIV can be used to increase the success of extubation after extubation in patients with OSA and to ensure airway patency [18].

Postoperative Extubation in OSA

In the perioperative setting, several factors have been identified that increase the risk of extubation failure. According to A Closed Claims Analysis of the American Society of Anesthesiologists, it has been shown that extubation failure is more common in patients with obesity or obstructive sleep apnea (OSA) [19]. In the report of the Fourth National Audit Project of the Royal College of Anesthetists and the Difficult Airway Society, the most common comorbidities associated with reintubation after anesthesia was reported to be obesity (46%) and OSA (13%) [20]. In extubation guidelines, OSA is defined among risk factors for extubation failure [7, 21].

Although OSA causes perioperative morbidity, more than half of the patients admitted for surgery are not diagnosed with OSA, causing difficulties in treatment (intubation and extubation). It is recommended that all adult obese patients be routinely asked about nocturnal snoring, apnea, and daytime sleepiness, as the definitive diagnosis of preoperative OSA will likely affect anesthetic management [22-24].

Before extubation, the patient should be fully awake. Postoperative OSA patients should be in an upright or semi-upright position, as the supine position worsens OSA [25]. Reverse Trendelenburg can be used as an alternative if the patient cannot tolerate the upright or semi-upright position. Reverse Trendelenburg or extubation in the semi-upright position minimizes compression of the diaphragm by the abdominal contents [26]. Studies have shown that in OSA patients, being in a semi-upright position instead of the supine position reduces the Apnea-Hypopnea Index (AHI) and increases oxygen saturation. In addition, the pharynx may collapse in the supine position, causing upper airway obstruction [27-29].

Routine use of positive airway pressure (PAP) therapy is recommended in the post-operative post-extubation period in compatible patients with a known diagnosis of OSA. Use of PAP is recommended when hypoxemia, airway obstruction, apnea, or hypoventilation occurs for patients with or without a diagnosis of OSA but who are not compatible or intolerant of PAP therapy. The use of PAP in OSA patients is safe in the perioperative period. Despite concerns that PAP therapy may lead to anastomotic leaks after upper gastrointestinal surgery, a systematic review of thirteen observational studies of 5500 patients undergoing gastric bypass surgery found that postoperative noninvasive positive ventilation did not increase the risk of anastomotic separation [30].

Although the use of postoperative PAP in OSA is recommended in the guidelines, it has been observed in studies that compliance with the guidelines is low [2, 31]. To increase the compliance of OSA patients using PAP at home in the preoperative period, they should be asked to bring their devices to the hospital to continue in the postoperative period. The general approach for postoperative PAP treatment is to start at the level used before. However, perioperative changes such as facial swelling, upper airway edema should be taken into account, and pressures should be adjusted again in patients who need to be considered [32]. If the previously specified level is unknown, it is recommended to begin PAP at an empirical level of 8 to 10 cm H_2O. The level should then be titrated until apneas, episodes of oxygen desaturation, and snoring disappear. Alternatively, PAP with automatic titration is increasingly used to eliminate the need for manual titration [33-35].

There are many studies supporting the routine use of continuous positive airway pressure (CPAP) in postoperative patients with OSA [36-38]. It has been reported that the use of CPAP for 24-48 hours postoperatively after extubation can reduce the risk of postoperative complications and extubation failure in severely obese OSA patients admitted to the intensive care unit, and also cause a decrease in mortality in patients with hypercapnia [39, 40].

Although guidelines recommend initiating PAP as soon as possible postoperatively, there are not enough studies on this subject [41]. The preferred mode of PAP is usually the one applied preoperatively. In most cases it is CPAP, but bi-level PAP (BPAP) can be used in patients with concomitant OHS or COPD. It is appropriate to switch to BPAP (with spontaneous/timed mode) in patients who develop hypoventilation as a complication of their surgery. For patients using an oral device for the treatment of OSA, the device should be administered in the postoperative anesthesia intensive care unit whenever possible.

Patients with OSA have a higher incidence of postoperative oxygen desaturations and respiratory complications compared with those without OSA. Therefore, after extubation, oxygen therapy is frequently used, and these patients need close follow-up with continuous pulse oximetry [18]. However, oxygen therapy in patients with OSA should be low- flow titrated to ensure adequate oxygenation (e.g., >90 percent) and prevent acute hypercapnia from hypoventilation. Oxygen therapy is gradually reduced until the patient can maintain adequate oxygenation in room air [42].

In postoperative patients receiving opioids and respiratory depression, nasal high-flow oxygen can provide airway support, improve oxygenation, and overcome obstructive hypopnea. Studies in patients with OSA suggest that high-flow nasal oxygen may be beneficial [43, 44].

It is recommended that patients with OSA who receive postoperative supplemental oxygen therapy should be followed closely in terms of ventilation requirements. Clinical evaluation of ventilation; Continuous measurement of respiratory rate or end-tidal carbon dioxide (CO_2) monitoring (i.e., capnography) can also be done with arterial blood gas monitoring. Oxygen saturation <90%, bradypnea <8 breaths/minute, and apnea ≥10 seconds are important indicators of hypoventilation in patients with postoperative OSA [45]. When the quantitative assessment is required, arterial blood gas measurement provides the most sensitive measurement of ventilation. OSA-Extubation recommendations are summarized in Table 3.

Table 3. OSA-Extubation recommendations

Should be in an upright or semi-upright position when extubating.
Patients who cannot tolerate these positions should be placed in the reverse trendelenburg position
It must be extubated when full awakening is achieved.
Early PAP treatment is recommended after extubation in patients with OSA
Oxygenation and ventilation should be continuously monitored
After extubation, oxygen therapy should be given at the lowest flow that will keep saturation above 90%.

Difficult intubation is more common in patients with OSA, so successful extubation is very important. In addition to general strategies (upright positioning, aspiration, secretion control.) in extubation in patients with OSA, post-extubation PAP application and preservation of airway patency are focused on.

Positive airway pressure therapy is used after extubation for airway safety in OSA. OSA itself and accompanying conditions such as obesity, large neck circumference, and snoring are risk factors for difficulty in airway management. PAP therapy is the mainstay of treatment for adults with OSA. The mechanism of CPAP involves maintaining positive pharyngeal transmural pressure so that the intraluminal pressure exceeds the ambient pressure [46]. CPAP also stabilizes the upper airway through increased expiratory lung volume. As a result, respiratory events due to upper airway collapse (e.g., apneas, hypopneas) are prevented.

Conclusion

In summary, Extubation failure is more common in patients with OSA, and difficult intubation is more common in patients with OSA. Therefore, a successful weaning period and timing of extubation are important to prevent extubation failure. Patients with OSA should be in an upright or semi-upright position when extubating. Patients who cannot tolerate these positions should be placed in the reverse Trendelenburg position. It must be extubated when full awakening is achieved. Early PAP treatment is recommended after extubation in patients with OSA. Oxygenation and ventilation should be continuously monitored. After extubation, oxygen therapy should be given at the lowest flow that will keep saturation above 90%. However, high-flow oxygen therapy may be beneficial in patients with OSA who use opioids and whose breathing may be depressed.

References

[1] Lechner M., Breeze C. E., Ohayon M. M., Kotecha B. Snoring and breathing pauses during sleep: interview survey of a United Kingdom population sample reveals a significant increase in the rates of sleep apnoea and obesity over the last 20 years - data from the UK sleep survey. *Sleep Med.* 2019; 54:250-256.

[2] Memtsoudis S. G., Besculides M. C., Mazumdar M. (2013). A rude awakening of the perioperative sleep apnea epidemic. *N Engl J Med,* 368(25), 2352-2353.

[3] Benjafield A. V., Ayas N. T., Eastwood P. R., Heinzer R., Ip M. S. M., Morrell M. J., Nunez C. M., Patel S. R., Penzel T., Pépin J. L., Peppard P. E., Sinha S., Tufik S., Valentine K., Malhotra A. Estimation of the global prevalence and burden of obstructive sleep apnoea: a literature-based analysis. *Lancet Respir Med.* 2019;7(8):687-689.

[4] Flegal K. M., Carroll M. D., Ogden C. L., Johnson C. L. Prevalence, and trends in obesity among US adults, 1999-2000. *JAMA*, 2002; 288(14):1723-1727.

[5] Peppard P. E., Young T., Barnet J. H., Palta M., Hagen E. W., Hla K. M. Increased prevalence of sleep-disordered breathing in adults. *Am J Epidemiol.* 2013; 177(9):1006-1014.

[6] Epstein S. K. (2009). Weaning from ventilatory support. *Current opinion in critical care*, 15(1), 36-43.

[7] Artime C. A., Hagberg C. A. (2014). Tracheal Extubation-Discussion. *Respiratory Care,* 59(6), 991-1005.

[8] Cavallone L. F., Vannucci A. (2013). Extubation of the difficult airway and extubation failure. *Anesthesia & Analgesia,* 116(2), 368-383.

[9] Epstein, S. (2002). Decision to extubate. *Intensive care medicine,* 28(5), 535-546.

[10] MacIntyre N. R., Cook D. J., Ely Jr E. W., Epstein S. K., Fink J. B., Heffner J. E., Hess D., Hubmayer R. D., Scheinhorn D. J. Evidence-based guidelines for weaning and discontinuing ventilatory support: a collective task force facilitated by the American College of Chest Physicians, the American Association for Respiratory Care, and the American College of Critical Care Medicine. *Chest* 2001; 120:375S-95S.

[11] Rothaar R. C., Epstein S. K. (2003). Extubation failure: magnitude of the problem, impact on outcomes, and prevention. *Current opinion in critical care,* 9(1), 59-66.

[12] Coplin W. M., Pierson D. J., Cooley K. D., Newell D. W., Rubenfeld G. D. Implications of extubation delay in brain-injured patients meeting standard weaning criteria. *Am J Respir Crit Care Med.* 2000; 161(5):1530-1536.

[13] Salam A., Tilluckdharry L., Amoateng-Adjepong Y., Manthous C. A. Neurologic status, cough, secretions and extubation outcomes. *Intensive Care Med.* 2004;30(7):1334-1339.

[14] Khamiees M., Raju P., DeGirolamo A., Amoateng-Adjepong Y., Manthous C. A. Predictors of extubation outcome in patients who have successfully completed a spontaneous breathing trial. *Chest.* 2001; 120(4):1262-1270.

[15] Beuret P., Roux C., Auclair A., Nourdine K., Kaaki M., Carton M. J. Interest of an objective evaluation of cough during weaning from mechanical ventilation. *Intensive Care Med.* 2009; 35(6):1090-1093.

[16] Thille A. W., Boissier F., Ben Ghezala H., Razazi K., Mekontso-Dessap A., Brun-Buisson C. Risk factors for and prediction by caregivers of extubation failure in ICU patients: a prospective study. *Crit Care Med.* 2015; 43(3):613-620.

[17] Namen A. M., Ely E. W., Tatter S. B., Case L. D., Lucia M. A., Smith A., Landry S., Wilson J. A., Glazier S. S., Branch C. L., Kelly D. L., Bowton D. L., Haponik E. F. Predictors of successful extubation in neurosurgical patients. *Am J Respir Crit Care Med.* 2001; 163(3):658-664.

[18] American Society of Anesthesiologists Task Force on Perioperative Management of patients with obstructive sleep apnea. Practice guidelines for the perioperative management of patients with obstructive sleep apnea: an updated report by the American Society of Anesthesiologists Task Force on Perioperative Management of patients with obstructive sleep apnea. *Anesthesiology.* 2014 Feb; 120(2):268-86.

[19] Peterson G. N., Domino K. B., Caplan R. A., Posner K. L., Lee L. A., Cheney F. W. Management of the difficult airway: a closed claims analysis. *The Journal of the American Society of Anesthesiologists,* 2005:103(1), 33-39.

[20] Cook T., Woodall N., Harper J., Benger J., Fourth National Audit Project. (2011) Major complications of airway management in the UK: results of the Fourth National Audit Project of the Royal College of Anesthetists and the Difficult Airway Society. Part 2: intensive care and emergency departments. *British journal of anesthesia*, 106(5), 632-642.

[21] Popat M., Mitchell V., Dravid R., Patel A., Swampillai C., Higgs A. Difficult Airway Society Guidelines for the management of tracheal extubation. *Anesthesia* 2012; 67(3):318–340.

[22] Singh M., Liao P., Kobah S., Wijeysundera D. N., Shapiro C., Chung F. Proportion of surgical patients with undiagnosed obstructive sleep apnoea. *Br J Anaesth.* 2013; 110(4):629-636.

[23] Lockhart E. M., Willingham M. D., Abdallah A. B., Helsten D. L., Bedair B. A., Thomas J., Duntley S., Avidan M. S. Obstructive sleep apnea screening and postoperative mortality in a large surgical cohort. *Sleep Med.* 2013 May;14(5):407-15.

[24] Chan M. T. V., Wang C. Y., Seet E., Tam S., Lai H. Y., Chew E. F. F., Wu W. K. K., Cheng B. C. P., Lam C. K. M., Short T. G., Hui D. S. C., Chung F., Postoperative Vascular Complications in Unrecognized Obstructive Sleep Apnea (POSA) Study Investigators. Association of Unrecognized Obstructive Sleep Apnea with Postoperative Cardiovascular Events in Patients Undergoing Major Noncardiac Surgery. *JAMA.* 2019; 321(18):1788-1798.

[25] Benumof J. L. (2002). Obstructive sleep apnea in the adult obese patient: implications for airway management. *Anesthesiology Clinics of North America,* 20(4), 789-811.

[26] Jokic R., Klimaszewski A., Crossley M., Sridhar G., Fitzpatrick M. F. Positional treatment vs continuous positive airway pressure in patients with positional obstructive sleep apnea syndrome. *Chest.* 1999; 115(3):771-781.

[27] Ong J. S., Touyz G., Tanner S., Hillman D. R., Eastwood P. R., Walsh J. H. Variability of human upper airway collapsibility during sleep and the influence of body posture and sleep stage. *J Sleep Res.* 2011 Dec; 20(4):533-537.

[28] Zaremba S., Mueller N., Heisig A. M., Shin C. H., Jung S., Leffert L. R., Bateman B. T., Pugsley L. J., Nagasaka Y., Duarte I. M., Ecker J. L., Eikermann M. Elevated upper body position improves pregnancy related OSA without impairing sleep quality or sleep architecture early after delivery. *Chest,* 2015; 148(4):936-944.

[29] Chung F., Liao P., Yegneswaran B., Shapiro C. M., Kang Postoperative changes in sleep-disordered breathing and sleep architecture in patients with obstructive sleep apnea. *Anesthesiology.* 2014;120(2):287-298.

[30] Tong S., Gower J., Morgan A., Gadbois K., Wisbach G. Noninvasive positive pressure ventilation in the immediate post-bariatric surgery care of patients with obstructive sleep apnea: a systematic review. *Surg Obes Relat Dis.* 2017;13(7):1227-1233.

[31] Chung F., Nagappa M., Singh M., Mokhlesi B. CPAP in the Perioperative Setting: Evidence of Support. *Chest.* 2016; 149(2):586-597.

[32] Chung F., Memtsoudis S. G., Ramachandran S. K., Nagappa M., Opperer M., Cozowicz C., Patrawala S., Lam D., Kumar A., Joshi G. P., Fleetham J., Ayas N., Collop N., Doufas A. G., Eikermann M., Englesakis M., Gali B., Gay P., Hernandez A. V., Kaw R., Kezirian E. J., Malhotra A., Mokhlesi B., Parthasarathy S., Stierer T., Wappler F., Hillman D. R., Auckley D. Society of Anesthesia and Sleep Medicine Guidelines on Preoperative Screening and Assessment of Adult Patients with Obstructive Sleep Apnea. *Anesth Analg* 2016; 123:452.

[33] Liao P., Luo Q., Elsaid H., Kang W., Shapiro C. M., Chung F. Perioperative auto-titrated continuous positive airway pressure treatment in surgical patients with obstructive sleep apnea: a randomized controlled trial. *Anesthesiology* 2013; 119:837-847.

[34] Proczko M. A., Stepaniak P. S., de Quelerij M., van der Lely F. H., Smulders J. F., Kaska L., Soliman Hamad M. A. STOP-Bang and the effect on patient outcome and length of hospital stay when patients are not using continuous positive airway pressure. *J Anesth* 2014; 28:891-897.

[35] O'Gorman S. M., Gay P. C., Morgenthaler T. I. Does auto titrating positive airway pressure therapy improve postoperative outcome in patients at risk for obstructive sleep apnea syndrome? A randomized controlled clinical trial. *Chest* 2013; 144:72-78.

[36] Nagappa M., Mokhlesi B., Wong J., Wong D. T., Kaw R., Chung F. The Effects of Continuous Positive Airway Pressure on Postoperative Outcomes in Obstructive Sleep Apnea Patients Undergoing Surgery: A Systematic Review and Meta-analysis. *Anesth Analg* 2015; 120(5):1013-1023.

[37] Mutter T. C., Chateau D., Moffatt M., Ramsey C., Roos L. L., Kryger M. A. matched cohort study of postoperative outcomes in obstructive sleep apnea: could

preoperative diagnosis and treatment prevent complications? *Anesthesiology* 2014; 121(4):707-718.

[38] Abdelsattar Z. M., Hendren S., Wong S. L., Campbell Jr. D. A., Ramachandran S. K. The Impact of Untreated Obstructive Sleep Apnea on Cardiopulmonary Complications in General and Vascular Surgery: A Cohort Study. *Sleep* 2015; 38(8):1205-1210.

[39] Rennotte M. T., Baele P., Aubert G., Rodenstein D. O. Nasal continuous positive airway pressure in the perioperative management of patients with obstructive sleep apnea submitted to surgery. *Chest.* 1995;107(2):367-74.

[40] El-Solh A. A., Aquilina A., Pineda L., Dhanvantri V., Grant B., Bouquin P. Noninvasive ventilation for prevention of post-extubation respiratory failure in obese patients. *Eur Respir J.* 2006;28(3):588-95. https://doi.org/10.1183/09031936.06.00150705.

[41] Weingarten T. N., Flores A. S., McKenzie J. A., Nguyen L. T., Robinson W. B., Kinney T. M., Sprung J. Obstructive sleep apnoea and perioperative complications in bariatric patients. *Br J Anaesth* 2011; 106(1):131-139.

[42] Fu E. S., Downs J. B., Schweiger J. W., Miguel R. V., Smith R. A. Supplemental oxygen impairs detection of hypoventilation by pulse oximetry. *Chest* 2004; 126(5):1552-1558.

[43] McGinley B. M., Patil S. P., Kirkness J. P., Smith P. L., Schwartz A. R., Schneider H. A nasal cannula can be used to treat obstructive sleep apnea. *Am J Respir Crit Care Med* 2007; 176(2):194-200.

[44] Hawkins S., Huston S., Campbell K., Halbower A. High-Flow, Heated, Humidified Air via Nasal Cannula Treats CPAP-Intolerant Children with Obstructive Sleep Apnea. *J Clin Sleep Med* 2017; 13(8):981-989.

[45] Gali B., Whalen F. X., Schroeder D. R., Gay P. C., Plevak D. J. Identification of patients at risk for postoperative respiratory complications using a preoperative obstructive sleep apnea screening tool and post anesthesia care assessment. *Anesthesiology* 2009; 110(4):869-877.

[46] Jordan A. S., McSharry D. G., Malhotra A. Adult obstructive sleep apnoea. *Lancet,* 2014; 383(9918):736. Epub 2013 Aug 2.

Chapter 16

Obstructive Sleep Apnea in Anesthesiology-Perioperative Medicine: Pathophysiology, Diagnosis and Treatment

Dipasri Bhattacharya[1,*], MD
and Mohanchandra Mandal[2], MD
[1]Department of Anesthesiology, Pain Medicine, and Critical Care,
R. G. Kar Medical College, Kolkata, West Bengal, India
[2]Department of Anesthesiology, Institute of Post Graduate Medical Education
and Research / S.S.K.M. Hospital, Kolkata, West Bengal, India

Abstract

Obstructive sleep apnea is characterized by periodic and variable degree of airway obstruction during sleep. This sleep-disordered breathing can invite many health hazards and if remain undiagnosed can further increase the adverse events during anesthesia care. Different pertinent issues during anesthesia care and the goals of anesthetic management have been mentioned. A brief outline regarding the role of non-invasive ventilation in the perioperative management of such patients is provided in this chapter.

Keywords: anesthesia, apnea, hypopnea, obesity, sleep-disordered breathing

---

[*] Dipasri Bhattacharya, MD, MNAMS, FIAPM;
Corresponding Author's Email: drmcmandal@gmail.com.

In: Obstructive Sleep Apnea in Pulmonary Critical Care
Editors: Antonio M. Esquinas and Takatoshi Kasai
ISBN: 979-8-88697-858-2

Introduction

Obstructive sleep apnea (OSA) is a syndrome that encompasses periodic, partial, or complete obstruction of upper airway during sleep [1]. The patient suffers from repetitive arousal from sleep to restore airway patency, which may result in daytime hypersomnolence or irritable behavior. OSA is the most common type of sleep-disordered breathing (SDB) with varying prevalence across age groups, ethnicities, and countries [2]. The prevalence of OSA is about one in every four men and one in every ten women [3].

The incidence of OSA increases with obesity and is of great concern for anesthesiologists [2]. A large number of surgical patients may have unrecognized OSA. These patients are at increased risk for perioperative complications. This increased risk is related to more difficult intubations, use of ventilator, use of respiratory depressant medications to minimize patient-ventilator asynchrony, and body positioning [2]. Besides the overweight patient, a leaner patient with significant craniofacial deformities, such as retrognathia or mid-facial hypoplasia, may also have OSA [4]. Asymptomatic patients can present special challenges that must be managed to minimize the risk of perioperative morbidity or mortality [1]. Patients who have difficulty in mask ventilation, laryngoscopy and tracheal intubation may have undiagnosed OSA [5].

Identification and perioperative management of patient with undiagnosed OSA is a bigger challenge than managing patient with a pre-existing diagnosis of sleep apnea [6]. Our primary goal is to identify the perioperative complications of OSA and discussing various interventions aimed at risk reduction in perioperative period and thus ensuring favourable outcome.

Pathophysiology

During inspiration, the negative pressures produced by the diaphragm and intercostal muscles cause a collapse of the oropharynx. Increased soft tissue around the airway and decreased tone of the oropharyngeal muscles aggravates the situation. Co-ordinated contraction of the oropharyngeal dilator and abductor muscles maintains the patency of the upper airway [7]. Any imbalance between collapsing forces and the dilating forces of upper airway can lead to airway obstruction in OSA patients [1, 7]. Airway obstruction causes oxygen desaturation, episodic hypercarbia, and cardiovascular dysfunction in the perioperative period. Increased adipose tissue in the pharynx will cause further narrowing of airway in obese patients, thereby demanding an increase in oropharyngeal muscle tone to maintain upper airway patency. Complete collapse results in obstruction and a period of apnea, whereas partial collapse results in snoring and hyperpnoea. Breathing resumes when there is arousal from sleep, because of increased oxygen and carbon dioxide chemo-receptor activity and an increased oropharyngeal muscle tone in response to an increased inspiratory effort [1, 7].

Diagnosis

Predisposing conditions for OSA: Obesity, Age 40-70 years, male gender, excessive alcohol intake, smoking, pregnancy, neck circumference > 40cm, tonsil or adenoid hypertrophy, craniofacial abnormality [1, 7]. *History and clinical examination*: The use of STOP-Bang questionnaire (Snoring, Tiredness, Observed apnea, high blood Pressure, BMI, Age, Neck circumference, and Gender). BMI > 35, age > 50 years, neck circumference > 40 cm and male gender are high risk patient with higher score. The obese patients with a STOP-Bang score of 0 to 2 can be considered as low-risk case whereas those with a score of 5 to 8 can be classified as high-risk for moderate to severe OSA [1]. The STOP-Bang questionnaire is reported to have a sensitivity of 100% with specificity of about 37% [7].

On physical examination the characteristic stigmata of OSA such as a short and thick neck, nasal obstruction, tonsillar hypertrophy, narrow oropharynx, and retrognathia may be found. Obesity hypoventilation syndrome increases the risk of OSA [8]. Obesity hypoventilation syndrome (OHS) remains to be one of the most important postoperative adverse events seen in patients with morbid obesity. OHS is defined by the triad of obesity (body mass index [BMI] $\geq$ 30 kg/m^2), daytime hypoventilation with hypercapnia (partial pressure of arterial carbon dioxide $PaCO_2 \geq 45$ mm Hg at sea level, and hypoxemia (partial pressure of arterial oxygen PaO_2 less than 70 mm Hg at sea level, and sleep-disordered breathing.[8] Patients with OHS usually suffers from several comorbidities which increases the risk for perioperative morbidity and mortality [8].

The following history may suggest the possibilities of undiagnosed OSA: difficulty in maintaining airway patency, difficulty in intubation, postoperative snoring, airway obstruction out of proportion to the apparent degree of sedation. The degree of difficulty in visualizing the faucial pillars, the soft palate, and the base of the uvula predicts difficulty with intubation and should increase the suspicion of OSA [9]. Clinical examination carries a diagnostic sensitivity and specificity of only 50% to 60% for sleep apnea [9].

Investigations: The gold standard investigation of OSA is full overnight polysomnography [10]. The equipment monitors heart, lung, and brain activity, breathing patterns, arm and leg movements, and blood oxygen levels during sleep. The apnea-hypopnea index is used to diagnose OSA. Apnea can be defined as a complete cessation of airflow, and hypopnea is defined as a partial reduction (at least 50%) of airflow; both lasting for a minimum of 10 seconds. Hypopneas are measured by oxygen desaturation of 3% or more or arousal from sleep. The Apnea-Hypopnea Index (AHI) is calculated by adding all apneas and hypopneas and then dividing by total sleep time. None/Minimal AHI < 5 per hour, Mild AHI ≥ 5, but < 15 per hour, Moderate AHI ≥ 15, but < 30 per hour, Severe AHI ≥ 30 per hour [10]. Reeder et al., [11] used preoperative overnight oximetry in 24 patients and demonstrated significant abnormalities of respiration (SARS) postoperatively in all patients with preoperative SARS.

Issues and Goals of Anaesthesia

1. To optimize the patient for surgery
2. To avoid hypoxemia
3. To avoid hypercapnia
4. To reduce postoperative pulmonary complications
5. To reduce cardiovascular complications

A. Preoperative Management

Multiple factors predispose to OSA patients to various airway management issues particularly when anaesthesia and opioids use are concerned. These factors include reduction in pharyngeal dilator muscle activation and lung volume, delayed or abolished upper airway muscle tone during inspiration [12], impaired upper airway neuromotor responses and variability in the collapsibility of upper airway [12]. During preoperative visit following entities should be enquired about such as presence of heavy snoring, sudden awakenings with a chocking sensation and incidences of apnea as witnessed by partner. Severity of these problems in the history directly correlates with the severity of sleep study proven OSA [12].

CPAP or BiPAP therapy should be utilized for perioperative optimization in severe OSA patients. Patients who use CPAP therapy at home should be advised to bring their devices for possible postoperative use with the advantage of familiarity. In addition to CPAP, other treatment modalities such as corrective surgery, mandibular advancement devices and oral appliances should be considered when feasible [12]. It is recommended that a patient who had corrective airway surgery should be assumed to remain at risk for OSA complications unless the sleep studies and symptoms have normalized [12].

Associated diseases: There is an association between the presence of OSA and the following diseases such as hypertension [13], obesity [14], coronary artery disease [15], myocardial dysfunction and arrhythmias [16], pulmonary arterial hypertension [17] and gastroesophageal reflux [18].

Decisions regarding surgical setting: Severity of OSA, type of surgery, need for postoperative narcotics and clinical course in the recovery room- all should be considered during preoperative evaluation. All these are important considerations to plan postoperative monitoring and management. Surgery requiring only regional anesthesia or a limited need for postoperative narcotic analgesia should be considered for outpatient surgery. These patients can be discharged when fully conscious if they are not snoring and no sign of airway obstruction exists in the recovery room. An inpatient monitoring is essential in following scenarios: (1) patients who are expected to have significant pain requiring high dose of opioid and narcotics, (2) those who have history of severe OSA requiring CPAP therapy at home, and (3) those who have an observed obstruction of episodes of desaturation in the recovery room [19].

B. Intraoperative Concerns in OSA Patients

Difficult airway - Patient with OSA often presents with difficulty in airway management. Kheterpal et al., [20] reported identical predictors like BMI > 30kg/m^2 and neck circumference > cm for both OSA and difficult intubation among a cohort of 50000 anesthetized patients. Considering the possibility of difficult intubation during general anesthesia, preparation for induction and intubation should follow ASA difficult airway guidelines [21]. The positioning of obese patients with known or suspected OSA includes positioning with a ramp of blankets to elevate the torso and head and achieve the sniffing position [21]. Upper body elevation relieves OSA by increasing upper airway stability and decreases passive airway closing pressure in OSA. Pharyngeal airway closure can be prevented by application of 10 cm of H_2O PEEP during positive pressure ventilation even in most severe cases of OSA.

Awake intubation and RSI are preferred when difficult intubation is suspected. ASA guidelines recommend a semi-upright position for extubation and recovery [21, 12]. Supine position should be avoided in the postoperative period as far as practicable [21].

Selecting sedation and analgesia- For previously undiagnosed OSA with high clinical suspicion, wherever possible, regional anesthesia and blocks are preferred and for general anesthesia, short acting agents like desflurane and propofol are recommended [22]. These techniques can reduce the threat of upper airway collapse during the procedures. ASA recommends general anesthesia with secure airway over sedation without airway particularly for procedures that may mechanically compromise airway. Use of regional anesthesia as an adjunct to general anesthesia also decreased use of opioids and other sedatives throughout the perioperative period [2]. Dosing of medications should also be adjusted for obese patients [22].

Reversal and postoperative analgesia - Full reversal from effects of muscle relaxants is important in these patients to avoid postoperative upper airway obstruction. Full reversal should be verified by a nerve stimulator prior to extubation [22]. It is also essential that the patient is fully awake, hemodynamically stable, normothermic and breathing spontaneously with adequate tidal volume before extubation [22]. Supplemental oxygen is often advisable after extubation in the recovery room until the patient can maintain baseline SpO_2 on room air. However supplemental oxygen may increase duration of apneic episodes and obscure detection of transient apnea, atelectasis, and hypoventilation [22]. Multimodal analgesia using non-steroidal anti-inflammatory drugs, acetaminophen, tramadol, ketamine, pregabalin and COX-2 inhibitors are used to minimize opioid requirement in postoperative period [23]. Opioids tend to decrease hypoxic and hypercapnic ventilatory drive [24]. Thus, even epidural, and intrathecal administration of opioids need caution and patients should be carefully monitored for obstruction and asynchrony of respiratory efforts in the postoperative period [24].

C. Perioperative Monitoring Protocols

An unsupervised holding area is inappropriate for a premedicated patient with OSA. ASA recommends continuous pulse oximetry monitoring in the immediate postoperative period in critical care or step-down unit for patients with increased risk from OSA. Patients with preclinical suspicion of OSA, undergoing invasive surgery and receiving postoperative narcotics should receive pulse oximetry monitoring for 24-48 hours postoperatively [2].

ASA recommends longer (3 hours) postoperative monitoring in OSA patients after ambulatory surgery [12, 25]. Close monitoring should be continued as long as the patient remains at high risk regarding maintaining the patent airway. If any episode of airway obstruction or hypoxemia is witnessed during postoperative observation, the monitoring should be continued for additional 7 hours. Application of nasal CPAP or non-invasive positive airway pressure (NIPPV) may be required and thereby monitoring period is extended accordingly [12, 25]. Transesophageal echocardiography is increasingly being used for noncardiac surgery and may be useful in selected patients with sleep apnea because it can provide insight into heart function and pulmonary artery pressures. If the patient with OSA has morbid obesity an intra-arterial catheter may be helpful as noninvasive blood pressure monitoring is unreliable or not possible for technical reasons [25].

D. Perioperative Interventions to Improve Oxygenation

Presently three approaches are suggested for improving ventilation and oxygenation in obese patients: High tidal volume, positive end expiratory pressure (PEEP) and vital capacity maneuver.

Reverse Trendelenburg position: This position improves oxygenation in anesthetized obese patients and allows better exposure of subdiaphragmatic region leading to mechanical ventilation with safe airway pressure [26]. It also improves functional residual capacity by lowering the abdominal contents from pushing on the diaphragm.

Preinduction and maintenance PEEP: Prevention and reduction of atelectasis from induction and maintenance of general anesthesia is accomplished by preoxygenation with 100% FiO_2 and PEEP at 10 cm of H_2O during bag mask ventilation and after intubation [26]. This maneuver significantly allows increase in the time before desaturation begins.

Perioperative CPAP: Prophylactic use of CPAP in first 24 hours after surgery significantly reduces risk of pulmonary restrictive syndrome [27]. However, it has also been postulated that postoperative use of CPAP carries theoretical risk of increased rate of anastomotic leaks resulting from increased flow of pressurized air into stomach and proximal anastomosis of Roux-en-Y gastric bypass. So, Jensen et al., [28] reported that CPAP or BiPAP may be omitted in laparoscopic Roux-en-Y Gastric bypass patients if proper monitoring facility is available and pulmonary status is optimized by aggressive incentive spirometry and early ambulation. However perioperative NIV overall improves lung function if initiated immediately after extubation in OSA patients. Patients are encouraged to bring their home mask to ensure the best fit. If frequent or severe airway obstruction or hypoxemia is noted in recovery room, consideration has to be made to initiate NIPPV. This is particularly useful for patients with OSA, and COPD overlap syndrome or patients with overt obesity-hypoventilation syndrome with worsening hypercapnia. The best studied postoperative use of NIPPV in patients with obesity and OSA is in the bariatric surgery population [29].

E. Role of NIV in the Perioperative Period

Surgical patients often experience profound changes of the respiratory system. General anesthesia reduces oropharyngeal tone and airway reflexes. Opioids and other anesthetic agents reduce minute ventilation by blunting central respiratory drive. Functional residual capacity declines, closing capacity approaches FRC during general anesthesia causing small airway closure and atelectasis, and ventilation-perfusion mismatch is exacerbated. Postoperative hypoxemia and/or acute respiratory failure (ARF) mainly develop after abdominal and thoracic surgery. NIV does not require an artificial airway like endotracheal tube or tracheostomy and its use is well established to prevent occurrence of ARF (prophylactic treatment) or treat ARF to avoid reintubation (curative treatment) [30].

NIV therapy is increasingly popular for treatment of fore cited pulmonary complications in high-risk patients like OSA and new indications such as improvement of preoxygenation before intubation. Patients with SDB who are already receiving long-term domiciliary CPAP can often be managed with ward-based NIV support instead of ICU care. In such types of patients preoperative CPAP therapy may have beneficial effects in terms attenuation of symptom severity and curtailing the incidence of postoperative pulmonary complications [30].

F. Beneficial Effects of Preventive and Curative NIV in the Perioperative Period

Major abdominal surgery. Current evidence suggests that both preventive and therapeutic uses of CPAP improve postoperative oxygenation, reduce atelectasis, decrease chance of reintubation, and reduce length of ICU stay after major abdominal surgery. The risk of upper digestive anastomotic leakage due to nonoptimal NIV setting (PSV+PEEP > 25cm of H_2O) can be avoided by preferring CPAP over PSV. If at all needed, PSV level must be maintained below 6-8cm of H_2O. However, CPAP therapy is easier to cater for in comparison with NIV using PSV + PEEP, especially outside of ICU and/or PACU settings. During NIV there is chance of air leak around the face mask owing to presence of nasogastric tube. Care should be taken in this aspect. It is always practicable to keep the nasogastric tube on a bag rather than in aspiration to detect deleterious gastric insufflations due to NIV use [31].

Thoracic and thoracoabdominal surgery. As compared with conventional management, the use of NIV after cardiothoracic surgery is found to yield benefits in terms of improved oxygenation and decreased incidence of re-intubation [32]. Evidence suggests that prophylactic nasal CPAP reduces the incidence of pulmonary complications and shortened hospital stay after thoracoabdominal aortic aneurysm repair [30]. PPC remains to be the most frequent cause of death in patients after lung resection, where re-intubation increases the mortality up to 60–80% [30]. NIV therapy after thoracic surgery has been found to be safe without an increase in bronchial stump disruption and persistent air leaks [30]. NIV yields benefit in terms of improved gas exchange, reduced need for invasive ventilation, and reduced mortality in patients with respiratory failure after lung resection [30].

Bariatric surgery. Morbidly obese patients, often with comorbid disease such as OSA and obesity-hypoventilation syndrome have high risk of postoperative pulmonary complication and restrictive ventilator pathology [31]. NIV has been utilized to improve preoxygenation before induction and for postoperative oxygen therapy and thereby can reduce critical care admission. Concerns over the increased risk of anastomotic disruption in Roux-en-Y gastric bypass have been allayed by recent literature [31].

G. Postoperative Complications in Patients with OSA

Postoperative adverse events in patients with OSA are influenced by several factors such as types and duration of surgical procedures, timing of surgery such as inpatient or outpatient, and many other factors.

Postoperative respiratory failure in OSA: Amongst various respiratory complications after noncardiac surgery in OSA patients, postoperative respiratory failure is most worrisome. Memtsoudis et al., [33] reported a five-fold increase in the incidence of intubation and mechanical ventilation after orthopaedic surgery in OSA patients (n = 66000) and that of two-fold increase after general surgery (n = 48000). In a matched cohort study [34] analysis of data (Manitoban health administrative data between 1987 to 2008) regarding the postoperative outcomes in adult OSA patients including data up to 5 years before (undiagnosed OSA, n = 1,571), and any time after polysomnography (diagnosed OSA, n = 2,640) in comparison with the matched controls at low risk of having sleep apnea (n = 16,277). It was found that diagnosis of OSA and use of CPAP therapy was associated with a reduction in postoperative cardiovascular complications. The postoperative respiratory failure after elective surgery is higher in patients with obesity hypoventilation syndrome as compared to OSA [35]. The reason may be that a higher number of medical morbidities are associated with those having obesity hypoventilation syndrome (OHS) compared with those having OSA alone [36].

Unanticipated ICU transfer after surgery: Unanticipated ICU transfer can be used as an outcome measure among patients OSA excluding observation transfers to ICU [37].

Cardiovascular complications: A higher incidence of atrial fibrillation has been observed after orthopaedic and prostate surgery in patients with OSA. But whether it is a new onset atrial fibrillation or chronic atrial fibrillation diagnosed for the first time in perioperative period is unclear. Among adults undergoing major noncardiac surgery, unrecognized severe OSA was found to be considerably associated with increased risk of 30-day postoperative cardiovascular complications [38]. In spite of the increased independent association of SDB with postoperative cardiopulmonary adverse events, the diagnosis of SDB was not independently associated with an increased rate of in-hospital death [39].

Several studies have demonstrated a high prevalence of SDB in patients undergoing cardiovascular interventions, but data demonstrating an impact on perioperative adverse events remains to be surprisingly inconclusive [40]. OSA remains to be an important risk factor for postoperative adverse events in patients undergoing cardiac surgery [41]. OSA is a strong predictor of new-onset atrial fibrillation in the postoperative CABG patients leading to longer hospital stay [42]. Incidence of cardiovascular complication is even higher in the undiagnosed cases of OSA [43].

Postoperative delirium: Preoperative SDB (undiagnosed OSA) was found to be associated with increased incidence of postoperative delirium. A preoperative AHI of 19 or higher was associated with a six-fold increased risk of postoperative delirium [44]. History of OSA has been associated with postoperative delirium in a study involving patients undergoing after knee transplant [45]. Postoperative delirium has been found to be associated with absolute decreases in postoperative cerebral oxygen saturation in older patients undergoing cardiac surgery. Higher age, history of smoking, nocturnal breathing disorders, and intraoperative transfusion-- all have been identified as independent risk factors for postoperative delirium after cardiac surgery [44, 46].

Postoperative mortality: Sudden cardiac death is more likely to occur during sleep hours among OSA patients [47]. Lowest nocturnal oxygen desaturation and AHI are independent predictors of sudden cardiac death [48]. Mortality in OSA patients is also associated with additional insults like failed airway, unmonitored respiratory depression from opioid and/or sedative administration especially with PCA infusions and others [49].

Conclusion

OSA is often undiagnosed in the surgical population and leads to higher postoperative complications. Early clinical recognition of OSA helps to design a safer anesthesia care plan. NIV should be used as a part complete perioperative strategy including early identification of patient, targeted intraoperative management, cautious use of opioids and sedatives and careful postoperative monitoring in appropriate environment. Encouragement of patients for participation in self-management may help shorten length of hospital stay, reduce cost of care, and improve patient independence after discharge from hospital.

References

[1] American Society of Anesthesiologists Task Force on Perioperative Management of patients with obstructive sleep apnea. Practice guidelines for the perioperative management of patients with obstructive sleep apnea: an updated report by the American Society of Anesthesiologists Task Force on Perioperative Management of patients with obstructive sleep apnea. *Anesthesiology.* 2014;120(2):268-86. https://doi.org/10.1097/ALN.0000000000000053.

[2] Kaw R, Gali B, Collop N A. Perioperative care of patients with obstructive sleep apnea. *Curr. Treat Options Neurol. 2011*;13(5):496-507. https://doi.org/10.1007/s11940-011-0138-5.

[3] Peppard P E, Young T, Barnet J H, Palta M, Hagen E W, Hla K M. Increased prevalence of sleep-disordered breathing in adults. *Am. J. Epidemiol.* 2013;177(9):1006-14. https://doi.org/10.1093/aje/kws342.

[4] Punjabi N M. The epidemiology of adult obstructive sleep apnea. *Proc. Am. Thorac. Soc.* 2008;5(2):136-43. https://doi.org/10.1513/pats.200709-155MG.

[5] Suzuki N, Isono S, Ishikawa T, Kitamura Y, Takai Y, Nishino T. Submandible angle in nonobese patients with difficult tracheal intubation. *Anesthesiology.* 2007;106(5):916-23. https://doi.org/10.1097/01.anes.0000265150.71319.91.

[6] Chung F, Yegneswaran B, Herrera F, Shenderey A, Shapiro C M. Patients with difficult intubation may need referral to sleep clinics. *Anesth Analg.* 2008;107(3):915-20. https://doi.org/10.1213/ane.0b013e31817bd36f.

[7] Martínez G, Faber P. Obstructive sleep apnoea. *Contin. Educ. Anaesth. Crit. Care Pain.* 2011;11(1):5-8. https://doi.org/10.1093/bjaceaccp/mkq042.

[8] Chau E H, Mokhlesi B, Chung F. Obesity Hypoventilation Syndrome and Anesthesia. *Sleep Med. Clin.* 2013;8(1):135-147. https://doi.org/10.1016/j.jsmc.2012.11.006.

[9] Kaw R, Gay P C. Perioperative Management of Obstructive Sleep Apnea. *Curr. Sleep Medicine Rep.* 2015; 1:251-256. https://doi.org/10.1007/s40675-015-0029-5.

[10] Sleep-related breathing disorders in adults: recommendations for syndrome definition and measurement techniques in clinical research. The Report of an American Academy of Sleep Medicine Task Force. *Sleep.* 1999;22(5):667-89. https://doi.org/10.1093/ sleep/22.5.667.

[11] Reeder M K, Goldman M D, Loh L, Muir A D, Casey K R, Lehane J R. Late postoperative nocturnal dips in oxygen saturation in patients undergoing major abdominal vascular surgery. Predictive value of pre-operative overnight pulse oximetry. *Anaesthesia.* 1992;47(2):110-5. https://doi.org/10.1111/j.1365-2044.1992.tb02005.x.

[12] Gross J B, Bachenberg K L, Benumof J L, Caplan R A, Connis R T, Coté C J, Nickinovich D G, Prachand V, Ward D S, Weaver E M, Ydens L, Yu S; American Society of Anesthesiologists Task Force on Perioperative Management. Practice guidelines for the perioperative management of patients with obstructive sleep apnea: a report by the American Society of Anesthesiologists Task Force on Perioperative Management of patients with obstructive sleep apnea. *Anesthesiology.* 2006;104(5):1081-93; quiz 1117-8. https://doi.org/10.1097/00000542-200605000-00026.

[13] Bixler E O, Vgontzas A N, Lin H M, Ten Have T, Leiby B E, Vela-Bueno A, Kales A. Association of hypertension and sleep-disordered breathing. *Arch. Intern. Med.* 2000;160(15):2289-95. https://doi.org/10.1001/archinte.160. 15.2289.

[14] Cherniack N S. Apnea and periodic breathing during sleep. *N. Engl. J. Med.* 1999;341(13):985-7. https://doi.org/10.1056/NEJM199909233411310.

[15] Chan J, Sanderson J, Chan W, Lai C, Choy D, Ho A, Leung R. Prevalence of sleep-disordered breathing in diastolic heart failure. *Chest.* 1997;111(6):1488-93. https://doi.org/10.1378/chest.111.6.1488.

[16] Fichter J, Bauer D, Arampatzis S, Fries R, Heisel A, Sybrecht G W. Sleep-related breathing disorders are associated with ventricular arrhythmias in patients with an implantable cardioverter-defibrillator. *Chest.* 2002;122(2):558-61. https://doi.org/10.1378/chest.122.2.558.

[17] Kessler R, Chaouat A, Weitzenblum E, Oswald M, Ehrhart M, Apprill M, Krieger J. Pulmonary hypertension in the obstructive sleep apnoea syndrome: prevalence, causes and therapeutic consequences. *Eur. Respir. J.* 1996;9(4):787-94. https://doi.org/10.1183/09031936.96.09040787.

[18] Gislason T, Janson C, Vermeire P, Plaschke P, Björnsson E, Gislason D, Boman G. Respiratory symptoms, and nocturnal gastroesophageal reflux: a population-based

study of young adults in three European countries. *Chest.* 2002;121(1):158-63. https://doi.org/10.1378/chest.121.1.158.

[19] Fouladpour N, Jesudoss R, Bolden N, Shaman Z, Auckley D. Perioperative Complications in Obstructive Sleep Apnea Patients Undergoing Surgery: A Review of the Legal Literature. *Anesth. Analg.* 2016;122(1):145-51. https://doi.org/10.1213/ANE.0000000000000841. Erratum in: Anesth Analg. 2016;122(4): 1228-9.

[20] Kheterpal S, Martin L, Shanks A M, Tremper K K. Prediction and outcomes of impossible mask ventilation: a review of 50,000 anesthetics. *Anesthesiology.* 2009;110(4):891-7. https://doi.org/10.1097/ALN.0b013e31819b5b87.

[21] Bolden N, Smith CE, Auckley D, Makarski J, Avula R. Perioperative complications during use of an obstructive sleep apnea protocol following surgery and anesthesia. *Anesth. Analg.* 2007;105(6):1869-70. https://doi.org/10.1213/01.ane.0000295223.31946.b5.

[22] Boushra N N. Anaesthetic management of patients with sleep apnoea syndrome. *Can J Anaesth.* 1996;43(6):599-616. https://doi.org/10.1007/BF03011774. Erratum in: *Can. J. Anaesth.* 1996;43(11):1184.

[23] Murphy G S, Szokol J W, Marymont J H, Greenberg S B, Avram M J, Vender J S. Residual neuromuscular blockade and critical respiratory events in the postanesthesia care unit. *Anesth. Analg.* 2008;107(1):130-7. https://doi.org/10.1213/ane.0b013e31816d1268.

[24] Bailey P L, Lu J K, Pace N L, Orr J A, White J L, Hamber E A, Slawson M H, Crouch D J, Rollins D E. Effects of intrathecal morphine on the ventilatory response to hypoxia. *N. Engl. J. Med.* 2000;343(17):1228-34. https://doi.org/10.1056/NEJM200010263431705.

[25] Rudra A, Chatterjee S, Das T, Sengupta S, Maitra G, Kumar P. Obstructive sleep apnoea and anaesthesia. *Indian J. Crit. Care Med.* 2008;12(3):116-23. https://doi.org/10.4103/0972-5229.43680.

[26] Kessler R, Chaouat A, Schinkewitch P, Faller M, Casel S, Krieger J, Weitzenblum E. The obesity-hypoventilation syndrome revisited: a prospective study of 34 consecutive cases. *Chest.* 2001;120(2):369-76. https://doi.org/10.1378/chest.120.2.369.

[27] Squadrone V, Coha M, Cerutti E, Schellino M M, Biolino P, Occella P, Belloni G, Vilianis G, Fiore G, Cavallo F, Ranieri V M; Piedmont Intensive Care Units Network (PICUN). Continuous positive airway pressure for treatment of postoperative hypoxemia: a randomized controlled trial. *JAMA.* 2005;293(5):589-95. https://doi.org/10.1001/jama.293.5.589.

[28] Jensen C, Tejirian T, Lewis C, Yadegar J, Dutson E, Mehran A. Postoperative CPAP and BiPAP use can be safely omitted after laparoscopic Roux-en-Y gastric bypass. *Surg. Obes. Relat. Dis.* 2008;4(4):512-4. https://doi.org/10.1016/j.soard.2008.05.003.

[29] Pérez de Llano L A, Golpe R, Ortiz Piquer M, Veres Racamonde A, Vázquez Caruncho M, Caballero Muinelos O, Alvarez Carro, C, Short-term and long-term effects of nasal intermittent positive pressure ventilation in patients with obesity-

hypoventilation syndrome. *Chest.* 2005;128(2):587-94. https://doi.org/10.1378/chest.128.2.587.

[30] Bauchmuller K, Glossop A J. Non-invasive ventilation in the perioperative period. *BJA Education* 2016;16(9):299-304. https://doi.org/10.1093/bjaed/mkw009.

[31] Adesanya A O, Lee W, Greilich N B, Joshi G P. Perioperative management of obstructive sleep apnea. *Chest.* 2010;138(6):1489-98. https://doi.org/10.1378/chest.10-1108. Erratum in: *Chest.* 2011;140(5):1393.

[32] Hu G, Huang Y, Wei D, Shi Y. Efficacy, and safety of noninvasive ventilation in patients after cardiothoracic surgery: A PRISMA-compliant systematic review and meta-analysis. *Medicine (Baltimore).* 2016;95(38):e4734. https://doi.org/10.1097/MD.0000000000004734.

[33] Memtsoudis S, Liu S S, Ma Y, Chiu Y L, Walz J M, Gaber-Baylis L K, Mazumdar M. Perioperative pulmonary outcomes in patients with sleep apnea after noncardiac surgery. *Anesth. Analg.* 2011;112(1):113-21. https://doi.org/10.1213/ANE.0b013e3182009abf.

[34] Mutter T C, Chateau D, Moffatt M, Ramsey C, Roos L L, Kryger M. A matched cohort study of postoperative outcomes in obstructive sleep apnea: could preoperative diagnosis and treatment prevent complications? *Anesthesiology.* 2014;121(4):707-18. https://doi.org/10.1097/ALN.0000000000000407.

[35] Berry R B, Chediak A, Brown L K, Finder J, Gozal D, Iber C, Kushida C A, Morgenthaler T, Rowley J A, Davidson-Ward S L; NPPV Titration Task Force of the American Academy of Sleep Medicine. Best clinical practices for the sleep center adjustment of noninvasive positive pressure ventilation (NPPV) in stable chronic alveolar hypoventilation syndromes. *J. Clin. Sleep Med.* 2010;6(5): 491-509.

[36] Kaw R, Bhateja P, Paz Y Mar H, Hernandez A V, Ramaswamy A, Deshpande A, Aboussouan LS. Postoperative Complications in Patients With Unrecognized Obesity Hypoventilation Syndrome Undergoing Elective Noncardiac Surgery. *Chest.* 2016;149(1):84-91. https://doi.org/10.1378/chest.14-3216.

[37] Abboud F, Kumar R. Obstructive sleep apnea and insight into mechanisms of sympathetic overactivity. *J. Clin. Invest.* 2014;124(4):1454-7. https://doi.org/10.1172/JCI70420.

[38] Chan M T V, Wang C Y, Seet E, Tam S, Lai H Y, Chew E F F, Wu W K K, Cheng BCP, Lam CKM, Short TG, Hui DSC, Chung F; Postoperative Vascular Complications in Unrecognized Obstructive Sleep Apnea (POSA) Study Investigators. Association of Unrecognized Obstructive Sleep Apnea with Postoperative Cardiovascular Events in Patients Undergoing Major Noncardiac Surgery. *JAMA.* 2019;321(18):1788-1798. https://doi.org/10.1001/jama.2019.4783.

[39] Mokhlesi B, Hovda M D, Vekhter B, Arora V M, Chung F, Meltzer D O. Sleep-disordered breathing and postoperative outcomes after elective surgery: analysis of the nationwide inpatient sample. *Chest.* 2013;144(3):903-914. https://doi.org/10.1378/chest.12-2905.

[40] Casey K R, Teodorescu M. Postoperative Complications in Patients with Obstructive Sleep Apnea: Where Do We Stand? *J. Clin. Sleep Med.* 2015;11(10):1081-2. https://doi.org/10.5664/jcsm.5074.

[41] Nagappa M, Ho G, Patra J, Wong J, Singh M, Kaw R, Cheng D, Chung F. Postoperative Outcomes in Obstructive Sleep Apnea Patients Undergoing Cardiac Surgery: A Systematic Review and Meta-analysis of Comparative Studies. *Anesth. Analg.* 2017;125(6):2030-2037. https://doi.org/10.1213/ANE.0000000000002558.

[42] Patel S V, Gill H, Shahi D, Rajabalan A, Patel P, Sonani R, Bhatt P, Rodriguez R D, Bautista M, Deshmukh A, Gonzalez J V, Patel S.. High risk for obstructive sleep apnea hypopnea syndrome predicts new onset atrial fibrillation after cardiac surgery: a retrospective analysis. *Sleep Breath.* 2018;22(4):1117-1124. https://doi.org/10.1007/s11325-018-1645-3.

[43] Gottlieb D J, Yenokyan G, Newman A B, O'Connor G T, Punjabi N M, Quan S F, Redline S, Resnick H E, Tong E K, Diener-West M, Shahar E. Prospective study of obstructive sleep apnea and incident coronary heart disease and heart failure: the sleep heart health study. *Circulation.* 2010;122(4):352-60. https://doi.org/10.1161/CIRCULATIONAHA.109.901801.

[44] Roggenbach J, Klamann M, von Haken R, Bruckner T, Karck M, Hofer S. Sleep-disordered breathing is a risk factor for delirium after cardiac surgery: a prospective cohort study. *Crit. Care.* 2014;18(5):477. https://doi.org/10.1186/s13054-014-0477-1.

[45] Flink B J, Rivelli S K, Cox E A, White W D, Falcone G, Vail T P, Young C C, Bolognesi M P, Krystal A D, Trzepacz P T, Moon R E, Kwatra M M. Obstructive sleep apnea and incidence of postoperative delirium after elective knee replacement in the nondemented elderly. *Anesthesiology.* 2012;116(4):788-96. https://doi.org/10.1097/ALN.0b013e31824b94fc.

[46] Eertmans W, De Deyne C, Genbrugge C, Marcus B, Bouneb S, Beran M, Fret T, Gutermann H, Boer W, Vander Laenen M, Heylen R, Mesotten D, Vanelderen P, Jans F. Association between postoperative delirium and postoperative cerebral oxygen desaturation in older patients after cardiac surgery. *Br. J. Anaesth.* 2020;124(2):146-153. https://doi.org/10.1016/j.bja.2019.09.042.

[47] Carr G E, Mokhlesi B, Gehlbach B K. Acute cardiopulmonary failure from sleep-disordered breathing. *Chest.* 2012;141(3):798-808. https://doi.org/10.1378/chest.11-1389.

[48] Kaw R, Chung F, Pasupuleti V, Mehta J, Gay P C, Hernandez AV. Meta-analysis of the association between obstructive sleep apnoea and postoperative outcome. *Br. J. Anaesth.* 2012;109(6):897-906. https://doi.org/10.1093/bja/aes308.

[49] Marin J M, Carrizo S J, Vicente E, Agusti A G. Long-term cardiovascular outcomes in men with obstructive sleep apnoea-hypopnoea with or without treatment with continuous positive airway pressure: an observational study. *Lancet.* 2005;365(9464):1046-53. https://doi.org/10.1016/S0140-6736(05)71141-7.

Chapter 17

Anesthesiology-Perioperative Medicine: Risk of Postoperative Complications in Patients with Obstructive Sleep Apnea Following Otorhinolaryngological Surgery

Andrea De Vito[1,*], MD, PhD
Massimo Terenzoni[2], MD
Stefano Oldani[3], MD
Tiziano Perrone[4], MD
Damiano Giardini[1], MD
Giorgia Ciammetti[1], MD
Francesco Moretti[4], MD
and Maurizio Fusari[2], MD

[1]Head and Neck Department, ENT Unit, Ravenna-Lugo Hospitals, Health Local Agency of Romagna, Italy
[2]Department of General Surgery, Anaesthesia and Critical Care Unit, Ravenna Hospital, Health Local Agency of Romagna, Italy
[3]Department Thoracic Diseases, Pulmonary Operative Unit, Forlì Hospital, Health Local Agency of Romagna, Italy
[4]Head and Neck Department, ENT Unit, Forlì – Faenza Hospitals, Health Local Agency of Romagna, Italy

[*] Corresponding Author's Email: dr.andrea.devito@gmail.com.

In: Obstructive Sleep Apnea in Pulmonary Critical Care
Editors: Antonio M. Esquinas and Takatoshi Kasai
ISBN: 979-8-88697-858-2

Abstract

Surgery of the upper airway performed in patients affected by obstructive sleep apnoea (OSA) could potentially cause peri-operative complications related to the specific surgical techniques, as well as the pathophysiology of OSA and could expose the patients at risk of respiratory failure more than other surgical procedures. The postoperative management should be the result of the protocols and strategies adopted in pre- and intra-operative steps. The severity of OSA is considered a significant factor in decision making procedures to adopt in postoperative period, considering that most of surgery of upper airway represents a relative or absolute contraindication for restarting the CPAP therapy at the end of the operation. Postoperative surveillance in the recovery room is recommended for OSA patients with low to medium risk of OSA, whereas the intensive care unit admission is recommended for severe OSA patients, who already apply CPAP. CPAP with full face mask could be a reasonable solution, to prevent dangerous apneas in postoperative period after nasal surgery, whereas CPAP treatment could not be applied after pharyngoplasty or functional sinus surgery. Patients with extremely severe grade of OSA could need prolonged tracheal intubation or the necessity of performing a temporary tracheotomy.

Keywords: obstructive sleep apnea, postoperative complication, postoperative respiratory failure, upper airway, pharyngoplasty, nasal surgery

Introduction

Obstructive sleep apnea (OSA) is characterized by repetitive complete (apnea) or partial (hypopnea) obstruction of upper airways (UA) during sleep. OSA represents the most common sleep-disordered breathing (SDB) disease, and its incidence rates between 5 and 17% in middle-aged population and 20 to 60% in people over 65yo [1-3].

OSA is associated with excessive daytime sleepiness, and several co-morbidities, including hypertension, myocardial infarction, stroke, hyperlipidemia, glucose intolerance and diabetes, arrhythmias, pulmonary hypertension, congestive heart failure and depression [4, 5].

Continuous positive airway pressure (CPAP) has been considered the gold standard for the treatment of OSA, decreasing apnea/hyopopnea events, hypoxia, and sleep disturbance [6]. However, surgery of the upper airways could represent a no-CPAP alternative if the apneas/hypopnea events are related to the preponderance of anatomical factors [7].

Hence, OSA patients who undergo surgery of the upper airway, could be potentially exposed to peri-operative complications related to the specific surgical techniques performed, as well as the pathophysiology of OSA and which could expose the patients at risk of respiratory failure more than other surgical procedures [8].

As a general view, the mechanism behind the increase in respiratory and cardiac complications in OSA patients in the postoperative period is quite complicated. It involves a complex interaction between the respiratory effect of drug-induced anesthesia and post-operative time and the UA pathological collapsibility, typical of OSA anatomical endotype (high Pcrit) [9].

General anesthesia (GA), narcotics and sedatives can worsen upper airway's collapse by enhancing pharyngeal muscle relaxation, reducing alveolar ventilation, and blunting arousal from sleep, increasing as a consequence the pathological effect of non-anatomical OSA endotypes on upper airway (muscular impairment, high loop gain, and low arousal threshold) [10].

Opioids depress the central response to hypoxia, producing a decrease of tidal volume at lower dosage, and an additional decrease of respiratory rate at higher dosage. These effects occur with both acute and chronic use of opioids [11].

Neuromuscular blocking drugs are widely used intraoperatively in order to facilitate tracheal intubation and surgical relaxation. However, these drugs decrease airway tone and blunt the protective airway reflex. Besides, it has been reported that they have residual effect also in the postoperative period, despite the administration of reversal agents, hence causing respiratory complications such as decreased inspiratory flow, upper airway obstruction, oxygen desaturation, impaired protection reflexes, respiratory muscle weakness, pneumonia and reintubation. Residual neuromuscular blockage is quite common and even mild levels might have serious effects [12].

Moreover, in the postoperative period some changes in rapid eye movement (REM) sleep have been documented, which could potentially worsen the grade of OSA severity. In fact, pain and postanesthetic effects can reduce REM sleep, leading to a rebound increase in REM sleep 3 to 5 days after surgery. This is a worsening factor for OSA, since REM sleep has more unstable breathing, less airways muscle tone, decreased arousal response to hypoxia, hypercapnia, and airway occlusion [9].

OSA is also an independent risk factor for difficult airway management. Intubation is reported to be difficult in 22-44% of OSA patients compared to 2-3% of patients without OSA. In 5% of cases the attempt to intubate OSA patients was not successful [13, 14].

The surgery of the upper airway represents a specific challenge for postoperative anaesthesiologic complications in OSA patients because its potential negative impact on upper airways patency in postoperative period, and consequently difficulty in applying PAP therapy [15].

Careful pre-operative, intra-operative and post-operative assessment, and management of OSA patients is of pivotal importance, aiming to a reduction of postoperative respiratory failure.

Preoperative Management

Identifying the presence of OSA in the preoperative setting is essential for the prevention of potential perioperative complications, especially in elective GA surgical procedures.

In absence of a prior diagnosis of OSA, attention should be paid to clues of OSA detectable in the patient's medical history, recorded from the patient and/or the bed partner, and in the clinical examination.

The risk of OSA is strongly related with BMI, and in most of obese OSA patients, obesity hypoventilation syndrome (OHS) is also reported [16]. The prevalence of OSA progressively increases up to the sixth-seventh decade and is up to two/three times more common in males than females. Family history of snoring or OSA could be due both to genetic predisposition, and behavioral or environmental factors. Smoking increases the risk or worsens OSA. Wetter et al. reported that current smokers were nearly three times more likely to have OSA than previous or non-smokers [16]. Moreover, the strong correlation between age (range 50-70 years), BMI>30 and severity of OSA should be considered [17].

In this patients' population at high risk of OSA, snoring history should be investigated, witnessed apneas, daytime sleepiness and other symptoms associated with OSA. A variety of substances and drugs, including alcohol, benzodiazepines, and sedatives, can exacerbate OSA. The risk of OSA has also increased in patients with a variety of cardiovascular medical conditions such as pulmonary hypertension, atrial fibrillation, heart failure. All these considerations are summarized in Table 1 [18, 19].

Clinical examination and UA evaluation allow the physician to recognize some typical anatomic patterns strongly related to OSA (palatine tonsils hypertrophy, base of the tongue hypertrophy, soft palate ptosis, micro-retrognatia) associated or not with other anatomical abnormalities, such as septal nasal deviation, inferior turbinates hypertrophy, limited mouth opening, which could represent also risk factors for difficult orotracheal and naso tracheal intubation [21, 22].

Table 1. Perioperative evaluation of patients with possible OSA

Past medical history	History from patient and bed partner	Physical findings
History of "difficult airway"	Loud snoring	"Suspect" airway, Mallampati score 3 or 4
Arterial hypertension	Witnessed periods of apnea	Neck circumference: >43 cm in men >40 cm in women
Other cardiovascular diseases	Repeated nocturnal awakening	Tonsillar enlargement
Prior evaluation in a sleep laboratory	Marked daytime sleepiness	Obesity, (Particularly BMI >35 kg/m^2)
Metabolic syndrome	Headache on awakening in the morning	

Table n 1 Adapted from ASA guidelines of perioperative management of patients with OSA.

Table 2. STOP-Bang questionnaire [25]

Snoring	Do you snore loudly (loudly enough to be heard through closed doors at night)?
Tiredness	Do you often feel tired or sleepy during the day?
Observed apnea	Has anyone observed you to stop breathing, choke, or gasp in your sleep?
Pressure	Do you have high blood pressure, or are you are being treated for it?
Body Mass Index (BMI)	Is the body-mass index over 35 kg/m^2?
Age	Is the patient over 50 years old?
Neck circumference	Is the patient's neck circumference >43 cm (men) or >40 cm (women)?
Gender	Is the patient male?
Low risk of OSA: yes to 0-2 questions Intermediate risk o OSA: yes to 3-4 questions High risk of OSA: yes to 5-8 questions, or yes to 2 or more STOP questions + male gender or BMI >35 or neck circumference (43 cm male, 41cm female)	

High risk patients should be referred to a sleep specialist to rule out OSA or other sleep breathing disorders or to begin the right treatment, such as continuous positive air pressure (CPAP) the first-line treatment in OSA patients.

Alternatively, if the procedure cannot be delayed the patients at high risk of OSA could be red-flagged for a proper management.

Intraoperative Management

Premedication

Sedatives such as benzodiazepines impair airway function, elevating arousal threshold. It is therefore recommended great attention in prescribing benzodiazepines preoperatively to OSA patients. No hard data exists to support this recommendation against sedatives, but potential alternatives should be used. For instance, centrally acting sedating α2-agonists such as clonidine and dexmedetomidine can be the sedative of choice in OSA patients [23].

Techniques of Anesthesia

As a general principle, the technique of anesthesia in OSA patients, as in any patient, should be tailored to the patient's comorbidities and to the type of procedure that is to be performed. In OSA patients, where appropriate, local or regional anesthesia techniques such as peripheral nerve blocks rather than general anesthesia are strongly recommended by both the American Society of Anesthesiologists and Society of Anesthesia and Sleep Medicine [18, 24].

If GA is required, short acting and easily managed drugs should be preferred. A combination of propofol and remifentanil, or of sevoflurane and remifentanil, are therefore suggested, since these drugs allow safe GA for OSA patients without elevating the postoperative AHI over its pre -operative value [18, 24].

If the patient is to be sedated, the potentially adverse effect of sedation on UA patency has to be carefully considered. CPAP could be provided intraoperatively by ventilating machine, which is available in any operating theater. However, every time the patient maintains spontaneous respiration during a mild or moderate sedation, oximetry and even capnography should be continuously monitored [18, 24].

Securing the Airway in Case of General Anesthesia

The anesthesiologist should be aware of the higher rate of difficult intubation in OSA patients and may choose among a broad series of intubation techniques, including the use of a video laryngoscope or fiber-optic awake intubation under surface anesthesia, in order to lessen the risk of an unsuccessful intubation attempt [25].

Preoxygenation with 100% oxygen in a 25° head-up position can extend the time to desaturation. During apnea, more oxygen is absorbed compared to the amount of carbon dioxide produced, leading to an intrapulmonary negative pressure, which augments ventilation, if the patency of the airway is pristine. Supplying CPAP up to 10 cm H_2O with oxygen for 5 minutes before intubation can also reduce the drop in functional residual capacity (FRC) consequent to change in body position, paralysis, and absorptive atelectasis from high concentration of oxygen, thereby helping to prolong nonhypoxic apnea up to a minute [26].

The head elevation laryngoscopy position (HELP) provides an improved laryngeal view by aligning the pharyngeal and laryngeal axis when the angle of neck flexion over the chest is about 35°. In morbid obese OSA patient, this can only be achieved by a 35° flexion of lower cervical spine on the chest and a 90° extension of the head on the neck at the atlanto-occipital joint also known as the ramp position [27].

Intraoperative Ventilation Strategies and Extubation

As soon as the patient is intubated, airway patency is secured. However, other aspects must be kept in mind while ventilating invasively, since the majority of OSA patients are also obese.

Tidal volumes (Vt) must be calculated on the basis of ideal body weight, since considering total body weight may overestimate Vt by 20%–50%. Such overdistension of the lungs might increase postoperative pulmonary complications.

Additionally, positive end-expiratory pressure (PEEP) titrated up to 10 cm H_2O can reduce the occurrence of atelectasis after laparoscopic bariatric surgery.

There is no strong evidence to recommend a specific ventilatory modality while ventilating OSA patients during GA. Nevertheless, in patients undergoing laparoscopic surgery, pressure control ventilation has been reported to result in better oxygenation when compared to volume-controlled ventilation [26, 28, 29].

At the end of the procedure, during the extubation, some review articles suggest that patients with OSA should be extubated only when fully awake. The patient should not only have an adequate spontaneous breath but should also be able to open the eyes when spoken to, and should be oriented. Whenever possible, the patient should be put in the lateral position or, if not feasible, the head of the bed should be raised, and this position maintained until recovery [30].

Lastly, before extubation, any clinically significant residual muscle relaxation must be ruled out by quantitative neuromuscular monitoring. Residual neuromuscular blockade should be antagonized with cholinesterase inhibitors or, even better, with sugammadex, since the first can impair neuromuscular transmission, threatening the integrity of the upper airway [12].

Upper Airways Surgery

It is possible distinguish three groups of OSA patients, who undergo surgery of the upper airway. The first group is represented by OSA patients surgically treated at the upper airway for several indications unrelated to sleep disturbances, without impact the respiratory patency of the upper respiratory tract, such as ear-surgery, thyroid, or neck surgery without alteration of the laryngotracheal tract. The second group is related to OSA patients, in whom surgery of the upper airways could alter the patency of the respiratory tract, such as oncological surgery, sinu-nasal surgery, or maxillo-facial surgery.

In the first case, post-operative care consists of general postoperative surgical management applied in all surgical patients affected by OSA. In the second case, the presence or absence of tracheostomy is fundamental, which allows direct support of the inferior respiratory tract and avoids the onset of apnoea events.

The third group is represented by OSA patients who undergo surgical therapy aimed at reducing or resolving apnoeic events. The most frequent surgical treatments include nasal surgery (septoplasty or endoscopic sinu-nasal functional surgery), surgery of the soft palate (pharyngoplasty in all its various techniques and modifications) and hypopharyngeal surgery (robotic surgery of the base of the tongue, epiglottoplasty, reduction of the tongue base by coblator or hypoglossal stimulation).

In these patients it will be necessary to adopt specific post-operative management manoeuvres, that consider the altered patency of the upper airways [15, 31, 32].

General Postoperative Management

The postoperative management should be the result of the protocols and strategies adopted in pre- and intra-operative steps. Indeed, the careful patient's preoperative clinical assessment, the right risk factors evaluation, and the intra-operative strategy, allow defining the postoperative algorithms and pharmacological schemes. For these reasons, postoperative surveillance in the recovery room is recommended for all patients with low to medium risk of OSA, whereas the intensive care unit admission is recommended for high-risk patients with severe OSA, even if already treated with CPAP at home. The main recommendations for post-operative management of OSA patients are:

1. Continuous monitoring of vital functions, especially respiratory rate and SPO2. Special attention is required to detect early signs of respiratory failure, such as bradypnea (FR $\leq$ 8 acts/min, at least three episodes), apnoea ($\geq$ 10", even a single episode), or major desaturation (<90%, at least three episodes).
2. Fluid management. OSA patients are often affected by cardiovascular comorbidities such as chronic congestive heart failure, arterial blood hypertension, atrial fibrillation, or ischemic coronary artery disease. In these patients, clinicians should consider cautious fluid administration to avoid life threatening events such as acute pulmonary edema. In addition, some experts suggest that patients with OSA may benefit from infusion of crystalloids with lower salt content (Ringer's Lactate for example) rather than normal saline (NaCl 0.9%). The rationale is that the infusion of fluids with high salt content, along with supine position typical of the postoperative

period, might result in rostral fluid shift, thereby worsening OSA [33].

3. Multimodal analgesic therapy, with combined loco-regional or plessic techniques. As aforementioned, some analgesic drugs, especially opioids, have a respiratory depressant effect. To avoid this detrimental effect, a valid strategy in the management of pain control in post-operative patients with OSA is the so-called multimodal analgesia. This is a combination of an opioid drug at the lowest needed dose with one or more other agents such as: nonsteroidal anti-inflammatory drugs (NSAIDs), cyclooxygenase-2 inhibitors (COX-2 inh), paracetamol, peripheral nerve blockers, glucocorticoids, gabapentin, pregabalin or even ketamine. In a large population based retrospective cohort study of postoperative analgesia in over 180.000 OSA patients who underwent hip or knee orthopaedic procedures, multimodal analgesia was associated with a decreased risk of critical care admission (OR 0.60), mechanical ventilation (OR 0.23), gastrointestinal complications (OR 0.65) and resulted in a 15% sparing of opioid prescriptions [34].
4. Absolute contraindication for the supine position. Postoperative OSA patients should be maintained in the upright or semi-upright position, or even in the lateral position, whenever feasible. In fact, supine position may worsen OSA especially in patients with positional OSA. Supine position also increases the passive pharyngeal collapsibility and rostral fluid shift, narrowing the upper airways' diameter [35, 36].
5. If necessary, administer opioid antagonists or benzodiazepines (naloxone- flumazenil) to clear the respiratory suppressant effects of these drugs.

The Role of Positive Airway Pressure (PAP) Therapies

PAP therapies, especially CPAP, are the cornerstone of treatment of OSA. It is therefore advisable that OSA patients already in nocturnal PAP therapy keep using their home devices in the postoperative period. Instead, for those patients without a previous diagnosis of OSA, or for OSA patients non-compliant to PAP therapies, PAP might be titrated as soon as apnoea, hypoxemia or hypoventilation occurs.

It is important to underline the role that PAP therapies play in the postoperative hours. PAP contrasts OSA but, at the same time, keeps the lung inflated, hence preventing atelectasis, especially when the patient becomes bed ridden or develops impairment in cough due to post procedural pain. Moreover, some small studies show a close interaction between nocturnal hypoxemia, sleep disruption from untreated OSA and pain sensitivity. According to these studies, intermittent hypoxia may worsen postoperative pain control; therefore, sleep restoration with CPAP treatment might improve pain control [37].

Despite these rationales, there is no strong evidence of improved outcomes for OSA patients treated with CPAP in the postoperative setting. For instance, one meta-analysis by Nagappa et al. reported no difference in postoperative complications with or without CPAP treatment, although treated patients showed a lower postoperative AHI and a trend toward a shorter hospital stay (-0.4 days). However, this analysis was limited by the small sample size and by the inclusion of both suspected and known OSA [41]. On the other hand, two large cohort studies, not included in the aforementioned analysis, showed that CPAP was associated with a reduction in cardiovascular complications and particularly unplanned reintubations [38, 39].

In addition, the Official European Respiratory Society/American Thoracic Society (ERS/ATS) clinical practice guidelines concerning non-invasive ventilation for acute respiratory failure (ARF) published in 2017, pointed out the pivotal role of PAP therapies in the treatment of postoperative ARF [40]. Physiological and imaging studies have shown that CPAP and NIV improve lung aeration, blood oxygenation, and reduce the occurrence of atelectasis without adverse haemodynamic effects during the post-operative period after extubation [36, 37]. Moreover, better outcomes were reported in postoperative patients promptly treated with PAP therapies for ARF. In fact, the pooled analysis of the data performed in the guidelines showed that PAP compared to standard oxygen therapy led to a decrease in mortality (RR 0.28), in need for intubation (RR 0.27) and even in the incidence of nosocomial pneumonia (RR 0.20). Both CPAP and bilevel NIV are therefore effective to improve outcomes in patients with post-operative ARF, particularly after abdominal and thoracic surgery, but also after cardiac surgery [41-43].

All these data suggest that PAP therapies are recommended in the treatment of postoperative ARF, whether the patient is affected by OSA or not. Additionally, in patients with OSA, PAP therapies might also prevent the development of postoperative ARF, hence being an effective tool in the postoperative setting.

Postopertive Management of Surgical OSA Patients

Most upper airway surgical procedures performed for OSA represents a relative or absolute contraindication for restarting the CPAP therapy at the end of the operation:

1. Nasal surgery is frequently performed in OSA patients as a single surgery or combined with oropharyngeal and/or hypopharyngeal surgical procedures [44]. In postoperative period, mucosal tears, nasal packing, and intranasal splints can represent a contraindication for the instant CPAP application in the postoperative period. Consequently, for simple septoplasty with or without turbinoplasty, observation in a medium or high care unit if the packs are in place is advisable, and in the case of severe OSA CPAP with full face mask could be a reasonable solution, to prevent dangerous apneas. The effectiveness of a therapeutic alternative, such as ventilation channel inside the nasal pack, is not feasible [15].
2. If functional endoscopic sinus surgery (FESS) or rhinoplasty is combined with septoplasty, major concerns in applying CPAP as postoperative care unit is justify by the performance of delicate surgical maneuvers such as pyramidal osteotomies and tip work in rhinoplasty or etmoidal deiscences in FESS. An early application of CPAP could alter the cosmetic results in rhinoplasty or determine the risk of pneumoencefalus or orbital complications in FESS.
3. Finally, pharyngoplasty with or without tonsillectomy and/or hypopahryngeal surgery represent a real challenge for the immediate application of CPAP. On one hand the postoperative edema and/or hematomas could temporally increase the AHI, because of the increasing of the upper airway narrowing; on the other hand, the early application of positive pressure during the CPAP could facilitate the risk of postoperative bleeding. Mortality rate of 0.2% at 30-day after pharyngoplasty has been reported [32, 45].

The severity of OSA was considered a significant factor in decision making procedure to adopt in postoperative period, considering that the higher a patient's AHI, the earlier one would recommend restarting CPAP. The possible solution to apply in relation to AHI grade and upper airway surgery could be the observation of patients in PACU or ICU until adequate control of breathing and oxygen saturations are documented, cardiac monitoring with continuous pulse oximetry and supplemental O2 as needed, and the positional therapy with head of bed elevation, and lateral decubitus positioning if possible.

Patients with extremely severe grade of OSA could need prolonged tracheal intubation or the necessity of performing a temporary tracheotomy. Supplemental oxygen should be administered with caution because the ventilation process may be dependent on its "hypoxic" drive and may increase the duration of apneic episodes and may hinder detection of atelectasis, transient apnea, and hypoventilation by pulse oximetry [46].

Conclusion

Identifying the presence of OSA in the preoperative setting is of pivotal importance for the prevention of potential perioperative complications, especially when the surgical procedure is elective. STOP-Bang questionnaire has shown to be accurate in predicting moderate to severe OSA in surgical patients (sensitivity of 100% predicting AHI >30 i.e., severe OSA). Great attention must be paid in prescribing benzodiazepines preoperatively to OSA patients. In OSA patients, where appropriate, local, or regional anesthesia techniques such as peripheral nerve blocks rather than GA are strongly recommended. If GA is required, short acting, easily managed drugs should be preferred. A combination of propofol and remifentanil, or of sevoflurane and remifentanil, are therefore suggested.

The anesthesiologist should be aware about the higher rate of difficult intubation in OSA patients and may choose among a broad series of intubation techniques in order to lessen the risk of an unsuccessful intubation attempt. Preoxygenation with 100% oxygen in a 25° head-up position can prolong the time to desaturation during the intubation timing. At the end of the procedure, during the extubation, some review articles suggest that patients with OSA should be extubated only when fully awake. The post-operative surveillance in OSA patients requires special attention to detect early signs of respiratory failure or episodes of bradypnea or apneas, or major desaturation episodes. Postoperative surveillance in the recovery room is recommended for OSA patients with low to medium risk of OSA, whereas the intensive care unit admission is recommended for severe OSA patients, who already apply CPAP. PAP therapies are recommended for the prevention and treatment of postoperative acute respiratory failure, hence being an effective tool in the postoperative setting. CPAP with full face mask could be a reasonable solution, to prevent dangerous apneas after nasal surgery, whereas prolonged intubation or temporary tracheotomy should be considered for extremely severe grade of OSA.

References

[1] Heinzer R, S Vat, P Marques-Vidal, H Marti-Soler, D Andries, N Tobback, V Mooser, M Preisig, A Malhotra, G Waeber, P Vollenweider, M Tafti, J Haba-Rubio. Prevalence of sleep-disordered breathing in the general population: the HypnoLaus study. *Lancet Respir Med*, 2015, 3(4), 310e8.

[2] Lee, JJ; Sundar, KM. Evaluation and Management of Adults with Obstructive Sleep Apnea Syndrome. *Lung*., 2021 Mar 13. doi: 10.1007/s00408-021-00426-w. Epub ahead of print. *PMID*: 33713177.

[3] Osman, AM, Carter, SG, Carberry, JC, Eckert, DJ. Obstructive sleep apnea: Current perspectives. *Nat. Sci. Sleep*., 2018, 10, 21–34. doi: 10.2147/NSS.S124657.

[4] Shahar, E, CW Whitney, S Redline, ET Lee, AB Newman, FJ Nieto, GT O'Connor, LL Boland, JE Schwartz, JM Samet. Sleep-disordered breathing and cardiovascular disease: cross-sectional results of the sleep heart health study. *Am J Respir Crit Care Med*, 2001, 163, 19-25.

[5] Bosi, M, De Vito, A, Gobbi, R, Poletti, V, Vicini, C. The importance of obstructive sleep apnoea and hypopnea pathophysiology for customized therapy. *Eur Arch Otorhinolaryngology*., 2017 Mar, 274(3), 1251-1261. doi: 10.1007/s00405-016-4223-y. Epub 2016 Jul 28. PMID: 27470114.

[6] CPAP Treatment for Adults with Obstructive Sleep Apnea: Review of the Clinical and Cost-Effectiveness and Guidelines [Internet]. Ottawa (ON): *Canadian Agency for Drugs and Technologies in Health*; 2013 Nov 18. PMID: 24741719.

[7] De Vito A, Woodson BT, Koka V, Cammaroto G, Iannella G, Bosi M, Pelucchi S, Filograna-Pignatelli GR, El Chater P, Vicini C. OSA Upper Airways Surgery: A Targeted Approach. *Medicina* (Kaunas). 2021 Jul 6;57(7):690. doi: 10.3390/medicina57070690. PMID: 34356971; PMCID: PMC8305825.

[8] Adesanya, AO, Lee W, Greilich NB, Joshi GP. Perioperative Management of Obstructive Sleep Apnea. *Chest*, 2010, 138, 1489–1498. doi:10.1378/chest.10-1108.

[9] Wolfe, RM, Pomerantz, J, Miller, DE, Weiss-Coleman, R, Solomonides, T. Obstructive Sleep Apnea: Preoperative Screening and Postoperative Care. *J. Am. Board Fam. Med.*, 2016, 29, 263–275. doi:10.3122/jabfm.2016.02.150085.

[10] Thomas J Altree, Frances Chung, Matthew TV Chan, Danny J Eckert. Vulnerability to postoperative complications in obstructive sleep apnea: importance of phenotypes. *Anesthesia & Analgesia*, 2021, 132(5), 13281337.

[11] Zutler, MC, Holty, JE. Opioids, Sleep, and Sleep-Disordered Breathing. *Curr. Pharm. Des*., 2011, 17, 1443–1449. doi:10.2174/138161211796197070.

[12] Khawaja Rashid Hafeez, Arvind Tuteja, Mandeep Singh, David T Wong, Mahesh Nagappa, Frances Chung, Jean Wong. Postoperative complications with

neuromuscular blocking drugs and/or reversal agents in obstructive sleep apnea patients: a systematic review. *BMC Anesthesiol.*, 2018, 18, 91. doi:10.1186/s12871-018-0549-x.

[13] Langeron O, E Masso, C Huraux, M Guggiari, A Bianchi, P Coriat, B Riou Prediction of Difficult Mask Ventilation. *Anesthesiology*, 2000, 92, 1229–1236. doi:10.1097/00000542-200005000-00009.

[14] Siyam, MA, Benhamou, D, Difficult Endotracheal Intubation in Patients with Sleep Apnea Syndrome. *Anesth. Analg.*, 2002, 95, 1098–1102. doi:10.1097/00000539-200210000-00058.

[15] Cohen JC, Larrabee YC, Weinstein AL, Stewart MG. Use of continuous positive airway pressure after rhinoplasty, septoplasty, and sinus surgery: A survey of current practice patterns. *Laryngoscope.* 2015 Nov;125(11):2612-6. doi: 10.1002/lary.25336. Epub 2015 May 6. PMID: 25946236.

[16] Wetter DW, TB Young, TR Bidwell, MS Badr, M Palta. Smoking as a risk factor for sleep-disordered breathing. *Arch Intern Med*, 1994, 154, 2219.

[17] Peppard, PE, Young, T, Barnet, JH, Palta, M, Hagen, EW, Hla, KM. Increased prevalence of sleep-disordered breathing in adults. *Am J Epidemiol*, 2013, 177(9), 1006–1014. 4.

[18] Practice Guidelines for the Perioperative Management of Patients with Obstructive Sleep Apnea. *Anesthesiology*, 2014, 120, 268–286. doi:10.1097/ ALN.0000000000000053.

[19] Flavia Petrini, Ida Di Giacinto, Rita Cataldo, Clelia Esposito, Vittorio Pavoni, Paolo Donato, Antonella Trolio, Guido Merli, Massimiliano Sorbello, Paolo Pelosi Obesity Task Force for the SIAARTI Airway Management Study Group. Obesity Task Force for the SIAARTI Airway Management Study Group. Perioperative and periprocedural airway management and respiratory safety for the obese patient: 2016 SIAARTI Consensus. *Minerva Anestesiol.*, 2016, 82 (12), 1314-1335.

[20] Luo, J, Huang, R, Zhong, X, Xiao, Y, Zhou, J. STOP-Bang questionnaire is superior to Epworth sleepiness scales, Berlin questionnaire, and STOP questionnaire in screening obstructive sleep apnea hypopnea syndrome patients. *Chin. Med. J. (Engl).*, 2014, 127, 3065–70.

[21] Chung, F, Yang, Y, Liao, P. Predictive Performance of the STOP-Bang Score for Identifying Obstructive Sleep Apnea in Obese Patients. *Obes. Surg.*, 2013, 23, 2050–2057. doi:10.1007/s11695-013-1006-z.

[22] Rundo, JV. Obstructive sleep apnea basics. *Cleve Clin J Med.*, 2019 Sep, 86(9 Suppl 1), 2-9. doi: 10.3949/ccjm.86.s1.02. PMID: 31509498.

[23] Chung, F, Ankichetty, S, Wong, J. A systematic review of the effects of sedatives and anesthetics in patients with obstructive sleep apnea. *J. Anaesthesiol. Clin. Pharmacol.*, 2011, 27, 447. doi:10.4103/0970-9185.86574.

[24] Stavros G Memtsoudis, Crispiana Cozowicz, Mahesh Nagappa, Jean Wong, Girish P Joshi, David T Wong, Anthony G Doufas, Meltem Yilmaz, Mark H Stein, Megan L Krajewski, Mandeep Singh, Lukas Pichler, Satya Krishna Ramachandran, Frances Chung. Society of Anesthesia and Sleep Medicine Guideline on Intraoperative Management of Adult Patients with Obstructive Sleep Apnea. *Anesth. Analg.*, 2018, 127, 967–987. doi:10.1213/ANE.0000000000003434.

[25] Fassbender, P, Herbstreit, F, Eikermann, M, Teschler, H, Peters, J. Obstructive Sleep Apnea: A Perioperative Risk Factor. *Dtsch. Aerzteblatt Online*, 2016, doi:10.3238/arztebl.2016.0463.

[26] Kaw, R, Wong, J, Mokhlesi, B. Obesity and Obesity Hypoventilation, Sleep Hypoventilation, and Postoperative Respiratory Failure. *Anesth. Analg.*, 2021, 132, 1265–1273. doi:10.1213/ANE.0000000000005352.

[27] Collins, JS, Lemmens, HJM, Brodsky, JB, Brock-Utne, JG, Levitan, RM. Laryngoscopy and Morbid Obesity: A Comparison of the 'Sniff' and 'Ramped' Positions. *Obes. Surg.*, 2004, 14, 1171–1175. doi:10.1381/0960892042386869.

[28] Hesham F Talab, Ibrahim Ali Zabani, Hassan Saad Abdelrahman, Waleed L Bukhari, Irfan Mamoun, Majed A Ashour, Bakr Bin Sadeq, Sameh Ibrahim El Sayed. Intraoperative Ventilatory Strategies for Prevention of Pulmonary Atelectasis in Obese Patients Undergoing Laparoscopic Bariatric Surgery. *Anesth. Analg.*, 2009, 109, 1511–1516. doi:10.1213/ANE.0b013e3181ba7945.

[29] Cadi, P, Guenoun, T, Journois, D, Chevallier, JM, Diehl, JL, Safran, D. Pressure-controlled ventilation improves oxygenation during laparoscopic obesity surgery compared with volume-controlled ventilation. *Br. J. Anaesth.*, 2008, 100, 709–716. doi:10.1093/bja/aen067.

[30] Vasu, TS, Grewal, R, Doghramji, K. Obstructive Sleep Apnea Syndrome and Perioperative Complications: A Systematic Review of the Literature. *J. Clin. Sleep Med.*, 2012, 08, 199–207. doi:10.5664/jcsm.1784.

[31] Gehrke T, Scherzad A, Hagen R, Hackenberg S. Risk factors for children requiring adenotonsillectomy and their impact on postoperative complications: a retrospective analysis of 2000 patients. *Anaesthesia.* 2019 Dec;74(12):1572-1579. doi: 10.1111/anae.14844. Epub 2019 Sep 11. PMID: 31508815.

[32] Huyett P, Soose RJ, Schell AE, Fernandez-Miranda JC, Gardner PA, Snyderman CH, Wang EW. Risk of Postoperative Complications in Patients with Obstructive Sleep Apnea following Skull Base Surgery. *Otolaryngol Head Neck Surg*. 2018 Jun;158(6):1140-1147. doi: 10.1177/0194599818771540. Epub 2018 Apr 24. PMID: 29688821.

[33] Lam, T, Singh, M, Yadollahi, A, Chung, F. Is Perioperative Fluid and Salt Balance a Contributing Factor in Postoperative Worsening of Obstructive Sleep Apnea? *Anesth. Analg.*, 2016, 122, 1335–1339. doi:10.1213/ANE.0000000000001169.

[34] Cozowicz C, J Poeran, N Zubizarreta, J Liu, S M Weinstein, L Pichler, M Mazumdar, SG Memtsoudis. non-opioid analgesic modes of pain management are associated with reduced postoperative complications and resource utilisation: a retrospective study of obstructive sleep apnoea patients undergoing elective joint arthroplasty. *Br. J. Anaesth.*, 2019, 122, 131–140. doi:10.1016/j.bja.2018.08.027).

[35] Ong, JSL, Touyz, G, Tanner, S, Hillman, DR, Eastwood, PR, Walsh, JH. Variability of human upper airway collapsibility during sleep and the influence of body posture and sleep stage. *J. Sleep Res.*, 2011, 20, 533–537. doi:10.1111/j.1365-2869.2011.00925.x.

[36] Chung, F, Liao, P, Yegneswaran, B, Shapiro, CM, Kang, W. Postoperative Changes in Sleep-disordered Breathing and Sleep Architecture in Patients with Obstructive

Sleep Apnea. *Anesthesiology*, 2014, 120, 287–298. doi:10.1097/ALN.0000000000000040.

[37] Khalid, I, Roehrs, TA, Hudgel, DW, Roth, T. Continuous Positive Airway Pressure in Severe Obstructive Sleep Apnea Reduces Pain Sensitivity. *Sleep*, 2011, 34, 1687–1691. doi:10.5665/sleep.1436.

[38] Nagappa, M, Mokhlesi, B, Wong, J, Wong, DT, Kaw, R, Chung, F. The Effects of Continuous Positive Airway Pressure on Postoperative Outcomes in Obstructive Sleep Apnea Patients Undergoing Surgery. *Anesth. Analg*., 2015, 120, 1013–1023. doi:10.1213/ANE.0000000000000634.

[39] Mutter, TC, Chateau, D, Moffatt, M, Ramsey, C, Roos, LL, Kryger, M. A Matched Cohort Study of Postoperative Outcomes in Obstructive Sleep Apnea. *Anesthesiology*, 2014, 121, 707–718. doi:10.1097/ALN.0000000000000407).

[40] Bram Rochwerg, Laurent Brochard, Mark W Elliott, Dean Hess, Nicholas S Hill, Stefano Nava, Paolo Navalesi Members Of The Steering Committee, Massimo Antonelli, Jan Brozek, Giorgio Conti, Miquel Ferrer, Kalpalatha Guntupalli, Samir Jaber, Sean Keenan, Jordi Mancebo, Sangeeta Mehta, Suhail Raoof Members Of The Task Force Official ERS/ATS clinical practice guidelines: Noninvasive ventilation for acute respiratory failure. *European Respiratory Journal*, 2017, doi:10.1183/13993003.02426-2016.

[41] Abdelsattar, ZM, Hendren, S, Wong, SL, Campbell, DA, Ramachandran, SK. The Impact of Untreated Obstructive Sleep Apnea on Cardiopulmonary Complications in General and Vascular Surgery: A Cohort Study. *Sleep*, 2015, 38, 1205–1210. doi:10.5665/sleep.4892.

[42] Jaber, S, Chanques, G, Jung, B, Riou, B. Postoperative Noninvasive Ventilation. *Anesthesiology*, 2010, 112, 453–461. doi:10.1097/ALN.0b013e3181c5e5f2.

[43] Chiumello, D, Chevallard, G, Gregoretti, C. Non-invasive ventilation in postoperative patients: a systematic review. *Intensive Care Med*., 2011, 37, 918–929. doi :10.1007/s00134-011-2210-8.

[44] Mansur Sufioğlu, Omer Afşin Ozmen, Fikret Kasapoglu, Uygar Levent Demir, Ahmet Ursavas, Levent Erişen, Selcuk Onart. The efficacy of nasal surgery in obstructive sleep apnea syndrome: a prospective clinical study. *Eur Arch Otorhinolaryngol* 2012;269:487–494.

[45] Kezirian EJ, Weaver EM, Yueh B, Deyo RA, Khuri SF, Daley J, Henderson W. Incidence of serious complications after uvulopalatopharyngoplasty. *Laryngoscope*. 2004 Mar;114(3):450-3. doi: 10.1097/00005537-200403000-00012. PMID: 15091217.

[46] Hai, F, Porhomayon, J, Vermont, L, Frydrych, L, Jaoude, P, El-Solh, AA. Postoperative complications in patients with obstructive sleep apnea: a meta-analysis. *J. Clin. Anesth*., 2014, 26, 591–600. doi:10.1016/j.jclinane.2014.05.010.

Chapter 18

Anesthesiology-Perioperative Medicine: Social Life Effects

Ahmet Cemal Pazarlı*, MD
and Handan İnönü Köseoğlu, MD
Gaziosmanpaşa University Faculty of Medicine,
Department of Pulmonary Diseases, Tokat,Turkey

Abstract

Obstructive sleep apnea is a chronic disease that is a significant cause of mortality and morbidity in the world. In parallel with its increasing recognition, the effects of the disease have started to be investigated thoroughly. The incidence of the disease rises with age, which also increases the tendency of the disease towards comorbid conditions. Despite many improvements and innovations presented in its diagnosis and treatment in recent years, especially the social effects of the disease are still tried to be investigated and resolved in all its aspects. Notwithstanding the disease causes adverse effects on the individuals' health, the impacts of the disease on social life also reduce the living standards of many people. For this reason, patients with obstructive sleep apnea syndrome should be evaluated not only by the natural course of the disease, but also by all aspects, and accordingly, treatment modalities and treatment management should be planned.

Keywords: obstructive sleep apnea, social life, traffic accidents, economic burden, continuous positive airway pressure

* Corresponding Author's Email: drcemalpazarli@gmail.com.

In: Obstructive Sleep Apnea in Pulmonary Critical Care
Editors: Antonio M. Esquinas and Takatoshi Kasai
ISBN: 979-8-88697-858-2

Introduction

Obstructive sleep apnea (OSA) syndrome is a life-threatening pathology with consequences such as hypertension, coronary artery disease, arrhythmia, stroke, and sudden death, characterized by recurrent respiratory arrest, oxygen desaturation, and arousals during sleep, associated with complete or partial airway obstruction [1]. It is the most commonly seen sleep breathing disorder type today. According to a recent analysis conducted worldwide, it is estimated that approximately 425 million adults with 30 – 69 years of age suffer from moderate-to-severe OSA [2]. Sleep interruptions due to repetitive apneas and hypopneas, and nighttime hypoxia prevent people from getting a healthy, uninterrupted and efficient sleep. Especially deep sleep and rapid eye movement (REM) sleep decline in OSA. Patients do not feel rested after waking up, tiredness continues throughout the day. Daytime symptoms include excessive sleepiness, loss of energy, irritability, withdrawal from social activities, difficulty concentrating, cognitive dysfunction, anxiety and depressive mood disorders, and psychomotor changes [3]. Apart from these, OSA is a significant public health issue that can also cause traffic and work accidents, marriage problems and serious economic losses.

OSA, which is a potentially life-threatening condition, significantly decreases the quality of life by also creating many adverse effects on the social life of individuals with the above-mentioned aspects. In this section, the effects of OSA on social life are discussed.

Discussion

The prevalence of psychiatric comorbidities such as mood disorders and anxiety are higher in OSA cases than in those without OSA [4]. A cohort study has showen a correlation between OSA and depressive disorders within one year after the onset of OSA [5]. It has been reported that depressive symptoms exist in more than 63% of patients with OSA. However, the association between OSA and affective disorders is yet to be fully understood. While it is stated that oxygen desaturation occurred during sleep may influence the emergence of psychological symptoms, there are also studies regarding that there is no relationship between OSA severity and psychological symptoms [6]. There are results in the literature that these symptoms are related to excessive daytime sleepiness rather than hypoxemia, and that reducing sleepiness decreases depressive symptoms [7, 8]. It has been reported that structural or metabolic changes in the brains of patients with OSA may be related to a high rate of depressive and anxiety disorders [9]. OSA itself is also regarded as a possible comorbidity of affective and cognitive disorders. If not diagnosed and treated, OSA can worsen the symptoms of comorbid psychiatric disorders and prevent remission and undermine the patient's compliance with medication. On the other hand, since the use of hypnotics and benzodiazepines is contraindicated in OSA, treatment with polypharmacy in a patient diagnosed with depression may cause rapid worsening of OSA symptoms [3]. Psychiatric comorbidities in patients with OSA may negatively affect their compliance with continuous Positive Airway Pressure (PAP) therapy, which takes a significant place in the treatment of these patients [6]. This is why: typical symptoms of depression such as depressed mood, sadness, emotional lethargy, anhedonia, hypobulia, loss of appetite, as well as other symptoms that are not particularly responsive to PAP treatment, such as hypoprosexia, fatigue, and sleep disturbance may be signs of a comorbid depressive disorder. The PAP treatment aimed at reducing apnea and hypopnea improves common symptoms, but it is unknown whether it will ameliorate the specific symptoms of depressive disorder [3]. Therefore, as OSA and depression share some common symptoms, it is of uttermost importance to recognize and treat both separately.

Another important impact of OSA on individuals' daily activities and social life is its neurocognitive effects. Deterioration in memory, concentration, vigilance, and executive functions can be listed among the neurocognitive symptoms of OSA [10]. Additionally, attention, working and episodic memory functions are reduced in patients with OSA [3]. It was stated in the review article published by Bucks et al. that while attention, long-term verbal and visual memory, and executive functions are impaired, visuospatial learning and immediate visual recall are intact [11]. It is difficult to differentiate the impairment in the cognitive (executive) functions in OSA from psychomotor retardation, attention deficit, depression and anxiety. Another difficulty that is widely ignored during revealing the effects of OSA on cognitive functions is that most of these patients have comorbidities such as obesity, hypertension, and diabetes associated with impaired performance [12]. Impairments in cognitive functions should be reevaluated following successful treatment of OSA, because the concentration loss developing after sleep deprivation and mimicking cognitive impairment are ameliorated after treatment. Some studies have demonstrated that cognitive performance in patients with OSA is not at the same level of healthy controls even after PAP treatment [13, 14]. This finding reinforces the idea that the brain damage induced by permanent hypoxemia causes cognitive impairment in untreated OSA patients [3]. One of the psychiatric diseases frequently accompanying sleep disturbances is eating disorders such as anorexia nervosa, bulimia nervosa, and night eating syndrome. In a study in which cases with and without OSA has been compared, the Eating Attitudes Test score has been found higher in the OSA group [15]. Since eating behavior disorders, and weight gain that may subsequently develop will create difficulties in the control of OSA symptoms, cases should be carefully evaluated from this point of view.

One other important factor that impacts the social life in individuals with OSA is the decrease in participating physical activities. Commonly seen clinical results of OSA, such as excessive daytime sleepiness, fatigue, exhaustion, lack of energy, depression, and functional and cognitive decline, may prolong the duration of sedentary time [16]. As well as studies reporting that low physical activity level is related to the severity of OSA [17], there are also findings that no relationship exists between the severity of OSA and exercise capacity [18]. Fatigue, a symptom that is frequently seen in patients with OSA, is of utmost importance on physical activity. Hong and Dimsdale emphasized that regardless of the severity of sleep apnea or body mass index in moderate-to-severe OSA patients, the physical activity level was significantly correlated to subjective well-being, and the perception of fatigue was negatively associated with physical activity [19].

OSA, which can cause many physical, psychological and social problems, adversely impacts the quality of life through all these aspects. Quality of life can be described as the person's subjective perception of own health and well-being in the sociocultural environment in which she/he lives. Health-related quality of life, on the other hand, is a phenomenon influenced by diseases and their treatment. The most commonly used scale in the assessment of life quality parameters in epidemiological and clinical studies in OSA is the Medical Outcomes Study Short-Form Health Survey (SF-36) [20]. It was found in the Wisconsin Sleep Cohort that in middle-aged men and women, even in a moderate degree OSA, quality of life was lower than those without OSA [21]. In that case, worsening in quality of life should not be just associated with determinants of OSA severity, such as apnea-hypopnea index and nocturnal hypoxemia. As daytime sleepiness reduces mobility and vigilance, quality of life is affected in a greater extent in individuals with OSA, especially those with excessive daytime sleepiness. The mechanism behind excessive daytime sleepiness observed in OSA has yet to be exactly explained, decreased oxygen saturation as well as sleep fragmentation can cause excessive daytime sleepiness. It has been reported that daytime sleepiness may also be associated with systemic inflammation [22]. In a study in which the factors correlated with daytime sleepiness and clinical outcomes have been examined, it has been detected that in patients with complaints of daytime sleepiness, the subjective sleep quality and daytime dysfunction parameters of the Pittsburgh Sleep Quality Index and the social function and emotional status assessed by the SF-36 Quality of Life Scale were poorer [23]. It has been found that the decrease in quality of life in moderate to severe OSA patients is correlated with physical functionality, and the Epworth sleepiness score (ESS) is associated with the physical and mental domains of quality of life [24].

Traffic and work accidents due to OSA is its another important social impact. Daytime sleepiness is responsible for one-fifth of traffic accidents. As well as daytime sleepiness may occur due to many reasons, it is also an important finding and outcome of sleep apnea syndrome, which is seen at a rate of 4% in the population. In addition, neurological sequelae including tendency to sleep, concentration impairment, loss of motor coordination, decrease in reflexes increase traffic and work accidents by causing failure in tasks requiring complex motor coordination such as concentration and hand-foot coordination. Driving is a complex task requiring perceptual, motor and decision-making abilities, as well as eye-hand coordination.

Regardless of the presence and intensity of the "sleepiness" symptom, patients diagnosed with OSA are under a risk of motor vehicle accidents at high extent while driving. The increased risk seems to be irrelevant to the symptom of excessive daytime sleepiness, and a clear dose-response relationship has not been revealed regarding the severity of apneas and hypopneas in many studies [25]. For this reason, it is very important in terms of public health that the inclusion of sleep apnea syndrome, which increases the risk of traffic accidents, is common in commercial vehicle drivers and can be ameliorated with treatment, in the driver's license regulations, and that the assessment of drivers and driver candidates with suspected OSA with a sleep test. It is recommended that people who arouse high clinical suspicion for OSA and who meet the definition of high-risk driver (with moderate or severe daytime sleepiness; who, due to sleepiness, fatigue or inattention, recently had an accident or narrowly escaped from an accident) should be evaluated by polysomnography, and PAP treatment should be started if OSA is detected [26].

The majority of adults sleep with a partner, and in a significant proportion of couples, sleep disturbances and relationship problems co-occur. A variety of physical health outcomes, including cardiovascular disease, chronic pain, and infectious diseases predict the quality of marriage. Among the potential mechanisms that link marital quality with health are behavioral, neuroendocrine, cardiovascular, and immune pathways. These conventional biopsychosocial mechanisms explain some part of the relationship between marital quality and health, not in entirety [27]. Nevertheless, although the facts that health-related consequences of sleep disturbances are well documented and most couples engage in this health behavior together, studies in which sleep is investigated as a potential mediator of the marital quality-health relationship are rare. It is likely that the link between sleep and marital relationships is bilateral and mutual. The impact of co-sleeping on the bed partner's sleep as well as the impact of sleep disturbance or sleep disorders on relationship functioning affect the quality of life of the partners [28]. That's why, the recognition of the social context of sleep and including this kind of knowledge into clinical practice and research activities in sleep medicine can shed light on key mechanisms in the etiology and maintenance of both sleep disorders and relationship issues and may consequently enhance quality of life and marriage.

Perhaps one of the most important impacts of OSA on social life is economic losses that may occur depending on the disease or the treatment burden brought by the disease. As well as there is a decrease in patients' capacity to work according to the severity of the disease, observational studies have indicated that OSA is correlated with increased comorbidities and health service costs. Obesity is considered a significant risk factor in OSA; related health expenses in obese people are 42% higher than in people with normal body weights, and about 9% of annual healthcare expenses in North America is pertinent to obesity [29].

It has been shown that undiagnosed and untreated OSA correlates with poor quality of life, cardiovascular diseases, and depression, and also causes the demand for physician services and medical services and costs to increase [30]. In addition to these, excessive daytime sleepiness and lack of attention induce reduced work performance, decreased productivity, absenteeism, and workplace and motor vehicle accidents. An increase in unemployment, underemployment and socioeconomic cost is present in OSA cases. OSA has been associated with many of the most common health conditions leading to morbidity, mortality and social and economic costs. Most data demonstrate that the cost of treating OSA is less than the human and economic cost of untreated OSA [31]. In meeting this global burden, sensible utilization of improvements in the awareness and comprehension of OSA, the technology to diagnose and manage OSA and its related comorbidities, and advancements in health infrastructure of the world for everyone's benefit would contribute to preventing economic losses linked to the disease.

Conclusion

Although OSA leads to many conditions of morbidity, while treating patients with OSA, rather than solely targeting at ameliorating sleep apnea, it should be aimed at improving their quality of life by addressing patients as a whole with their psychological, social, economic and physical functions. In summary, a) OSA, a chronic disease with an important cause of mortality and morbidity, is a serious public health issue with all its impacts, b) As well as many pathophysiological negative effects, the disease has also reflection in social life with its significant outcomes, c) To minimize its negative effects on social life, OSA should be addressed with all its aspects and treated effectively, d) It should be kept in mind that the effective treatment of OSA will enhance the quality of life and have positive impacts on social life, besides improving the person's health status and e) It should be known that the most valid and effective treatment method for OSA is positive airway pressure therapy, and the acceptability of this treatment method by the patients should be increased.

References

[1] Aslan G, Afsar B, Siriopol D, Kanbay A, Sal O, Benli C, Okcuoglu J, Covic A, Kanbay M. Cardiovascular Effects of Continuous Positive Airway Pressure Treatment in Patients With Obstructive Sleep Apnea: A Meta-Analysis. *Angiology* 2018; 69(3): 195-204.

[2] Benjafield A V, Ayas N T, Eastwood P R, Heinzer R, Ip M S M, Morrell M J, Nunez CM, Patel S R, Penzel T, Pépin J L, Peppard P E, Sinha S, Tufik S, Valentine K, Malhotra A. Estimation of the global prevalence and burden of obstructive sleep apnoea: a literature-based analysis. *Lancet Respir. Med.* 2019; 7(8): 687-98.

[3] Vanek J, Prasko J, Genzor S, Ociskova M, Kantor K, Holubova M, Slepecky M, Nesnidal V, Kolek A, Sova M. Obstructive sleep apnea, depression and cognitive impairment, Review Article. *Sleep Medicine* 2020; 72: 50-58.

[4] Sharafkhaneh A, Giray N, Richardson P, Young T, Hirshkowitz M. Association of psychiatric disorders and sleep apnea in a large cohort. *Sleep* 2005; 28(11): 1405-1411.

[5] Chen Y H, Keller J K, Kang J H, Hsieh H J, Lin H C. Obstructive sleep apnea and the subsequent risk of depressive disorder: a population-based follow-up study. *J. Clin. Sleep Med.* 2013; 9(5): 417-23.

[6] Kim J Y, Ko I, Kim D K. Association of Obstructive Sleep Apnea With the Risk of Affective Disorders. *JAMA Otolaryngol. Head Neck Surg.* 2019; 145(11): 1020-26.

[7] Lee S A, Han S H, Ryu H U. Anxiety and its relationship to quality of life independent of depression in patients with obstructive sleep apnea. *J. Psychosom. Res.* 2015; 79(1): 32-36.

[8] Ishman S L, Benke J R, Cohen A P, Stephen M J, Ishii L E, Gourin C G. Does surgery for obstructive sleep apnea improve depression and sleepiness? *Laryngoscope* 2014; 124(12): 2829-36.

[9] Yadav S K, Kumar R, Macey P M, Woo M A, Yan-Go F L, Harper R M. Insular cortex metabolite changes in obstructive sleep apnea. *Sleep* 2014; 37(5): 951-58.

[10] Ekici A, Ekici M, Oğuztürk O, Karaboğa I, Cimen D, Senturk E. Personality profiles in patients with obstructive sleep apnea. *Sleep Breath* 2013; 17:305–310.

[11] Bucks R S, Olaithe M, Rosenzweig I, Morrell M J. Reviewing the relationship between OSA and cognition: Where do we go from here? *Respirology* 2017; 22: 1253–1261.

[12] Borges J G, Ginani G E, Hachul H, Cintra F D, Tufik S, Pompéia S. Executive functioning in obstructive sleep apnea syndrome patients without comorbidities: Focus on the fractionation of executive functions. *Journal of Clinical and Experimental Neuropsychology* 2013; 35(10): 1094–1107.

[13] Salorio C F, White D A, Piccirillo J, Duntley S P, Uhles M L. Learning, memory, and executive control in individuals with obstructive sleep apnea syndrome. *J. Clin. Exp. Neuropsychol.* 2002; 24: 93-100.

[14] Lau EY, Eskes GA, Morrison DL, Rajda M, Spurr KF. Executive function in patients with obstructive sleep apnea treated with continuous positive airway pressure. *J. Int. Neuropsychol. Soc.* 2010; 16: 1077-88.

[15] Gulec Balbay E, Yildiz P, Elverisli MF, Cangur S, Erçelik M.The eating attitudes in patients with obstructive sleep apnea syndrome. *The Aging Male* 2020; 23(5): 1170-75.

[16] Çalışkan H, Ertürk N, Kütükçü EÇ, Calik E,Arikan H,Yagli N.V,Saglam M,Fırat H,Ardic S Ince D.I, Ege M.Y. The Relationship Between the Physical Activity Level and Fatigue Perception, Quality of Life and Psychological Status in Patients with Obstructive Sleep Apnea Syndrome. *Journal of Turkish Sleep Medicine* 2019; 6: 1-6.

[17] Verwimp J, Ameye L, Bruyneel M. Correlation between sleep parameters, physical activity and quality of life in somnolent moderate to severe obstructive sleep apnea adult patients. *Sleep Breath* 2013; 17: 1039-46.

[18] Butner KL, Hargens TA, Kaleth AS, Miller LE, Zedalis D, Herbert WG. Association of Obstructive Sleep Apnea Severity with Exercise Capacity and Health-related Quality of Life. *N. Am. J. Med. Sci.* 2013; 5: 362-6.

[19] Hong S, Dimsdale J E. Physical activity and perception of energy and fatigue in obstructive sleep apnea. *Med. Sci. Sports Exerc.* 2003; 35: 1088-92.

[20] Ware J E Jr, Sherbourne C D. The MOS 36-item short-form health survey (SF-36). I. Conceptual framework and item selection. *Medical Care* 1992; 30(6):473–83.

[21] Finn L, Young T, Palta M, Fryback D G. Sleep-disordered breathing and self-reported general health status in the Wisconsin Sleep Cohort Study. *Sleep* 1998; 21(7):701–6.

[22] Vqontzas A N, Bixler E O, Chrousos G P. Sleep apnea is a manifetation of the metabolic syndrome. *Sleep Med. Rev.* 2005;9:211-24.

[23] Çiğdem Berkeşoğlu. The Relation Between Daytime Sleepiness and Clinical Outcomes in Patients with Obstructive Sleep Apnea Syndrome. *Journal of Turkish Sleep Medicine* 2014; 3:71-6.

[24] Asghari A, Mohammadi F, Kamrava SK, Jalessi M, Farhadi M. Evaluation of quality of life in patients with obstructive sleep apnea. *Eur. Arch. Otorhinolaryngol.* 2013; 270: 1131-6.

[25] Tregear S, Reston J, Schoelles K, Phillips B. Continuous positive airway pressure reduces risk of motor vehicle crash among drivers with obstructive sleep apnea: systematic review and meta-analysis. *Sleep* 2010; 33: 1373-1380.

[26] Strohl K P, Brown D B, Collop N, George C, Grunstein R, Han F, Kline L, Malhotra A, Pack A, Phillips B, Rodenstein D, Schwab R, Weaver T, Wilson K. An official American Thoracic Society Clinical Practice Guideline: sleep apnea, sleepiness, and driving risk in noncommercial drivers. An update of a 1994 Statement. *Am. J. Respir. Crit Care Med.* 2013; 187: 1259-1266.

[27] Kiecolt-Glaser J K, Newton T L. Marriage and health: His and hers. *Psychological Bulletin* 2001;127(4):472–503.

[28] Beninati W, Harris C D, Herold D L, Shepard J W Jr. The effect of snoring and obstructive sleep apnea on the sleep quality of bed partners. *Mayo Clin. Proc.* 1999 Oct;74(10):955-8. doi: 10.4065/74.10.955. PMID: 10918859.

[29] Finkelstein E A, Trogdon J G, Cohen J W, Dietz W. Annual medical spending attributable to obesity: payer-and service-specific estimates. *Health Aff (Millwood)* 2009; 28: 822–831.

[30] Wickwire E M, Tom S E, Vadlamani A, Diaz-Abad M, Cooper L M, Johnson A M, Scharf S M, Albrecht J S. Older adult US Medicare beneficiaries with untreated obstructive sleep apnea are heavier users of health care than matched control patients. *J. Clin. Sleep Med* 2020; 16: 81–9.

[31] Lyons M M, Bhatt N Y, Pack A I, Magalang U J. Global burden of sleep-disordered breathing and its implications. *Respirology* 2020 Jul;25(7):690-702. doi: 10.1111/resp.13838. Epub 2020 May 21. PMID: 32436658.

Chapter 19

Postoperative Management of Obstructive Sleep Apnea following Abdominal Surgery

Dipasri Bhattacharya[1*], MD
Antonio M. Esquinas[2,†], MD, PhD
and Mohanchandra Mandal[3], MD
[1]Department of Anesthesiology, Pain Medicine, and Critical Care, R. G. Kar Medical College, Kolkata, West Bengal, India
[2]Intensive Care Unit, Hospital Morales, Meseguer, Murcia, Spain
[3]Department of Anesthesiology and Critical Care, Institute of Post Graduate Medical Education and Research/S.S.K.M. Hospital, Kolkata, West Bengal, India

Abstract

Obstructive sleep apnea (OSA), a common form of sleep disordered breathing seen in all age groups. These patients have been recognized as potential independent risk factors for adverse perioperative outcome. They are at increased risk of developing postoperative pulmonary complications after general anesthesia [1]. They very often remain undiagnosed before operation. Mortality rate after upper abdominal operation in OSA patient is higher than non-OSA patient. Upper abdominal operation reduces lung volume, leading to hypoxaemia. Proper preoperative screening and management reduces the risk of postoperative problems.

---

* Dipasri Bhattacharya, MD, MNAMS, FIAPM
† Antonio M. Esquinas, MD, PhD, FCCP, FNIV, FAARC;
Corresponding Author's Email: antmesquinas@gmail.com.

In: Obstructive Sleep Apnea in Pulmonary Critical Care
Editors: Antonio M. Esquinas and Takatoshi Kasai
ISBN: 979-8-88697-858-2

Keywords: obstructive sleep apnea, functional residual capacity, STOP-Bang questionnaire, abdominal surgery, noninvasive ventilation

Introduction

The incidence of OSA in general population is 2 to 26% [1]. In another study 70% of patient undergoing bariatric surgery were found to have OSA and 30% of OSA patient has obesity hypoventilation syndrome [2]. In the Wisconsin Sleep Cohort Study, the percentage of obese individuals (with a BMI > 40) with an apnea-hypopnea index (AHI) of 15 or higher is 42% to 55% in men and 16% to 24% in women [3, 4].

Pulmonary Consequences of OSA Patient

Pulmonary changes in OSA patient include a reduction in functional residual capacity (FRC) at the expense of expiratory reserve volume (ERV). FRC falls below closing capacity during tidal ventilation and premature airway closure occurs. Adoption of supine position causes further decrease (10 to 40%) in FRC [5]. Hypoxaemia results from increased venous mixture. Under anesthesia FRC is reduced resulting in marked deterioration in oxygenation, alveolar arterial oxygen tension difference and hypoxemia. Results demonstrated that venous admixture can be reduced by application of CPAP/PEEP [5].

Classification of OSA Patient

Obstructive sleep apnea (OSA) is a syndrome characterized by periodic, partial, or complete obstruction of upper airway during sleep. This causes repetitive arousal from sleep to restore airway patency resulting in daytime hypersomnolence or aggressive behavior particularly in children [6] and is diagnosed by polysomnography (PSG). The apnea-hypopnea index is used to diagnose OSA. Apnea can be defined as a complete cessation of airflow, and hypopnea is defined as a partial reduction (at least 50%) of airflow; both lasting for a minimum of 10 seconds. Hypopneas are measured by oxygen desaturation of 3% or more or arousal from sleep. Apnoea hypopnea Index

(AHI) is categorized as Minimal AHI < 5 per hour, Mild AHI ≥ 5, but < 15 per hour, Moderate AHI ≥ 15, but < 30 per hour, Severe AHI ≥ 30 per hour. American Society of Anaesthesiologists recommends early identification and appropriate preparation of suspected OSA patient to avoid complications [7]. Overnight oximetry is another tool that has been used to screen OSA patient. The predictive power of the STOP-Bang questionnaire for obstructive sleep apnea screening in obese patients has been validated and is found to be a high sensitivity and appropriate screening test [8]. The STOPBANG questionnaire Score comprises of parameters such as Snoring, Tiredness during daytime, Observed apnea, high blood Pressure, Body mass index, Age, Neck circumference, Gender. A score of 3 or more is usually indicative of high risk and less than 3 is indicative of low risk. The cut off value of the score has important influence on the sensitivity and specificity. The sensitivity of STOP-Bang score ≥ 3 to detect moderate to severe OSA (apnea-hypopnea index [AHI] > 15) and severe OSA (AHI > 30) has been found to be 93% and 100%, respectively [9]. Another study reports that, a STOP-Bang score of 4 has high sensitivity of 88% to identify sever OSA while a score of 6 is more specific for confirming the severe OSA cases [10].

Problems of OSA in Perioperative Period

OSA patients have reduced lung volume with mismatched ventilation and perfusion. Increased pulmonary venous admixture and lower arterial oxygen tension than predicted for age. Preoperative hypoxemia can easily occur. Continuous preoperative monitoring of oxygen should be considered as an integral component of care [5]. The combined effect of supine posture and anesthetic induction further reduces FRC. Trendelenburg position further reduces FRC accentuating arterial hypoxemia. Residual effects of anesthetics further aggravate decrease in functional residual capacity and oxygenation, potentially leading to more apneic events and hypoxemia [11]. Surgical exposure with laparotomy, packs and retractors further reduces lung volume and impair venous return leading to further reduction of cardiac output. OSA patients undergoing surgical procedure are prone to develop postoperative airway obstruction, myocardial ischemia, congestive heart failure, stroke, and oxygen desaturation [1]. Those patients who are undiagnosed during surgery are more vulnerable to develop postoperative pulmonary complications.

Risk Factors for Postoperative Complications

OSA with comorbidities including hypothyroidism, coronary artery disease, diabetes, heart failure, asthma, chronic obstructive airway disease, ASA Physical Status III and IV and BMI>35 kg, upper abdominal surgery are important risk factors for post operative pulmonary complications [12]. The combination of obesity, OSA and supine positioning reduce lung volume, increasing chance of upper airway collapse and worsen gas exchange [13]. Intra operative use of sedatives, induction agents, opioid analgesics and topical anesthetics impairs protective upper airway reflexes [14].

Effect of Abdominal Operation on OSA

General or regional anesthesia is administered in OSA patients undergoing abdominal surgery. General anesthesia is usually administered in upper abdominal surgery. Endotracheal intubation or Laryngeal Mask Airway can be used for airway control in such population. Regional anesthesia, central blocks, can be used either as a sole anesthetic technique or combined with general anesthesia in lower abdominal surgery. Sedation is often used when regional techniques are used alone. Pulmonary function is impaired after abdominal surgery more severely than after non-thoracic, non-abdominal surgery in all patients, the effect is more pronounced in OSA patient [5]. A higher incidence of postoperative pulmonary complications has been observed after upper abdominal procedures. Adequate postoperative pain control improves ventilation. Epidural administration of opioids or patient-controlled analgesia is recommended for postoperative pain management.

Preoperative Assessment and Preparation

Thorough history and physical examination with the special emphasis on the evaluation of sleep apnea are encouraged. In history, sleep apnea including snoring, excessive daytime sleepiness, witnessed apneas, frequent awakenings at night, and morning headaches are important clues to OSA [4]. A focused physical examination should be done to note neck circumference, body mass index, Mallampati score, size and volume of tongue and nasopharyngeal characteristics. ASA, or STOP-Bang questionnaire to identify high risk OSA patient. Polysomnography is advised for all OSA patient posted for bariatric surgery. Preoperative initiation of CPAP should be considered, if OSA is severe. Patients who do not respond to CPAP adequately, the application of NIPPV should be considered. Patients with known or suspected OSA may have difficult airways, so difficult airway cart should be kept ready during intubation.

Intra Operative Clinical Suspicion of OSA [11]

We consider that there are five main aspects: a) Problems with maintenance of the airway, b) Airway obstruction out of proportion to the apparent degree of sedation, c) Proves difficult to intubate- difficulty in visualizing the faucial pillars, the soft palate, and the base of the uvula and d) Observed to be snoring or having airway obstructions after extubation in the immediate postoperative period.

Intra Operative Management

Judicious use of premedication, sedatives, analgesics, induction agent, and difficult intubation measures reduce postoperative complications. Muscle relaxation should be guided by neuromuscular monitoring. Extubation should be done awake [11].

Postoperative Adverse Events [1, 12]

Early

We consider that there are five main aspects: 1). Upper airway obstruction; 2). Mild to moderate hypoxemia (SpO_2 90-95%). Oxygenation with nasal cannula with 3l/minute, if the patient does not respond, flow should be increased to more than 3l/minute or high flow facemask can be used [1], 3). Severe hypoxemia (SpO_2< 90%) and or PaO_2<60%. High flow face mask or High flow nasal cannula may be used. Noninvasive ventilation (NIV) improves oxygenation if other devices fail, 4). Impending ventilator failure (respiratory rate >20/minute, accessory muscles working, tracheal tug). NIV use is recommended, 5) NIV failure and patient requiring reintubation, 6) Pulmonary aspiration after extubation, 7) Cardiac arrhythmias and 8). Myocardial infarction.

Late

OSA is associated with a hypercoagulable state, may increase risk of cardiovascular events, increase thromboembolism in the postoperative period [15]. Other postoperative adverse events that have been recognized in patients with OSA are atelectasis, pneumonia, pulmonary embolism, increased propensity for infection and sepsis, and prolonged hospital stays [16, 17].

Perioperative Interventions to Improve Oxygenation

Close observation of high risk OSA patients is the key to the perioperative management. In ambulatory surgery these patients should be observed for an extended period before being discharged to home [18]. Following major surgery OSA patient should be admitted in ICU [4]. In the immediate postoperative period monitoring of respiratory obstruction and asynchrony of respiratory efforts should be detected. Management of postoperative pain in patients with OSA can be a challenging task. Opioids, the gold standard analgesic, decrease hypoxic and hypercapnic ventilatory drive. Non opioid analgesics are preferred [4].

Postoperative Management

The recent ASA practice guideline for peri operative management of OSA patient recommends preoperative and postoperative use of NIV to OSA patient depending on severity. Patient preoperatively may receive continuous positive airway pressure (CPAP) in home or nasal intermittent positive pressure ventilation (NIPPV). They should be routinely advised to receive CPAP after surgery [19]. Nasal continuous positive airway pressure (NCPAP) can be a fruitful method to provide respiratory support after extubation [20].

There is no randomized control trial to prove efficacy of CPAP therapy to be beneficial in the postoperative setting. Rather routine use of CPAP in the immediate postoperative period in CPAP-native or previously noncompliant patients is discouraged. In presence of frequent episodes of severe obstruction occur, CPAP use should be considered [4] . Body posture has some effect on pharyngeal shape and size in adult in patient with OSA. Sleep disorders worsen in supine position. Lateral recumbent position does not alter cross sectional area of airway and is beneficial in OSA patient [21]. Head of bed elevation 30 to 60 degree effectively reduce OSA related problems, but patient may not tolerate it in postoperative period [22].

A recent study [23] suggest that use of high flow nasal cannula and upper body elevation to 30 degrees can be an alternative to CPAP application, and that may be utilized in patients who refuse CPAP. High flow nasal cannula significantly improves nocturnal hypoxemia and OSA frequency. Combination of high flow nasal cannula and upper body elevation decrease apnea hypopnea index [24]. OSA patient have been effectively treated with auto-titrated continuous positive airway pressure (APAP) in the postoperative period with less hypoxemia and less apnea hypopnea index [25].

Conclusion

OSA in abdominal surgery is really a challenge to an anesthesiologist. Proper history taking and clinical examination lead to early diagnosis before surgery. Patient most often suffers from hypoxemia of varying degree in the postoperative period. Recent treatment modalities in peri operative period like application of preoperative CPAP, postoperative head of bed elevation, high flow nasal oxygen therapy or APAP should be applied judiciously to reduce postoperative pulmonary complications.

References

[1] Xará D, Mendonça J, Pereira H, Santos A, Abelha F J. Adverse respiratory events after general anesthesia in patients at high risk of obstructive sleep apnea syndrome. *Braz. J. Anesthesiol.* 2015 Sep-Oct;65(5):359-66. doi: 10.1016/j.bjane.2014.02.008. Epub 2014 Mar 12. PMID: 26323734.

[2] Romero-Corral A, Caples S M, Lopez-Jimenez F, Somers V K. Interactions between obesity and obstructive sleep apnea: implications for treatment. *Chest.* 2010 Mar;137(3):711-9. doi: 10.1378/chest.09-0360. PMID: 20202954; PMCID: PMC3021364.

[3] Thompson J, Bordi S, Boytim M, Elisha S, Heiner J, Nagelhout J. Anesthesia case management for bariatric surgery. *AANA J.* 2011 Apr;79(2):147-60. PMID: 21560977.

[4] Kaw R, Gali B, Collop N A. Perioperative care of patients with obstructive sleep apnea. *Curr. Treat. Options Neurol*. 2011 Oct;13(5):496-507. doi: 10.1007/s11940-011-0138-5. PMID: 21769651; PMCID: PMC4452109.

[5] Nagappa M, Ho G, Patra J, Wong J, Singh M, Kaw R, Cheng D, Chung F. Postoperative Outcomes in Obstructive Sleep Apnea Patients Undergoing Cardiac Surgery: A Systematic Review and Meta-analysis of Comparative Studies. *Anesth. Analg*. 2017 Dec;125(6):2030-2037. doi: 10.1213/ANE.0000000000002558. PMID: 29049073.

[6] Seet E, Chung F. Management of sleep apnea in adults - functional algorithms for the perioperative period: Continuing Professional Development. *Can. J. Anaesth*. 2010 Sep;57(9):849-64. doi: 10.1007/s12630-010-9344-y. Epub 2010 Aug 4. PMID: 20683690.

[7] American Academy of Sleep Medicine Task Force. Sleep-related breathing disorders in adults: Recommendations for syndrome definition and measurement techniques in clinical research. *Sleep*. 1999;22:667-89 https://doi.org/10.1093/sleep/22.5.667, PMID:10450601.

[8] Mergen H, Altındağ B, Zeren Uçar Z, Karasu Kılıçaslan I. The Predictive Performance of the STOP-Bang Questionnaire in Obstructive Sleep Apnea Screening of Obese Population at Sleep Clinical Setting. *Cureus*. 2019 Dec 29;11(12):e6498. doi: 10.7759/cureus.6498. PMID: 32025419; PMCID: PMC6986466.

[9] hung F, Abdullah H R, Liao P. STOP-Bang Questionnaire: A Practical Approach to Screen for Obstructive Sleep Apnea. *Chest*. 2016 Mar;149(3):631-8. doi: 10.1378/chest.15-0903. Epub 2016 Jan 12. PMID: 26378880.

[10] Chung F, Abdullah H R, Liao P. STOP-Bang Questionnaire: A Practical Approach to Screen for Obstructive Sleep Apnea. *Chest*. 2016 Mar;149(3):631-8. doi: 10.1378/chest.15-0903. Epub 2016 Jan 12. PMID: 26378880.

[11] Auckley D. Perioperative Complications in Obstructive Sleep Apnea Patients. *Curr. Sleep Medicine Rep*. 2016;2:87–98. https://doi.org/10.1007/s40675-016-0040-5.

[12] Liao P, Yegneswaran B, Vairavanathan S, Zilberman P, Chung F. Postoperative complications in patients with obstructive sleep apnea: a retrospective matched cohort study. *Can. J. Anaesth*. 2009 Nov;56(11):819-28. https://doi.org/10.1007/s12630-009-9190-y. PMID: 19774431.

[13] McIsaac D I, Gershon A, Wijeysundera D, Bryson G L, Badner N, van Walraven C. Identifying Obstructive Sleep Apnea in Administrative Data: A Study of Diagnostic Accuracy. *Anesthesiology*. 2015 Aug;123(2):253-63. doi: 10.1097/ALN.0000000000000692. PMID: 26200178.

[14] Hai F, Porhomayon J, Vermont L, Frydrych L, Jaoude P, El-Solh A A. Postoperative complications in patients with obstructive sleep apnea: a meta-analysis. *J. Clin. Anesth*. 2014 Dec;26(8):591-600. doi: 10.1016/j.jclinane.2014.05.010. Epub 2014 Oct 16. PMID: 25439403.

[15] Liak C, Fitzpatrick M. Coagulability in obstructive sleep apnea. *Can. Respir. J*. 2011 Nov-Dec;18(6):338-48. doi: 10.1155/2011/924629. PMID: 22187690; PMCID: PMC3267624.

[16] Adesanya A O, Lee W, Greilich N B, Joshi G P. Perioperative management of obstructive sleep apnea. *Chest*. 2010 Dec;138(6):1489-98. doi: 10.1378/chest.10-1108. Erratum in: Chest. 2011 Nov;140(5):1393. PMID: 21138886.

[17] Vasu T S, Grewal R, Doghramji K. Obstructive sleep apnea syndrome and perioperative complications: a systematic review of the literature. *J. Clin. Sleep Med.* 2012 Apr 15;8(2):199-207. doi: 10.5664/jcsm.1784. PMID: 22505868; PMCID: PMC3311420.

[18] Hillman D R, Platt P R, Eastwood P R. Anesthesia, sleep, and upper airway collapsibility. *Anesthesiol. Clin.* 2010 Sep;28(3):443-55. doi: 10.1016/j.anclin.2010.07.003. PMID: 20850076.

[19] Kaw R, Pasupuleti V, Walker E, Ramaswamy A, Foldvary-Schafer N. Postoperative complications in patients with obstructive sleep apnea. *Chest*. 2012 Feb;141(2):436-441. doi: 10.1378/chest.11-0283. Epub 2011 Aug 25. PMID: 21868464.

[20] Davis P G, Lemyre B, de Paoli A G. Nasal intermittent positive pressure ventilation (NIPPV) versus nasal continuous positive airway pressure (NCPAP) for preterm neonates after extubation. *Cochrane Database Syst. Rev*. 2001;(3):CD003212. doi: 10.1002/14651858.CD003212. Update in: *Cochrane Database Syst. Rev*. 2014;9: CD003212. PMID: 11687052.

[21] Walsh J H, Leigh M S, Paduch A, Maddison K J, Armstrong J J, Sampson D D, Hillman D R, Eastwood P R. Effect of body posture on pharyngeal shape and size in adults with and without obstructive sleep apnea. *Sleep*. 2008 Nov;31(11):1543-9. doi: 10.1093/sleep/31.11.1543. PMID: 19014074; PMCID: PMC2579983.

[22] Souza F J F B, Genta P R, de Souza Filho A J, Wellman A, Lorenzi-Filho G. The influence of head-of-bed elevation in patients with obstructive sleep apnea. *Sleep Breath*. 2017 Dec;21(4):815-820. doi: 10.1007/s11325-017-1524-3. Epub 2017 Jun 24. PMID: 28647854; PMCID: PMC5700252.

[23] Sakaguchi Y, Nozaki-Taguchi N, Hasegawa M, Ishibashi K, Sato Y, Isono S. Combination Therapy of High-flow Nasal Cannula and Upper-body Elevation for Postoperative Sleep-disordered Breathing: Randomized Crossover Trial. *Anesthesiology*. 2022 Jul 1;137(1):15-27. doi: 10.1097/ALN.0000000000004254. PMID: 35471655.

[24] Nishimura M. High-Flow Nasal Cannula Oxygen Therapy in Adults: Physiological Benefits, Indication, Clinical Benefits, and Adverse Effects. *Respir. Care*. 2016 Apr;61(4):529-41. doi: 10.4187/respcare.04577. PMID: 27016353.

[25] Liao P, Luo Q, Elsaid H, Kang W, Shapiro C M, Chung F. Perioperative auto-titrated continuous positive airway pressure treatment in surgical patients with obstructive sleep apnea: a randomized controlled trial. *Anesthesiology*. 2013 Oct;119(4):837-47. doi: 10.1097/ALN.0b013e318297d89a. Erratum in: *Anesthesiology*. 2014 May;120(5):1302. Erratum in: *Anesthesiology*. 2014 May;120(5):1302. PMID: 24195872.

Chapter 20

Postoperative Key Recommendations in Orthopedic Surgery

Gokce Selcuk Sert*, MD
Department of Anesthesiology, Ankara City Hospital, Ankara, Turkey

Abstract

Obstructive sleep apnea in patients undergoing orthopedic surgery bears additional risks than normal population, particularly including postoperative respiratory complications. Therefore, preoperative diagnosis, perioperative anesthesia management and postoperative follow-up gain utmost importance. Detection of undiagnosed patients with obstructive sleep apnea in the preoperative evaluation, fluid management and anesthesia preference in the perioperative period, and initiation of continue positive aieway pressure therapy with early diagnosis in the postoperative period reduce the need for intubation in the postoperative follow-up and increase early discharge and patient comfort.

Keywords: orthopedic surgery, positive airway pressure, regional anesthesia, analgesia, respiratory complication

Introduction

Obstructive sleep apnea (OSA) is a syndrome characterized by recurrent complete or partial obstructions of the upper airway during sleep, often

* Corresponding Author's Email: gokcesert83@gmail.com.

In: Obstructive Sleep Apnea in Pulmonary Critical Care
Editors: Antonio M. Esquinas and Takatoshi Kasai
ISBN: 979-8-88697-858-2

accompanied by a decrease in blood oxygen saturation and arousals. Obesity, age, male gender, endocrine disorders, craniofacial abnormalities, family history, sedative-hypnotics, smoking, and alcohol consumption are risk factors [1, 2]. The typical presentation is when an overweight male patient presents with a history of loud snoring, choking on sleep, excessive daytime sleepiness, and witnessed apnea. Nevertheless, OSA is a heterogeneous disorder with many nocturnal and daytime symptoms. Obesity and upper airway narrowing should be noted in the physical examination. Early diagnosis gains importance because of the cardiovascular, metabolic, and neurocognitive consequences of OSA. In addition to the evaluation of clinical features in the diagnosis, sleep breathing disorder should be demonstrated objectively with an appropriate sleep test. Although laboratory polysomnography is the "gold standard" for objective evaluation, there is increasing evidence that home sleep tests are sufficient in many cases.

OSA is a common sleep-related breathing disorder with an estimated prevalence of 2% to 25% in the general population. It has been found to have a higher incidence in patients undergoing elective surgery, ranging from 40% to 70%, depending on the planned procedure [3–4]. The presence of OSA in surgical patients has recently attracted attention due to numerous studies showing increased perioperative complication rates in OSA patients. These side effects include hypoxemia, difficult intubation, myocardial infarction, pulmonary embolism, cardiac arrhythmias, longer length of hospital stay, and unplanned intensive care unit (ICU) admission [5].

These adverse outcomes in OSA patients are attributable to the effects of anesthetics in OSA patients. Surgical patients often take various forms of sedation, opioids, and other drugs that affect the airway. These drugs increase pharyngeal collapse, decrease ventilatory response, impair arousal, and worsen sleep apnea in the perioperative period [6].

It is well known that patients with OSA have high pharyngeal closure pressures as well as decreased velopharyngeal and oropharyngeal cross-sectional areas, and this leads to increased upper airway instability in the postoperative setting compared to age- and BMI-matched controls. It is thought that the need for postoperative endotracheal intubation may be more frequent due to these reasons [7]. Another possibility is that clinicians have a lower threshold to intubate patients with known OSA in the event of post-operative respiratory complications. There is a significant difference in postoperative complications in patients with OSA compared to patients without OSA. The need for endotracheal intubation is much more common in emergency conditions.

Due to the increase in collapsibility of the upper airway, OSA patients are more likely to experience dangerous respiratory side effects of anesthetic drugs. As a result of the increasing adverse outcomes in surgical patients with OSA, many hospitals are intensively examining OSA patients prior to elective surgery, particularly in the outpatient setting. However, most of the available literature examines patients undergoing various inpatient procedures that require general anesthesia, as opposed to outpatient surgery, which can usually be performed under varying levels of regional anesthesia and sedation. For example, knee arthroscopy is one of the most performed orthopedic outpatient surgeries in the United States, with more than 1 million procedures performed each year, with more than half of them performed in an outpatient setting. Most of the orthopedic surgeries can be performed in centers where short hospitalization surgeries are performed. Anesthesia management is also performed with a combination of regional block and sedation. However, in surgeries requiring general anesthesia, it is a matter of debate whether OSA patients should be operated on in day surgery hospitals or not [8].

Liu et al., reviewed 206 patients who underwent outpatient orthopedic procedures and were followed up with continuous pulse oximetry for 24 hours postoperatively. They suggested that 34% of patients in the postoperative care unit had hypoxemia and that these episodes were not associated with any increase in adverse outcomes or unplanned hospitalization, suggesting that overnight observation was unnecessary after such procedures.

A study examining more than 4,500 patients with OSA who underwent rotator cuff replacement (RCR) reported a significantly increased risk of hospital admission and emergency room admission within 30 days in patients with OSA who underwent ambulatory RCR compared with those without OSA. Postoperative OSA treatment of the patient gains importance. It has gained importance both to ensure patient safety and to reduce hospital costs by reducing postoperative hospitalizations.

Management

Management after orthopedic surgery in patients with OSA is a continuation of preoperative and intraoperative management. Preoperative evaluation of the patient correctly, determination of risk factors, perioperative management, postoperative analgesic, and intensive care process play an important role. For these reasons, postoperative follow-up of patients with low or moderate OSA requires regular and strict service follow-up, while patients with severe and home CPAP therapy should be followed-up in the intensive care unit.

Recommendations for the management of patients with OSA after orthopedic surgery are as follows:

1. Continuous monitoring of vital functions, especially respiratory rate and SPO2. Treatment options and intervention should be considered in the presence of bradypnea (FR $\leq$ 8 /min, at least three times), apnea ($\geq$ 10", even once), or major desaturation (< 90%, at least three measurements).
2. Fluid management. OSA patients often have cardiovascular comorbidities such as chronic congestive heart failure, hypertension, atrial fibrillation, or ischemic coronary artery disease. In these patients, clinicians require careful fluid administration to avoid life-threatening events such as fluid overload and acute pulmonary edema. In addition, some experts suggest that patients with OSA may benefit from infusion of crystalloids with a relatively lower salt content (e.g., Ringer's Lactate) instead of normal saline (NaCl 0.9%). The rationale for this is that infusion of fluids with a high salt content can cause rostral fluid shift and thus worsening of OSA, in addition to the supine position typical for the postoperative period [9]. In patients with kidney failure, congestive heart failure or known lung disease with OSA, fluid management and analgesic management should be determined and started in the initial period, preoperatively and perioperatively.
3. Multimodal analgesic therapy with combined local-regional or plexic techniques may be necessary for postoperative follow-up. As mentioned earlier, some analgesic drugs, especially opioids, have a respiratory depressant effect. To avoid this detrimental effect, a viable strategy in the management of pain control in patients with postoperative OSA is termed multimodal analgesia. This is the combination of an opioid drug at the lowest required dose with one or more other agents such as: nonsteroidal anti-inflammatory drugs (NSAIDs), cyclooxygenase-2 inhibitors (COX-2-inh), paracetamol, peripheral nerve blockers, glucocorticoids, gabapentin, pregabalin and even ketamine. At the same time, postoperative pain triggers sleep disorders and worsens respiratory tract diseases due to sleep disorders. Therefore, pain control becomes particularly important after orthopedic surgeries with intense pain potential.

4. The supine position should be avoided absolutely. Postoperatively, OSA patients should be kept in an upright or semi-upright position or even in a lateral position whenever possible. In fact, the supine position may worsen OSA, especially in patients with positional OSA. The supine position also narrows the diameter of the upper airways, increasing passive pharyngeal collapsibility and rostral fluid shift [10,11].
5. If opioid and hypnotic effects are thought to continue, opioid antagonists or benzodiazepines (naloxone-flumazenil) can be applied to clear the respiratory suppressive effects of these drugs.
6. Positive Airway Pressure (PAP)

Positive airway pressure (PAP) treatments, especially CPAP, are the mainstay of OSA treatment. Therefore, it is recommended that OSA patients who are already on nocturnal PAP therapy continue to use home appliances in the postoperative period. Instead, for patients without a previous diagnosis of OSA, or for patients with OSA who are not compliant with PAP therapies, it would be appropriate to switch to PAP therapy as soon as apnea, hypoxemia, or hypoventilation occurs.

PAP treatments can be particularly useful in terms of preventing atelectasis in the early postoperative period after orthopedic surgery or in the return of the inability to move and cough due to pain.

Among various administrations, CPAP has been reported to be the most effective and widely used treatment for OSA. It has been shown to effectively reduce nocturnal events and improve daytime sleepiness, cognitive function, and general well-being in patients with OSA.

The impact of preoperative CPAP use on perioperative adverse events after inpatient procedures has been well studied. A recent meta-analysis examining six studies and more than 900 patients concluded that there was no appreciable difference in such events between patients who received and did not receive perioperative CPAP therapy [12].

In contrast, the available literature does not evaluate the impact of perioperative CPAP therapy and postoperative adverse events after outpatient surgery. There are publications in the literature showing that it is possible to alleviate adverse events, including emergency room visit, re-admission, and respiratory arrest, with a CPAP prescription in the perioperative period [9].

Physiological and imaging studies have shown that CPAP and NIV improve lung aeration, blood oxygenation, and reduce the occurrence of atelectasis in the postoperative period after extubation without adverse hemodynamic effects [13, 14]. In addition, we know that CPAP therapy to prevent acute respiratory failure is effective and curative in postoperative surgical patients.

Both CPAP and NIV are effective in improving outcomes, especially after abdominal and thoracic surgery, as well as after cardiac surgery [15]. These studies suggest that CPAP and NIV will also be effective after orthopedic surgery.

Conclusion

Patients with OSAS should be monitored after orthopedic surgery, and their conditions such as hypoxemia and tachypnea should be followed closely. Since patients undergoing orthopedic surgery are of high general age and BMI and have multiple comorbidities, postoperative intensive care needs should be examined in detail and the appropriate analgesic method should be selected. Prevention of atelectasis and prevention of hypoxemia should be ensured by making the patient cough, control of pain, intravenous, regional, or peripheral nerve blocks and preventing movement limitation. Patients with OSA are more likely to have difficult intubation compared to the normal population, and the anesthetist's good preoxygenation practice in orthopedic surgeries under general anesthesia will prolong the time until desaturation in the presence of difficult intubation. Before intubation, preparation for difficult intubation should be made, and a video-laryngoscope and fiberoptic bronchoscope should be readily available. If general anesthesia is necessary, short-acting, easily manageable drugs should be preferred. Therefore, a combination of propofol and remifentanil or sevoflurane and remifentanil is recommended. Patients with severe OSA preoperatively should be followed in the early postoperative intensive care unit and PAP treatments should be initiated in the initial period. Postoperative regional analgesia and peripheral nerve blocks should be preferred for orthopedic surgery patients with OSA, and regional anesthesia should be preferred to general anesthesia perioperatively. Early detection of post-operative respiratory failure or episodes of bradypnea or apnea or episodes of desaturation in patients with OSA requires special attention. Post-operative follow-up in the recovery room is recommended for OSA patients at low to moderate risk of OSA, while intensive care unit follow-up is recommended for patients with severe OSA currently undergoing CPAP. PAP therapies are recommended for the prevention and treatment of postoperative acute respiratory failure.

References

[1] Hwang D, Shakir N, Limann B, Sison C, Kalra S, Schulman L, Souza A, Greenberg H. Association of sleep- disordered breathing with postoperative complications. *Chest.* 2008;133(5):1128-1134.

[2] Gross J B, Bachenberg K L, Benumof J L, Caplan R A, Connis R T, Coté C J, Nickinovich DG, Prachand V, Ward DS, Weaver EM, Ydens L, Yu S; *American Society of Anethesiologists Task Force on Perioperative Management. Practice guidelines for the perioperative management.*

[3] Kaw R, Pasupuleti V, Walker E, Ramaswamy A, Foldvary- Schafer N. Postoperative complications in patients with obstructive sleep apnea. *Chest.* 2012;141(2):436-441.

[4] Mador M J, Goplani S, Gottumukkala V A, El-Solh A A, Akashdeep K, Khadka G, Abo-Khamis M. Postoperative complications in obstructive sleep apnea. *Sleep Breath*. 2012; 17(2):727-734.

[5] Healthcare Cost and Utilization Project; Agency for Healthcare Research and Quality. What is the NIS? *Health Cost and Utilization Project website.* http://www.hcup-us.ahrq.gov/ nisoverview.jsp#Whatis. Accessed November 10, 2012.

[6] Isono S. Obstructive sleep apnea of obese adults: pathophysiology and perioperative airway management. *Anesthesiology*. 2009;110(4):908-921.

[7] Golaz R, Tangel V, Lui B, Albrecht E, Pryor K, White R. Post-operative outcomes and anesthesia type in total hip arthroplasty in patients with obstructive sleep apnea: A retrospective analysis of the State Inpatient Databases. *Journal of Clinical Anesthesia* 69 (2021) 110159.

[8] Jourdan m. Cancienne, Brockmeier, SF, Deasey, MJ, Werner, BC. Obstructive Sleep Apnea and Arthroscopic Rotator Cuff Repair—Are Complication Rates Really Increased? Post-operative outcomes and anesthesia type in total hip arthroplasty in patients with obstructive sleep apnea: A retrospective analysis of the State Inpatient Databases. *J. Am. Acad. Orthop. Surg.* 2019;27: 486-492.

[9] Liu S S, Chisholm M F, John R S, Ngeow J, Ma Y, Memtsoudis SG: Risk of postoperative hypoxemia in ambulatory orthopedic surgery patients with diagnosis of obstructive sleep apnea: A retrospective observational study. *Patient Saf. Surg.* 2010; 4:9.

[10] Lam, T; Singh, M; Yadollahi, A; Chung, F. Is Perioperative Fluid and Salt Balance a Contributing Factor in Postoperative Worsening of Obstructive Sleep Apnea? *Anesth. Analg*., 2016, 122, 1335–1339. doi:10. 1213/ANE.0000000000001169.

[11] Ong, J S L; Touyz, G; Tanner, S; Hillman, D R; Eastwood, P R; Walsh, J H. Variability of human upper airway collapsibility during sleep and the influence of body posture and sleep stage. *J. Sleep Res.,* 2011, 20, 533–537. doi:10.1111/j.1365-2869.2011.00925.x.

[12] Nagappa M, Mokhlesi B, Wong J, Wong D T, Kaw R, Chung F: The effects of continuous positive airway pressure on postoperative outcomes in obstructive sleep apnea patients undergoing surgery. *Anesth. Analg.* 2015;120: 1013-1023.

[13] Abdelsattar, Z M; Hendren, S; Wong, S L; Campbell, D A; Ramachandran, S K. The Impact of Untreated Obstructive Sleep Apnea on Cardiopulmonary Complications in General and Vascular Surgery: A Cohort Study. *Sleep,* 2015, 38, 1205–1210. doi:10.5665/sleep.4892.

[14] Jaber, S; Chanques, G; Jung, B; Riou, B. Postoperative Noninvasive Ventilation. *Anesthesiology*, 2010, 112, 453–461. doi:10.1097/ALN. 0b013e3181c5e5f2.

[15] Chiumello, D; Chevallard, G; Gregoretti, C. Non-invasive ventilation in postoperative patients: a systematic review. *Intensive Care Med.*, 2011, 37, 918–929. doi:10.1007/s00134-011-2210-8.

Chapter 21

Postoperative Neurosurgery

Remi Okwechime[1,*], MD, MPH
Peter J. Papadakos[2], MD
Fahad J. Laghari[3], MD
and Jenna Gonillo Davis[4]

[1]Neurosurgery and Medicine, University of Rochester Medical Center, Rochester, New York, USA
[2]Neurosurgery, Surgery, and Anesthesia and Perioperative Medicine, University of Rochester Medical Center, Rochester, New York, USA
[3]Neurocritical Care, University of Rochester Medical Center, Rochester, New York, USA
[4]Neuromedicine Intensive Care Unit, University of Rochester Medical Center, Rochester, New York, USA

Abstract

Obstructive sleep apnea (OSA) is an independent risk factor of stroke and a complex global health issue. Patients may present for elective or emergent surgeries with prior diagnosis of OSA. However, patients with undiagnosed or untreated OSA present unique challenges for the clinical teams caring for them. Patients with OSA may be at increased risk for postoperative cardiac events and respiratory failure which may require reintubation. Tools such as the STOP-Bang score can assist with identifying high risk OSA patients. Through careful assessment of patient specific risk factors, preoperative and postoperative evaluation, unplanned intensive care unit (ICU) admissions can be avoided thus decreasing length of hospital stay and overall cost of care. This chapter will discuss considerations and treatment options for the neurosurgical patient preoperatively, postoperatively, and while in the ICU.

* Corresponding Author's Email: remi_okwechime@urmc.rochester.edu.

In: Obstructive Sleep Apnea in Pulmonary Critical Care
Editors: Antonio M. Esquinas and Takatoshi Kasai
ISBN: 979-8-88697-858-2

Keywords: obstructive sleep apnea, neurosurgery, cerebrovascular disease, stroke, obesity, hypertension, atrial fibrillation, continuous positive airway pressure, STOP-Bang questionnaire, intensive care unit, post anesthesia care unit

Introduction

Obstructive sleep apnea (OSA) is an independent risk factor of stroke and a complex global health issue [1, 2]. Patients may present for elective or emergent surgeries, who may have previously diagnosed OSA. However, patients with undiagnosed or untreated OSA present unique challenges for the clinical teams caring for them. Patients with OSA may be at increased risk for postoperative cardiac events, Intensive Care Unit (ICU) transfers and respiratory failure which may require reintubation [3]. Tools such as the STOP-Bang score can assist with identifying high risk OSA patients [4].

Through careful assessment of patient specific risk factors, preoperative and postoperative evaluation, planned ICU admissions can be avoided thus decreasing length of hospital stay and overall cost of care. This chapter will discuss considerations and treatment options for the neurosurgical patient preoperatively, postoperatively, and while in the ICU.

Sleep Apnea

Sleep apnea is a chronic sleep-related breathing disorder characterized by repetitive reduced to absent ventilation during sleep. The disorder can be diagnosed by taking history, performing a physical examination, and obtaining an apnea-hypopnea index (AHI) from polysomnography or respiratory polygraphy [5]. The index is measured per hour of recording, providing useful data that helps diagnose and characterize the severity of sleep apnea. According to the American Academy of Sleep Medicine, a symptomatic patient can be diagnosed with sleep apnea if they have five or greater events per hour. Furthermore, the severity is characterized as: 5 - < 15 = mild sleep apnea, 15 – 30 = moderate sleep apnea, > 30 events =severe sleep apnea [5].

Types of Sleep Apnea

The absence of airflow in sleep apnea may be centrally mediated, resulting in a lack of attempt at respiration which is called central sleep apnea. Central sleep apnea (CSA) is less prevalent and is often seen in patients with heart failure. Cheyne-Stokes breathing is a common manifestation of CSA. Other risk factors for CSA include age, acute stroke, male sex, and opioid dependence [6].

Sleep apnea can also be caused by upper airway collapse during respiratory effort known as obstructive sleep apnea. OSA is the most common subtype of sleep apnea and is the most prevalent of sleep-related breathing disorders [6]. Approximately 15 to 30 percent of males in North America may have OSA while 10 to 15 percent of females may have OSA [6]. Risk factors for OSA include age, obesity, family history, nasal congestion, and facial features that increase the risk of upper airway collapse.

Complications

All sleep apneas lead to hypoxia. Recurrent hypoxia not only worsens the quality of sleep but also puts an individual at risk of severe complications. OSA has been identified as an independent risk factor for cerebrovascular morbidity [1, 2, 7]. It also increases the risk for systemic hypertension, cardiac arrhythmias including atrial fibrillations, insulin resistance, metabolic syndrome, and both ischemic and hemorrhagic cerebrovascular events [7].

Association with Cerebrovascular Diseases

OSA has been identified as an independent risk factor for cerebrovascular disease, while CSA has been frequently observed in the acute phase after cerebrovascular events [8]. Uncontrolled OSA has been shown to be associated with intracranial aneurysmal complications including rupture, vasospasm, and poorer outcome [9]. After controlling for risk factors such as atrial fibrillation, hypertension, hyperlipidemia, diabetes mellitus, age, race, and smoking status, a significant association between OSA and stroke was found [10, 11, 12]. Most importantly, a dose-response effect was also observed with increased severity of sleep apnea found to be associated with an increased risk of stroke [10].

A limitation in these data is the inclusion of females. Most studies available are less inclusive of female patients with OSA. Although limited data suggests that female patients have similar risk patterns for cerebrovascular events in untreated OSA [13], further research should explore this relationship in order to present a complete picture of the disease process.

Diagnosis and Treatment

Diagnosis and treatment of sleep apnea can decrease morbidity and mortality within the neurosurgical patient population as a stroke prevention measure. Sleep apnea can be diagnosed by obtaining AHI from performing polysomnography or respiratory polygraphy. The STOP-Bang score is derived from a set of questions and objective measurements that works as an initial screening tool for patients and has a high negative predictive value for moderate to severe OSA [14]. This questionnaire consists of four self-reportable measures- (STOP- Snoring, Tiredness, Observed Apnea and High-blood pressure) and four demographic measures (BANG- Body Mass Index {BMI; calculated with the formula weight in kilograms divided by height in meters squared}, age, neck circumference and gender) [14]. Positive airway pressure therapies are used to treat sleep apneas [5]. Treatment of patients with OSA with CPAP may decrease the risk of stroke, recurrence of stroke and death [15, 16]. Treatment can be started with low settings on continuous positive airway pressure during sleep and can be titrated according to symptoms and sleep study results.

Choosing a CPAP mask and device is a collaborative effort between the patient and care team. Synthesizing the patient's subjective and objective symptoms and patient feedback regarding device comfort can improve compliance. While admitted to the hospital, patients with known sleep apnea should be provided positive pressure ventilation. Recognizing that the patient's admitting diagnosis may change their needs, provider teams can begin CPAP support with their outpatient prescription and titrate as needed. Auto-titrating CPAP machines may be available to provide increased comfort to patients with fluctuating requirements.

Other measures to improve OSA include lifestyle modifications such as weight loss, avoidance of alcohol and sedatives, sleeping in a lateral position, and a trial of oral appliances if needed. For refractory patients with obstructive tissue in upper airway, surgical correction may also be an option.

Post Anesthesia Care Unit and Intensive Care Unit Considerations

Neurosurgical emergencies such as ischemic stroke and ruptured intracranial aneurysms are complex diseases which are affected by patient comorbidities and access to healthcare. Increased risk for the neurosurgical patient with OSA may be due to the hypoxemic episodes initiating the inflammatory cascade which damages the vascular endothelium. The damage activates platelet aggregation thus continuing the oxidative stress and perpetuating injury to the endothelium. This is the foundation of cardiovascular disease which is a risk factor for stroke. Patients with OSA are more likely to have cardiac arrythmias, such as atrial fibrillation, which also increases the risk of thrombo-embolic stroke [17]. Treatment of moderate to severe OSA with CPAP showed a decrease in new vascular events in patients with a history of ischemic stroke [18], as well as a reduction in mortality [19]. The relationship between OSA and ruptured intracranial aneurysms (RIA) is evolving. OSA has been identified as a positive predictor of unfavorable outcomes for patients with RIAs [20]. Many of these patients spend a significant amount of their hospital stay in the ICU for frequent neurological assessments, however evaluation and treatment of OSA should be considered during their hospitalization.

A thorough patient assessment should be completed prior to extubation in the post anesthesia care unit (PACU) and unique factors to the patient case should be considered. For example, patients who have undergone extensive spinal surgery requiring prone positioning may not be able to be extubated due to facial or laryngeal edema. Other components of the evaluation should include but are not limited to difficulty of initial intubation, trauma during intubation, patient-specific blood pressure or intracranial pressure goals for concurrent traumatic brain injury management, and other injuries in a patient with polytrauma. Assessment of a cuff leak prior to extubation can assist in identifying patients who are at higher risk for laryngeal edema or stridor [21] and allow for multi-dose treatment of laryngeal edema with dexamethasone [22]. Positioning prior to and immediately following extubation is a key to success in neurosurgical patients with OSA. The head of bed should be elevated to at least 30 degrees and ensure that the patient's neck remains midline. Oral suction and supplemental oxygen which can be delivered via face mask or nasal cannula should be readily available. Continuous pulse oximetry should be used in the immediate post-extubation period in the PACU or ICU with frequent vital signs and nursing assessments. A common cause of reintubation is laryngospasm which may be prevented with pretreatment with lidocaine and magnesium [23]. Although uncommon, vocal cord paralysis due to vagal nerve trauma should be assessed in the post-operative neurosurgical patient. Patients with unilateral paralysis may require further speech language therapy or ear, nose, and throat specialist consultations, however patients that experience bilateral paralysis will require immediate reintubation.

References

[1] Jehan, S., Farag, M., Zizi, F., Pandi-Perumal, S. R., Chung, A., Truong, A., Jean-Louis, G., Tello, D., & McFarlane, S. I. (2018). Obstructive sleep apnea and stroke. *Sleep medicine and disorders: international journal*, *2*(5), 120–125.

[2] Arzt, M., Young, T., Finn, L., Skatrud, J. B., & Bradley, T. D. (2005). Association of sleep-disordered breathing and the occurrence of stroke. *American journal of respiratory and critical care medicine*, *172*(11), 1447–1451. https://doi.org/10.1164/rccm.200505-702OC.

[3] Kaw, R., Chung, F., Pasupuleti, V., Mehta, J., Gay, P. C., & Hernandez, A. V. (2012). Meta-analysis of the association between obstructive sleep apnoea and postoperative outcome. *British journal of anaesthesia*, *109*(6), 897–906. https://doi.org/10.1093/bja/aes308.

[4] Pereira, H., Xará, D., Mendonça, J., Santos, A., & Abelha, F. J. (2013). Patients with a high risk for obstructive sleep apnea syndrome: postoperative respiratory complications. *Revista portuguesa de pneumologia*, *19*(4), 144–151. https://doi.org/10.1016/j.rppneu.2013.01.003.

[5] Epstein, L. J., Kristo, D., Strollo, P. J., Jr, Friedman, N., Malhotra, A., Patil, S. P., Ramar, K., Rogers, R., Schwab, R. J., Weaver, E. M., Weinstein, M. D., & Adult Obstructive Sleep Apnea Task Force of the American Academy of Sleep Medicine (2009). Clinical guideline for the evaluation, management and long-term care of obstructive sleep apnea in adults. *Journal of clinical sleep medicine : JCSM : official publication of the American Academy of Sleep Medicine*, *5*(3), 263–276.

[6] Baillieul, S., Dekkers, M., Brill, A. K., Schmidt, M. H., Detante, O., Pépin, J. L., Tamisier, R., & Bassetti, C. L. A. (2022). Sleep apnoea and ischaemic stroke: current knowledge and future directions. *The Lancet. Neurology*, *21*(1), 78–88. https://doi.org/10.1016/S1474-4422(21)00321-5.

[7] Drager, L. F., McEvoy, R. D., Barbe, F., Lorenzi-Filho, G., Redline, S., & INCOSACT Initiative (International Collaboration of Sleep Apnea Cardiovascular Trialists) (2017). Sleep Apnea and Cardiovascular Disease: Lessons From Recent

Trials and Need for Team Science. *Circulation*, *136*(19), 1840–1850. https://doi.org/10.1161/CIRCULATIONAHA.117.029400.

[8] Siccoli, M. M., Valko, P. O., Hermann, D. M., & Bassetti, C. L. (2008). Central periodic breathing during sleep in 74 patients with acute ischemic stroke - neurogenic and cardiogenic factors. *Journal of neurology*, *255*(11), 1687–1692. https://doi.org/10.1007/s00415-008-0981-9.

[9] Bir, S. C., Nanda, A., Cuellar, H., Sun, H., Guthikonda, B., Liendo, C., Minagar, A., & Chernyshev, O. Y. (2018). Coexistence of obstructive sleep apnea worsens the overall outcome of intracranial aneurysm: a pioneer study. *Journal of neurosurgery*, *128*(3), 735–746. https://doi.org/10.3171/2016.10.JNS162316.

[10] Yaggi, H. K., Concato, J., Kernan, W. N., Lichtman, J. H., Brass, L. M., & Mohsenin, V. (2005). Obstructive sleep apnea as a risk factor for stroke and death. *The New England journal of medicine*, *353*(19), 2034–2041. https://doi.org/10.1056/NEJMoa043104.

[11] Valham, F., Mooe, T., Rabben, T., Stenlund, H., Wiklund, U., & Franklin, K. A. (2008). Increased risk of stroke in patients with coronary artery disease and sleep apnea: a 10-year follow-up. *Circulation*, *118*(9), 955–960. https://doi.org/10.1161/CIRCULATIONAHA.108.783290.

[12] Loke, Y. K., Brown, J. W., Kwok, C. S., Niruban, A., & Myint, P. K. (2012). Association of obstructive sleep apnea with risk of serious cardiovascular events: a systematic review and meta-analysis. *Circulation. Cardiovascular quality and outcomes*, *5*(5), 720–728. https://doi.org/10.1161/CIRCOUTCOMES.111.964783.

[13] Campos-Rodriguez, F., Martinez-Garcia, M. A., Reyes-Nuñez, N., Caballero-Martinez, I., Catalan-Serra, P., & Almeida-Gonzalez, C. V. (2014). Role of sleep apnea and continuous positive airway pressure therapy in the incidence of stroke or coronary heart disease in women. *American journal of respiratory and critical care medicine*, *189*(12), 1544–1550. https://doi.org/10.1164/rccm.201311-2012OC.

[14] Tan, A., Yin, J. D., Tan, L. W., van Dam, R. M., Cheung, Y. Y., & Lee, C. H. (2016). Predicting obstructive sleep apnea using the STOP-Bang questionnaire in the general population. *Sleep medicine*, *27-28*, 66–71. https://doi.org/10.1016/j.sleep.2016.06.034.

[15] Kim, Y., Koo, Y. S., Lee, H. Y., & Lee, S. Y. (2016). Can Continuous Positive Airway Pressure Reduce the Risk of Stroke in Obstructive Sleep Apnea Patients? A Systematic Review and Meta-Analysis. *PloS one*, *11*(1), e0146317. https://doi.org/10.1371/journal.pone.0146317.

[16] Haba-Rubio, J., Vujica, J., Franc, Y., Michel, P., & Heinzer, R. (2019). Effect of CPAP Treatment of Sleep Apnea on Clinical Prognosis After Ischemic Stroke: An Observational Study. *Journal of clinical sleep medicine : JCSM : official publication of the American Academy of Sleep Medicine*, *15*(6), 839–847. https://doi.org/10.5664/jcsm.7832.

[17] Mansukhani, M. P., Calvin, A. D., Kolla, B. P., Brown, R. D., Jr, Lipford, M. C., Somers, V. K., & Caples, S. M. (2013). The association between atrial fibrillation and stroke in patients with obstructive sleep apnea: a population-based case-control study. *Sleep medicine*, *14*(3), 243–246. https://doi.org/10.1016/j.sleep.2012.08.021.

[18] Martínez-García, M. A., Galiano-Blancart, R., Román-Sánchez, P., Soler-Cataluña, J. J., Cabero-Salt, L., & Salcedo-Maiques, E. (2005). Continuous positive airway pressure treatment in sleep apnea prevents new vascular events after ischemic stroke. *Chest*, *128*(4), 2123–2129. https://doi.org/10.1378/chest.128.4.2123.

[19] Martínez-García, M. A., Soler-Cataluña, J. J., Ejarque-Martínez, L., Soriano, Y., Román-Sánchez, P., Illa, F. B., Canal, J. M., & Durán-Cantolla, J. (2009). Continuous positive airway pressure treatment reduces mortality in patients with ischemic stroke and obstructive sleep apnea: a 5-year follow-up study. *American journal of respiratory and critical care medicine*, *180*(1), 36–41. https://doi.org/10.1164/rccm.200808-1341OC.

[20] Chernyshev, O. Y., Bir, S. C., Maiti, T. K., Patra, D. P., Sun, H., Guthikonda, B., Kelley, R. E., Cuellar, H., Minagar, A., & Nanda, A. (2019). The Relationship Between Obstructive Sleep Apnea and Ruptured Intracranial Aneurysms. *Journal of clinical sleep medicine : JCSM : official publication of the American Academy of Sleep Medicine*, *15*(12), 1839–1848. https://doi.org/10.5664/jcsm.8096.

[21] Jaber, S., Chanques, G., Matecki, S., Ramonatxo, M., Vergne, C., Souche, B., Perrigault, P. F., & Eledjam, J. J. (2003). Post-extubation stridor in intensive care unit patients. Risk factors evaluation and importance of the cuff-leak test. *Intensive care medicine*, *29*(1), 69–74. https://doi.org/10.1007/s00134-002-1563-4.

[22] Lee, C. H., Peng, M. J., & Wu, C. L. (2007). Dexamethasone to prevent postextubation airway obstruction in adults: a prospective, randomized, double-blind, placebo-controlled study. *Critical care (London, England)*, *11*(4), R72. https://doi.org/10.1186/cc5957.

[23] Difficult Airway Society Extubation Guidelines Group, Popat, M., Mitchell, V., Dravid, R., Patel, A., Swampillai, C., & Higgs, A. (2012). Difficult Airway Society Guidelines for the management of tracheal extubation. *Anaesthesia*, *67*(3), 318–340. https://doi.org/10.1111/j.1365-2044.2012.07075.x.

Chapter 22

Discharge from the Intensive Care Unit

Nicola Launaro*, MD
Respiratory Intensive Care Unit, Saluzzo Civil Hospital, ASLCN1, Italy

Abstract

Patients with Obstructive Sleep Apnea Syndrome (OSAS) have an increased risk of being admitted to the ICU. This condition is a consequence of both the intrinsic characteristics of the pathology and the numerous co-morbidities such as COPD, Cardiovascular, Metabolic. This chapter presents various scenarios for managing the discharge of patients with OSAS from a protected environment such as Intensive Care to inpatient wards where patient monitoring and surveillance are inevitably less thorough, and to their homes. Each path is defined according to the condition responsible for admission. The first subdivision will be between patients hospitalized following surgery or trauma and those who have developed an aggravation of co-morbidities or an acute pathology.

Keywords: obstructive sleep apnea syndrome, obesity-hypoventilation syndrome, monitoring, STOP-Bang questionnaire, health care organization

* Corresponding Author's Email: nicola.launaro@gmail.com.

In: Obstructive Sleep Apnea in Pulmonary Critical Care
Editors: Antonio M. Esquinas and Takatoshi Kasai
ISBN: 979-8-88697-858-2

Introduction

From the analysis of the literature, no specific guidelines or indications regarding the topic of this chapter emerge. The discussion that follows therefore represents a compromise between various expert opinions and clinical practice.

The prevalence of OSA among patients admitted to intensive care is not known [1, 2]. As regards patients hospitalized after surgery, we do not want to define criteria for admission to intensive care because they present significant differences between the various centers. The purpose of the chapter will be exclusively that of defining a path of discharge from intensive care for all those who will be hospitalized according to the indications of each facility.

In this chapter we will try to provide indications for the safe discharge of patients with OSA who are admitted to intensive care. Many of these patients are admitted to the ICU without a diagnosis of OSA being established prior to admission. In the latter, it will be necessary, as we will see below, to make the diagnosis, define the severity of OSA and, when indicated, start treatment already during hospitalization in intensive care.

We thought of dividing patients into two large groups in relation to the causes that led to the need for admission to intensive care. In fact, we believe that patients who undergo scheduled surgery are always evaluated for any OSA whenever they present symptoms or signs that could lead to suspicion of this pathology. The use of the STOP-Bang questionnaire developed by Chung in 2008 [3] as a preoperative assessment tool for the screening of undiagnosed obstructive sleep apnea is now widespread [1, 4, 5]. This allows to adequately prepare patients with OSA and possibly plan hospitalization in an intensive setting for those cases that present an increased risk of developing apneas in the postoperative period [6, 7].

Risk factors for postoperative respiratory depression are defined by the severity of sleep apnea, intra and postoperative treatment with systemic opioids, the use of sedatives, and finally the location and invasiveness of the surgical procedure. There is also a known risk of developing apneas during REM sleep on the third or fourth postoperative day ("REM rebound"), when the physiological structure of sleep is re-established.

On the other hand, patients who are hospitalized for complications of OSA or for worsening of OSA comorbidities may arrive in intensive care without a specific diagnosis and above all still present an aggravation of the disease with the need for an overall re-evaluation of the patient's clinical condition.

OSA Undergoing Surgery

Patients with OSA who undergo surgery have an increased risk of developing complications in the peri-operative period [3, 8, 9, 10]. The incidence and severity of these adverse events depends on both the severity of OSA and the type of surgery performed on the patient [5, 11].

OSA patients present:

1) Difficulty in ventilation
2) Difficulty in oro-tracheal intubation maneuvers which may be responsible for an increased risk of difficult intubation up to ten times compared to the general population
3) Increased risk of pulmonary complications mainly as a result of hypoventilation
4) Increased risk of respiratory depression
5) Increased risk of cardiovascular complications, especially due to the increase in sympathetic tone

Furthermore, patients with OSA present an increased operative risk due to the presence of numerous co-morbidities

1) Diabetes mellitus
2) COPD
3) Dyslipidemia
4) Cardiovascular diseases: Severe arterial hypertension, Ischemic heart disease, Chronic heart failure
5) Liver disease
6) Obesity
7) Obesity-hypoventilation syndrome and hypoxemic and hypercapnic respiratory insufficiency

The risk of postoperative complications also correlates with the surgery and with the anesthesia that is applied to the patient. General anesthesia increases the risk of developing apneas in the postoperative period [12]. Treatment of pain with opioid drugs significantly increases the number of central apneas in these patients. Long-lasting interventions can be responsible for the development of areas of sloping atelectasis that can increase with postoperative hypoventilation.

According to what has been said, it is necessary to plan an intensive care hospitalization in patients with very severe OSA who must undergo major and long-lasting surgery under general anesthesia or who have serious comorbidities. The hospital stay must be related to the recovery of normal sleep or the restoration of OSA therapy [13].

The American Society of Anesthesiologists recommends carrying out a specific evaluation whenever there is a suspicion of a patient with OSA who needs to undergo surgery [14].

Interventions

A. Bariatric Surgery [15, 16]

These patients present for surgery with a diagnosis of OSA also defined by the level of severity. If positive for OSA they are already being treated with CPAP or other ventilation modalities. Admission to an Intensive Care Unit should be reserved only for patients who have very severe OSA, which is not adequately corrected by CPAP treatment or who have severe co-comorbidities with an increased risk of developing cardiovascular complications in the postoperative period.

If the surgery was performed with a laparoscopic technique, avoid the administration of opiates in the postoperative period [17].

Monitor ECG, SaO2, Post-operative blood pressure. The patient will have to be discharged from the ICU when:

1. has recovered an adequate level of consciousness
2. there is no severe deficit in arterial saturation during sleep during treatment with CPAP

After discharge, the patient will have to continue treatment with CPAP as defined before the surgery. Provide a new evaluation with cardiorespiratory monitoring during sleep in relation to the loss of body weight and in any case no later than 90 days.

B. Upper Airways Surgery, Maxillofacial Surgery [2, 18]

Often after these surgeries, CPAP treatment cannot be applied postoperatively. These patients will need to be closely monitored. The treatment of desaturations during sleep can be treated with low-flow oxygen, paying particular attention to the possible occurrence of central apneas.

Upon discharge, patients will be able to resume treatment with CPAP following the instructions of the surgeon who performed the surgery. Within 15 days, especially in the case of a failure to resume specific therapy, they will have to carry out an evaluation with cardiorespiratory monitoring during sleep to evaluate the appropriateness of continuing treatment with CPAP and in the case of the continued indication to carry out a new titration.

1. Non-OSA Related Scheduled Surgery

These patients, as mentioned above, will be admitted to intensive care only if they undergo major surgery, if they have severe OSA, if they have severe co-morbidities.

In the postoperative period they will have to be treated with the CPAP that they use daily without changing its setting. They will have to be discharged from intensive care when it is certain that they do not present an increased risk of developing complications related to OSA. In particular, the onset of central apneas related to postoperative pain relief, respiratory failure due to an aggravation of obstructive apneas must be excluded. In the latter case, it will be necessary to modify the treatment with CPAP by adjusting the pressure level until the arterial desaturations are corrected. Discharge when correction of arterial desaturations is detected.

At discharge, they will continue treatment with CPAP according to the parameters defined during hospitalization. Schedule a follow-up visit at your Sleep Medicine Center within 15 days.

2. Surgery in an Emergency/Trauma Regime

Hospitalization will depend on the criticality of the patient's clinical condition. During the ICU course, these patients may resume spontaneous breathing without the need for ventilatory support or develop conditions that will require prolonged ventilatory treatment.

If the patient is extubated, it is advisable to resume treatment with CPAP, where possible, which will continue even after discharge from the intensive care unit. As before, these patients will still have to undergo an evaluation at the Sleep Medicine Center at least 15 days after discharge.

In patients who will undergo tracheostomy and prolonged ventilation treatment, it will not be necessary to provide for an evaluation until a resumption of autonomous respiratory activity occurs. In this case, if a closure of the tracheostomy is foreseen, it is advisable to plan an evaluation with cardiorespiratory monitoring during sleep and possible new CPAP titration.

If the diagnosis of OSA is made during the hospital stay in intensive care, it is necessary to define the type of apnea and the severity of the condition with cardiorespiratory monitoring during sleep. Before discharge, the CPAP pressure value must be titrated. Upon discharge, these patients will have to continue CPAP therapy until the check-up visit at the Sleep Medicine Center which will have to be carried out as soon as possible depending on the patient's clinical condition. *Summary in Figure 1. OSA patients undergoing surgery from ICU.*

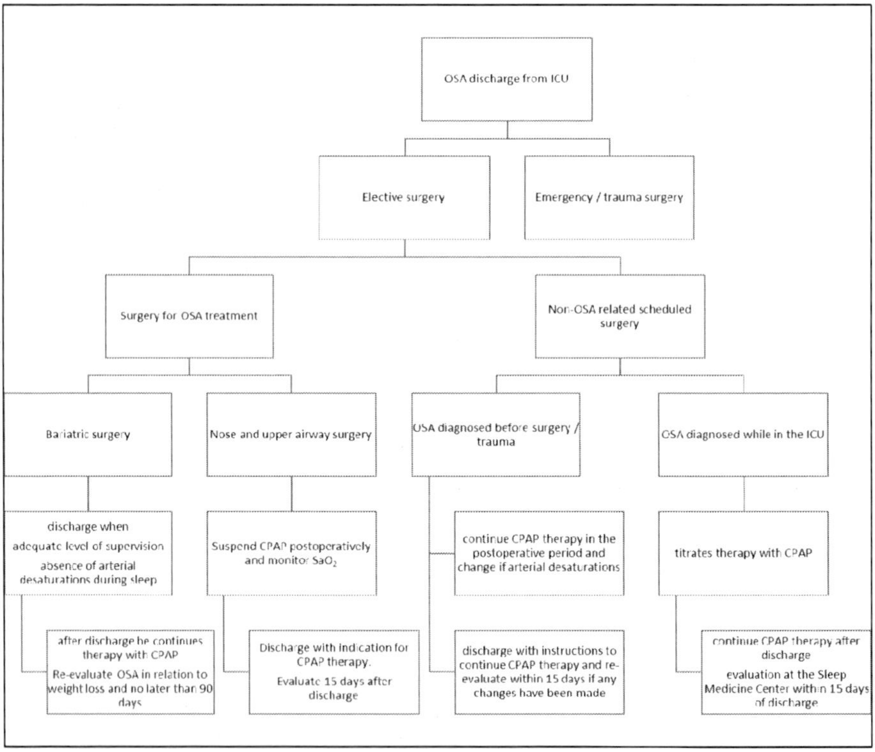

Figure 1. OSA patients undergoing surgery discharge from ICU.

OSA with Non-Surgical Diseases

The presence of numerous and often complex and severe comorbidities exposes patients with OSA to an increased risk of admission to intensive care units [19, 20, 21].

In particular, severe obesity (BMI > 40 kg / m^2) is an independent risk factor for an increased risk of admission to intensive care. Various studies have shown that patients with OSA have a reduced mortality in intensive care compared to patients without this disease [22, 23, 24, 25]. The obesity paradox has therefore been defined for a lower mortality probably linked to the nutritional reserve provided by excess lipids capable of compensating for the catabolism of the critically ill patient. On the contrary, in patients who develop an obesity hypoventilation syndrome (defined by a combination of BMI > 30 kg / m^2, sleep-disordered breathing (SDB), and daytime hypercapnia, $PaCO_2$ $\geq$ 45 mm Hg) an increase ICU lehngt of stay could be found. without increasing mortality [26, 27].

The prevalence of OSA is very high in patients admitted to the ICU for COPD exacerbation [28, 29, 30, 31, 32]. Among individuals with COPD, undiagnosed OSA is associated with a worse prognosis while COPD patients who present with OSA and are already being treated for it have a better prognosis. This leads to search for the association between the two diseases even during hospitalization in the ICU or before hospital discharge [33].

OSA is associated with an increased risk of developing severe airway infections following viral infections (Influenza and recently SARS COVID 19). The association with influenza has been demonstrated in large cohorts of patients, prompting the authors to recommend close monitoring of clinical conditions and early use of Oseltamivir in these patients [34].

In the case of pneumonia, the association with OSA seems to reduce the risk of hospital mortality, probably due to an increase in non-routine discharge [35].

Heart failure is a frequent cause of ICU admission for patients with obstructive sleep apnea [36]. There are several alterations induced by apneas that can determine or aggravate heart failure, such as:

Hypoxemia and hypercapnia responsible for pulmonary vasoconstriction with increased afterload of the right ventricle (cor pulmonale), oxidative stress and inflammation that can induce endothelial damage with consequent coronary atherosclerosis (ischemic heart disease) and arrhythmias. Finally, the reduced supply of oxygen to the myocardium increases the risk of acute ischemia and chronically induces left ventricle hypertrophy.

The arousals cause an increase in sympathetic tone and a reduction in the parasympathetic tone with an increase in heart rate, blood pressure and oxygen requirements.

Patients with OSA and severe obesity have an increased risk of developing myocardial infarction. Even in this condition, various studies have shown a reduced in-hospital mortality probably linked to various factors such as relatively younger age and major comorbidities can induce an early and more thorough treatment in these patients [6]. Given the greater severity, these patients are usually treated in hospital centers with more equipment and a higher level of skills.

Other causes of hospitalization in intensive care are related to oxidative stress which can induce severe cardiovascular damage, thus increasing the incidence of stroke.

OSA is responsible for the development of a metabolic syndrome which in turn increases oxidative stress and vascular damage [25, 37].

OSA patients admitted to the ICU have an increased risk of developing acute renal failure [38].

The main causes of hospitalization in the ICU of patients with OSA are

1. Hypoxic-hypercapnic respiratory failure in exacerbated COPD
2. Heart failure
3. Heart attack
4. Hypoxic-hypercapnic respiratory failure in hypoventilation obesity syndrome
5. Atrial fibrillation and arrhythmias [38]
6. Stroke
7. Aortic dissection
8. Pneumonia

These conditions can occur in patients with a sleep apnea syndrome already known and under treatment but often during the first admission to the intensive care unit it is possible to diagnose this pathology. The discharge program will therefore be diversified between these two categories of patients.

In these patients it is necessary to carefully diagnose and define the comorbidities and the cause of the current hospitalization. Evaluate whether it is the first ICU admission for this cause or whether others have already occurred.

1. Patients with OSA Diagnosed before Admission to the ICU

During hospitalization in intensive care, the disease in progress will have to be treated by assessing whether it is to be considered related to OSA and in this case, cardiorespiratory monitoring during sleep or a polysomnography during ventilatory treatment must be carried out to define its effectiveness. This evaluation appears necessary to define the program of discharge from the intensive care and the treatment of apneas. It is advisable to carry out a new titration of the ventilatory treatment in place before admission to intensive care. Such titration would be preferable to perform in a high-level monitoring setting such as an intensive care unit to reduce the risk of cardiovascular or respiratory complications. Discharge when the correct ventilation program has been defined.

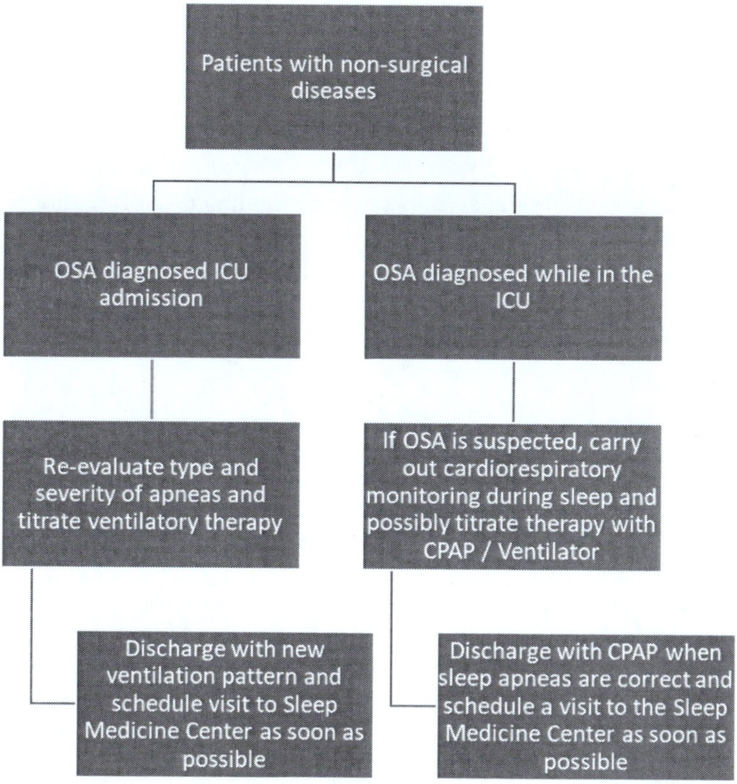

Figure 2. OSA-patients undergoing non-surgery from ICU.

2. Patients with Undiagnosed OSA Prior to ICU Admission

The diagnosis of OSA in these patients is often a consequence of the evaluation of the disease that induced admission, the comorbidities, the finding of arterial desaturations that occur when the patient sleeps. In these cases it is necessary to carry out a monitoring during sleep that can define the type of disturbance (Obstructive, Central, Mixed) and its severity (AHI, ODI).

The examination must be carried out after removing the possible causes of apnea (therapy with opioids and / or sedatives for example, delirium). Once the diagnosis has been made, also in this case, it is preferable to titrate the therapy with CPAP before discharge from the intensive care unit.

In both conditions, patients discharged from intensive care and from the hospital will then have to be referred to a center for the treatment of respiratory disorders during sleep to continue the checkups and treatment of their apneas.

Conclusion

Obstructive Sleep Apnea Syndrome (OSAS) have an increased risk in ICU from medicial or surgery interventions, related with inestable pathophysiology and numerous co-morbidities. Its necesary a great protocol for dicharge planning from ICU to conventional wards with a multidisciplinary team.

References

[1] Woodling K, Fiorda-Diaz J, Otto B A, Barnes C A, Uribe A A, Bergese S D, Yildiz V, Stoicea N, Guertin MG. A retrospective analysis on patients at high-risk for obstructive sleep apnea undergoing ear, nose, and throat surgeries. Laryngoscope Investig *Otolaryngol.* 2017 Dec 29;3(1):16-21. doi: 10.1002/lio2.131. PMID: 29492464; PMCID: PMC5824111.

[2] Cozowicz C, Memtsoudis SG. Perioperative Management of the Patient With Obstructive Sleep Apnea: A Narrative Review. *Anesth. Analg.* 2021 May 1;132(5):1231-1243. doi: 10.1213/ANE.0000000000005444. PMID: 33857965.

[3] Chung F, Yegneswaran B, Liao P, Chung S A, Vairavanathan S, Islam S, Khajehdehi A, Shapiro CM. STOP questionnaire: a tool to screen patients for obstructive sleep apnea. *Anesthesiology.* 2008 May;108(5):812-21. doi: 10.1097/ALN.0b013e31816d83e4. PMID: 18431116.

[4] Bryson G L, Gomez C P, Jee R M, Blackburn J, Taljaard M, Forster A J. Unplanned admission after day surgery: a historical cohort study in patients with obstructive

sleep apnea. *Can. J. Anaesth.* 2012 Sep;59(9):842-51. doi: 10.1007/s12630-012-9746-0. Epub 2012 Jul 6. PMID: 22766625.

[5] Practice Guidelines for the Perioperative Management of Patients with Obstructive Sleep Apnea: An Updated Report by the American Society of Anesthesiologists Task Force on Perioperative Management of Patients with Obstructive Sleep Apnea. *Anesthesiology* 2014; 120:268–286 doi: https://doi.org/10.1097/ALN.0000000000000053.

[6] Suen, C; Wong, J.; Ryan, C. M.; Goh, S.; Got, T.; Chaudhry, R.; Lee, D. S.; Chung, F. Prevalence of Undiagnosed Obstructive Sleep Apnea Among Patients Hospitalized for Cardiovascular Disease and Associated In-Hospital Outcomes: A Scoping Review. *J. Clin. Med.* 2020, 9, 989. https://doi.org/10.3390/jcm9040989.

[7] Ahmed Brgdar, Jin Yi, Ahmad Awan, Mohamed Taha, Richard Ogunti, John Gharbin, Mehrotra Prafulla, Isaac Opoku. (December 28, 2021) Impact of Obstructive Sleep Apnea On In-Hospital Outcomes in Patients With Atrial Fibrillation: A Retrospective Analysis of the National Inpatient Sample. *Cureus* 13(12): e20770. DOI 10.7759/cureus.20770.
[Cite this article as: Brgdar A, Yi J, Awan A, et al. (December 28, 2021) Impact of Obstructive Sleep Apnea On In-Hospital Outcomes in Patients With Atrial Fibrillation: A Retrospective Analysis of the National Inpatient Sample. *Cureus* 13(12): e20770. doi:10.7759/cureus.2077]

[8] Roop Kaw, Bhargavi Gali, Nancy A. Collop, Perioperative Care Of Patients With Obstructive Sleep Apnea Onwochei D N, Fabes J, Walker D, Kumar G, Moonesinghe SR. Critical care after major surgery: a systematic review of risk factors for unplanned admission. *Anaesthesia* 2020; 75(Suppl 1): e62– e74.

[9] Reis R, Antunes A. Obstructive sleep apnea prevalence and adverse respiratory events in surgical patients. *Rev. Port. Pneumol.* 2014 Jan-Feb;20(1):50-1. doi: 10.1016/j.rppneu.2013.08.003. Epub 2013 Dec 15. PMID: 24342229.

[10] ASMBS Clinical Issues Committee. *Surgery for Obesity and Related Diseases* 8 (2012) e27–e32.

[11] Xin Xi, Yu Chen, Wei-Guo Ma, Jiang Xie, Yong-Min Liu, Jun-Ming Zhu, Ming Gong, Guang-Fa Zhu, Li-Zhong Sun. Is obstructive sleep apnoea associated with hypoxaemia and prolonged ICU stay after type A aortic dissection repair? A retrospective study in Chinese population BMC Cardiovasc. Disord. (2021) 21:421. [Cite this article as: Xi, X., Chen, Y., Ma, WG. et al. Is obstructive sleep apnoea associated with hypoxaemia and prolonged ICU stay after type A aortic dissection repair? A retrospective study in Chinese population. *BMC Cardiovasc. Disord.* 21, 421 (2021). https://doi.org/10.1186/s12872-021-02226-9].

[12] Jean R E, Gibson C D, Jean R A, Ochieng P. Obstructive sleep apnea and acute respiratory failure: An analysis of mortality risk in patients with pneumonia requiring invasive mechanical ventilation. *J. Crit. Care.* 2015 Aug;30(4):778-83. doi: 10.1016/j.jcrc.2015.03.016. *Epub* 2015 Mar 20. PMID: 25862071.

[13] Vgontzas A N, Bixler E O, Chrousos G P. Sleep apnea is a manifestation of the metabolic syndrome. *Sleep Med. Rev.* 2005 Jun;9(3):211-24. doi: 10.1016/*j.smrv.*2005.01.006. PMID: 15893251.

[14] Kapur V K, Auckley D H, Chowdhuri S, Kuhlmann D C, Mehra R, Ramar K, Harrod C G. Clinical practice guideline for diagnostic testing for adult obstructive sleep apnea: an American Academy of Sleep Medicine clinical practice guideline. *J. Clin. Sleep Med.* 2017;13(3):479–504.

[15] Morgan D J, Ho K M, Armstrong J, Baker S. Incidence and risk factors for intensive care unit admission after bariatric surgery: a multicentre population-based cohort study. *Br. J. Anaesth.* 2015 Dec;115(6):873-82. doi: 10.1093/bja/aev364. PMID: 26582848.

[16] Han L. W., W. Chen, S. J. Lian, Y. C. Lin, C. Y. Tu, H. J. Chen, K. L. Chiu . Clinical characteristics and outcomes of patients with obstructive sleep apnoea requiring intensive care. *Anaesthesia and Intensive Care,* Vol. 38, No. 3, May 2010.

[17] Lee Y J, Lee J, Lee S M, Cho J. Postextubation respiratory events in patients admitted to the intensive care unit: a prospective pilot study using overnight respiratory polygraphy. *Acute Crit. Care.* 2020 Nov;35(4):271-278. doi: 10.4266/acc.2020.00479. Epub 2020 Nov 12. PMID: 33176403; PMCID: PMC7 808846.

[18] Wilson K., I. Lakheeram, A. Morielli, R. Brouillette, K.Brown . Can Assessment for Obstructive Sleep Apnea Help Predict Postadenotonsillectomy Respiratory Complications? *Anesthesiology*, V 96, No 2, Feb 2002.

[19] Walter T. McNicholas, *COPD-OSA Overlap Syndrome: Evolving Evidence Regarding Epidemiology, Clinical Consequences, and Management*, Chest, Volume 152, Issue 6, 2017, Pages 1318-1326, ISSN 0012-3692, https://doi.org/ 10.1016/j.chest.2017.04.160.

[20] anderath W, Verbraecken J, de Raaff CAL, Hedner J, Herkenrath S, Hohenhorst W, Jakob T, Marrone O, Marklund M, McNicholas WT, Morgan RL, Pepin JL, Schiza S, Skoetz N, Smyth D, Steier J, Tonia T, Trzepizur W, van Mechelen PH, Wijkstra P. European Respiratory Society guideline on non-CPAP therapies for obstructive sleep apnoea. *Eur. Respir. Rev.* 2021 Nov 30;30(162):210200. doi: 10.1183/16000617.0200-2021. PMID: 34853097; PMCID: PMC9489103.

[21] Prajapat B, Sandhya A S, Chaudhry D, Esquinas AM. Opioids in intensive care unit (ICU): causal agent for sleep apnea, unmasking the undiagnosed sleep apnea or both in the ICU. *Sleep.* 2018 Jul 1;41(7). doi: 10.1093/sleep/zsy081. PMID: 29788470.

[22] Bolona E, Hahn P Y, Afessa B. Intensive care unit and hospital mortality in patients with obstructive sleep apnea. *J. Crit. Care.* 2015 Feb;30(1):178-80. doi: 10.1016/j.jcrc.2014.10.001. *Epub* 2014 Oct 8. PMID: 25457113.

[23] Lin P, Li X, Zhang J, Liang Z. Association Between Obstructive Sleep Apnea and Reduced Mortality in Critically Ill Patients: A Propensity Score-Based Analysis. Int *J. Gen. Med.* 2021 Aug 21;14:4723-4729. doi: 10.2147/IJGM.S330752. PMID: 34456584; PMCID: PMC8387641.

[24] Dou L, Lan H, Reynolds D J, Gunderson T M, Kashyap R, Gajic O, Caples S, Li G, Kashani K B. Association between Obstructive Sleep Apnea and Acute Kidney Injury in Critically Ill Patients: A Propensity-Matched Study. Nephron. 2017;135(2):137-146. doi: 10.1159/000453367. *Epub* 2016 Dec 13. PMID: 27951 537.

[25] Divyanshu Mohananey; Pedro A. Villablanca, M D; Tanush Gupta; Sahil Agrawal,; Michael Faulx, Venugopal Menon, Samir R. Kapadia; Brian P. Griffin, Stephen G.

Ellis, Milind Y. Desai. Recognized Obstructive Sleep Apnea is Associated With Improved In-Hospital Outcomes After ST Elevation Myocardial Infarction. *J. Am. Heart Assoc.* 2017;6:e006133. DOI: 10.1161/JAHA.117.006133.

[26] Singh S, Kaur H, Singh S, Khawaja I. *The Overlap Syndrome. Cureus.* 2018 Oct 15;10(10):e3453. doi: 10.7759/cureus.3453. PMID: 30564532; PMCID: PMC62 98617.

[27] Shah, Amar J., et al. "Cardiovascular outcomes in patients with COPD-OSA overlap syndrome: A systematic review and meta-analysis." *Sleep Medicine Reviews* (2022): 101627.

[28] Adler D, Bailly S, Benmerad M, Joyeux-Faure M, Jullian-Desayes I, Soccal PM, Janssens JP, Sapène M, Grillet Y, Stach B, Tamisier R, Pépin JL. Clinical presentation and comorbidities of obstructive sleep apnea-COPD overlap syndrome. *PLoS One.* 2020 Jul 9;15(7):e0235331. doi: 10.1371/journal.pone.0235331. PMID: 32645005; PMCID: PMC7347183.

[29] Donovan L M, Feemster L C, Udris E M, Griffith M F, Spece L J, Palen B N, He K, Parthasarathy S, Strohl K P, Kapur V K, Au D H. Poor Outcomes Among Patients With Chronic Obstructive Pulmonary Disease With Higher Risk for Undiagnosed Obstructive Sleep Apnea in the LOTT Cohort. *J. Clin. Sleep Med.* 2019 Jan 15;15(1):71-77. doi: 10.5664/jcsm.7574. PMID: 30621828; PMCID: PMC6329538.

[30] Brennan M, McDonnell M J, Walsh S M, Gargoum F, Rutherford R. Review of the prevalence, pathogenesis and management of OSA-COPD overlap. Sleep Breath. 2022 Jan 16. doi: 10.1007/s11325-021-02540-8. *Epub ahead of print.* PMID: 35034250.

[31] Opperer M, Cozowicz C, Bugada D, Mokhlesi B, Kaw R, Auckley D, Chung F, Memtsoudis SG. Does Obstructive Sleep Apnea Influence Perioperative Outcome? A Qualitative Systematic Review for the Society of Anesthesia and Sleep Medicine Task Force on Preoperative Preparation of Patients with Sleep-Disordered Breathing. *Anesth Analg.* 2016 May;122(5):1321-34. doi: 10.1213/ANE.0000000 000001178. PMID: 27101493.

[32] Voulgaris, A.; Archontogeorgis, K.; Pataka, A.; Flaris, A.N.; Ntolios, P.; Bonsignore, M.R.; Schiza, S.; Steiropoulos, P. Burden of Comorbidities in Patients with OSAS and COPD-OSAS Overlap Syndrome. *Medicina* 2021, 57, 1201. https://doi.org/10.3390/medicina57111201.

[33] Wang H, Shao G, Rong L, Ji Y, Zhang K, Liu M, Ma L. Association between comorbid sleep apnoea-hypopnoea syndrome and prognosis of intensive care patients: a retrospective cohort study. *BMJ Open.* 2021 Jun 23;11(6):e048886. doi: 10.1136/bmjopen-2021-048886. PMID: 34162653; PMCID: PMC8230938.

[34] Sheikh M, Kuperberg S. An organ systems-based review of outcomes associated with sleep apnea in hospitalized patients. *Medicine (Baltimore).* 2021 Aug 27;100(34):e26857. doi: 10.1097/MD.0000000000026857. PMID: 34449455; PMCID: PMC8389950.

[35] Karamichali S, Sclifò F, Piroddi I M, Esquinas A M, Nicolini A. Obstructive sleep apnea and acute respiratory failure due to pneumonia: Is truly a protective factor to mortality risk? *J. Crit. Care.* 2015 Oct;30(5):1139. doi: 10.1016/j.jcrc.2015.06.002. Epub 2015 Jun 10. PMID: 26105746.

[36] Arnaud W. Thille, Ana Córdoba-Izquierdo, Bernard Maitre, Laurent Boyer, Laurent Brochard, Xavier Drouot. High prevalence of sleep apnea syndrome in patients admitted to ICU for acute hypercapnic respiratory failure: a preliminary study. *Intensive Care Med* 44, 267–269 (2018). https://doi.org/10.1007/s00134-017-4998-3.

[37] Sébastien Bailly, Louis-Marie Galerneau, Stéphane Ruckly, Nicolas Terzi, Carole Schwebel, Claire Dupuis, Renaud Tamisier, Bruno Mourvillier, Jean-Louis Pépin, Jean-François Timsit Impact of obstructive sleep apnea on ICU patient's prognosis – insights from a French ICU cohort. *European Respiratory Journal* Sep 2019, 54 (suppl 63) PA866; DOI: 10.1183/13993003.congress-2019.PA866.

[38] Tsai MS, Chen HC, Li HY, Tsai YT, Yang YH, Liu CY, Lee YC, Hsu CM, Lee LA. Sleep Apnea and Risk of Influenza-Associated Severe Acute Respiratory Infection: Real-World Evidence. *Nat Sci Sleep*. 2022 May 10;14:901-909. doi: 10.2147/NSS.S346984. PMID: 35586456; PMCID: PMC9109977.

Chapter 23

Critical Care: Determinants in Mortality

Chantal Cortesão[1,*], MD
and Pedro Silva Santos[1], MD
[1]Pneumology Service, Coimbra Hospital and University Center,
Coimbra, Portugal

Abstract

Obstructive sleep apnea (OSA) is a common condition, frequently found in patients admitted to intensive care units (ICU). OSA's effect on ICU patient's prognosis is controversial. OSA does not increase the length of ICU stay, ICU or hospital mortality and ventilator associated pneumonia, with exception of patients with OSA and morbid obesity, that have significantly longer ICU stay. Recent data on the context of the COVID-19 pandemic has shown that OSA can be associated with poor outcome on COVID-19 patients. Awareness for the impact of OSA on the prognosis of severely ill patients and patients admitted to the ICU is essential.

Keywords: obstructive sleep apnea, mortality, critical care, prognosis

Introduction

Obstructive sleep apnea (OSA) is a common condition characterized by repetitive upper airway obstruction during sleep. This promotes intra-thoracic pressure variation, intermittent hypoxia, and sleep fragmentation, associated with increased cardiovascular risk [1, 2].

---

[*] Corresponding Author's Email: rcchantal @gmail.com.

In: Obstructive Sleep Apnea in Pulmonary Critical Care
Editors: Antonio M. Esquinas and Takatoshi Kasai
ISBN: 979-8-88697-858-2

Patients admitted to intensive care units are typically male, older, have higher BMI and multiple chronic diseases, including OSA. The prevalence of OSA in the ICU population is estimated to be between 7.8% and 10.3% and some small studies point to a prevalence up to 61% of patients. In patients that present with acute hypercapnic respiratory failure, the prevalence of OSA increases to 65% [3].

Other sleep disturbances present in ICU patients, in relation to a combination of factors, such as noise, light, and clinical interventions happening in the ICU, abnormal melatonin secretion, mechanical ventilation, various medications, and critical illness itself, seeming to lead to delirium, prolonged ICU stay, and increased mortality. Sufficient and good quality sleep is important for good outcome in critically ill patients [4].

Determinants of Mortality in OSA Patients in Critical Care

OSA is associated with an elevated risk of cardiovascular and metabolic comorbidities, along with an overall increased risk of mortality. Despite this, known OSA is not an independent risk factor for adverse outcomes in ICU patients and OSA's effect on ICU patient's prognosis remains controversial [3].

OSA is generally considered to not worsen the prognosis of patients admitted to the ICU. Studies found that OSA did not increase the length of ICU stay, ICU or hospital mortality and ventilator associated pneumonia (VAP), while others even reported a significantly lower 28-day mortality, 90-day mortality, ICU mortality, and in-hospital mortality, as well as shorter ICU stay. Uncertainty remains on the cause of this apparent protective effect: is OSA a protective factor on severely ill patients or if this phenomenon linked to limitations inherent to observational research, namely the lack of assessment of potential confounders such as obesity and other comorbidities? [5, 6].

Obesity

The prevalence of obese patients in critical care units reaches 25%, with increasingly greater proportion of patients with morbid obesity. In general, obesity is associated with lower ICU mortality, including in patients presenting with acute respiratory distress syndrome (ARDS) or acute lung injury, illustrating the obesity paradox. This phenomenon is reportedly due to an increased metabolic reserve and more intense monitoring of obese patients, perceived to require more complex management. Obese patients are also at greater risk of infectious complications and other adverse events such as decubitus complications, eschars, or thrombotic events. While obesity in ICU patients is not systematically associated with an increase in mortality, obese patients have longer lengths of ICU stay than non-obese patients [7].

As the majority of OSA patients are obese, the obesity paradox may contribute to better ICU outcomes and should be considered as an important confounding factor, possibly explaining the lower mortality found in OSA patients.

However, some studies found that morbid obesity, i.e., a BMI over 40 kg/m^2, had significant impact on length of ICU stay of OSA patients. Adipose tissue exerts anatomic and physiological effects, such as changes in respiratory mechanics that cause expiratory flow limitation, atelectasis, and $\dot{V}/\dot{Q}$ mismatch with resultant hypoxemia. Altered work of breathing and obesity hypoventilation syndrome may cause hypercapnia. Challenging mask ventilation and peri-intubation hypoxemia may complicate intubation. Overall, obese patients are at risk of respiratory, infectious, and other complications with significant implications for critical illness [3].

Infections

Sleep apnoea and poor sleep quality might impair immune responses. In influenza patients, OSA was found to be a significant contributor for ICU admission [3].

Recent data on the context of the COVID-19 pandemic has shown that OSA can be associated with poor outcome on COVID-19 patients. OSA seems to be associated with a higher risk of severe COVID-19, ICU admission, need for mechanical ventilation, and mortality from COVID-19 infection. This could be due to comorbid conditions, such as weight excess or obesity, hypertension, cardiovascular disease, and diabetes, strongly associated with OSA as well as with severe COVID-19 and mortality outcomes from COVID-19. Another possible factor in this association is the dysregulation of the renin–angiotensin system (RAS) pathway found in OSA and obese patients, causing higher levels of angiotensin II and aldosterone and an increased angiotensin-converting enzyme (ACE) activity. Severe acute respiratory syndrome coronavirus 2 (SARS-CoV-2), the causative agent of COVID-19, uses ACE2 as their entry receptor into host cells. As such, the RAS dysregulation present in OSA patients can promote SARS-CoV-2 entry into host cells, increasing viral load and infectivity, while also contributing to cardiovascular and cerebrovascular disease, that factor in the severe outcome and mortality of COVID-19. Sleep fragmentation increases interleukin-6 (IL-6) and tumor necrosis factor-α (TNF-α), which promote the inflammatory activity in neutrophils, possibly exacerbating the cytokine storm in COVID-19, which can cause ARDS and multiorgan failure. Finally, repetitive airway collapse causes hypoxia during sleep, contributing to worsening of the hypoxia in COVID-19 pneumonia and increasing the likelihood of poor outcomes [8].

Surgery

OSA is a comorbidity of high prevalence in the surgical population. Sedation and anesthesia, as well as REM sleep rebound have been shown to cause worsening of sleep apnoea in the perioperative period [9] and extensive data has demonstrated that undiagnosed OSA syndrome is associated with an increased risk of poor outcomes and higher mortality in the postoperative period [3].

In the specific case of the post-surgery of type A aortic dissection repair, severe OSA was also associated with postoperative hypoxaemia and prolonged ICU stay [10].

Conclusion

Patients admitted to intensive care units frequently suffer from multiple chronic diseases, including obstructive sleep apnea The effect of OSA in ICU patient's prognosis has been controversial. It is mostly found that OSA does not worsen the prognosis of ICU admitted patients, with exception of patients with comorbid obesity and a BMI over 40kg/m2, associated with significantly longer ICU stay. Recent data on the context of the COVID-19 pandemic has shown that OSA can also be associated with poor outcome on COVID-19 patients. Awareness for the impact of OSA on the prognosis of severely ill patients and patients admitted to the ICU is essential. Extra care and close monitoring should be provided to patients with OSA, and simple questionnaires such as the STOP-Bang questionnaire can be used for screening patients, particularly morbidly obese patients, and surgical patients, to minimize OSA associated risk of prolongation of their ICU stay.

References

[1] Embarak S, Zake LG, Abd-El-Azem W, Sileem AE. Awareness of obstructive sleep apnea among critical care physicians in Sharkia Governorate, Egypt.

[2] Hoyos CM, Drager LF, Patel SR. OSA and cardiometabolic risk: What's the bottom line? *Respirology,* 2017; 22(3):420-9.

[3] Bailly Bailly S, Galerneau LM, Ruckly S, Seiller A, Terzi N, Schwebel C, Dupuis C, Tamisier R, Mourvillier B, Pepin JL, Timsit JF. Impact of obstructive sleep apnea on the obesity paradox in critically ill patients. *J Crit Care,* 2020; 56:120-4.

[4] Boyko Y, Ording H, Jennum P. Sleep disturbances in critically ill patients in ICU: How much do we know? *Acta Anaesthesiol Scand*, 2012; 56(8):950-8.

[5] Lin P, Li X, Zhang J, Liang Z. Association between Obstructive Sleep Apnea and Reduced Mortality in Critically Ill Patients: A Propensity Score-Based Analysis. *Int J Gen Med*, 2021; 14:4723-9.

[6] Bolona E, Hahn PY, Afessa B. Intensive care unit and hospital mortality in patients with obstructive sleep apnea. *J Crit Care*, 2015; 30(1):178-80.

[7] Imber DA, Pirrone M, Zhang C, Fisher DF, Kacmarek RM, Berra L. Respiratory Management of Perioperative Obese Patients. *Respir Care,* 2016; 61(12):1681-92.

[8] Hariyanto TI, Kurniawan A. Obstructive sleep apnea [OSA] and outcomes from coronavirus disease 2019 [COVID-19] pneumonia: A systematic review and meta-analysis. *Sleep Med,* 2021; 82:47-53.

[9] Vasu TS, Grewal R, Doghramji K. Obstructive sleep apnea syndrome and perioperative complications: A systematic review of the literature. *J Clin Sleep Med,* 2012; 8(2):199-207.

[10] Xi X, Chen Y, Ma WG, Xie J, Liu YM, Zhu JM, Gong M, Zhu GF, Sun LZ. Is obstructive sleep apnoea associated with hypoxaemia and prolonged ICU stay after type A aortic dissection repair? A retrospective study in Chinese population. *BMC Cardiovasc Disord*, 2021; 21(1):421.

Chapter 24

Critical Care: Outcome

Sibel Ocak Serin[1,*], MD
and Yıldız Okuturlar[2], MD

[1]Department of Internal Medicine, University of Health Sciences, Umraniye Training and Research Hospital, Istanbul, Turkey
[2]Department of Internal Medicine, Acibadem University School of Medicine, Atakent Hospital,Istanbul, Turkey

Abstract

Obstructive sleep apnea (OSA) is the most prevalent form of sleep-disordered breathing. It is characterized by recurring episodes of total and partial upper airway obstruction and can lead to intermittent hypoxemia. Despite the fact that a significant proportion of patients who present for surgery have a known diagnosis of OSA, more than half do not have a diagnosis in place which creates management challenges. As they are susceptible to cardiopulmonary complications, the need for intensive care, and unexpected death, OSA patients should undergo a rigorous risk assessment for the perioperative condition. This chapter will discuss the impact of OSA on perioperative evaluation, outcomes and management in patients with OSA.

Keywords: obstructive sleep apnea, obesity, perioperative evaluation, perioperative outcome, perioperative management

* Corresponding Author's Email: rdsibelocak@gmail.com.

In: Obstructive Sleep Apnea in Pulmonary Critical Care
Editors: Antonio M. Esquinas and Takatoshi Kasai
ISBN: 979-8-88697-858-2

Introduction

OSA is a complex disorder characterized by wide variation in severity, comorbid conditions, and risk of complications. In the general surgical population, 23 to 38% of patients have moderate-severe OSA, and 60 to 90% of these patients are undiagnosed before evaluation. > 70% of obese patients presenting for bariatric or other major non-cardiac surgery have some form of OSA [1].

The gold standard test for the diagnosis of obstructive sleep apnea (OSA) is polysomnography. Alternative questionnaires for the preoperative evaluation of OSA syndrome have been developed. According to reports, nocturnal pulse oximetry and ambulatory home monitoring tests are useful for detecting OSA patients. Before undergoing surgery, a significant number of patients are identified as having a high probability of OSA after undergoing preoperative screening for OSA in several health centers. Recent research has focused on the acute clinical effects of OSA, specifically the impact of OSA on surgical outcomes, where a variety of perioperative factors, such as anesthetics and opioids, can affect breathing [2].

We will review the preoperative identification of these patients and the steps that can be taken for their perioperative care.

Mechanisms for Perioperative Complications

Intraoperative Pulmonary Changes

In patients with OSA, the upper airway is frequently obstructed by excessive adipose tissue or by craniofacial abnormalities. Additionally, sedation and anesthetics for induction can increase the collapsibility of upper airways resulting in difficulty inintubation and airway management. Both the use of topical anesthetics during intubation and the impairment of protective upper airway reflexes may precipitate apnea during induction. Severe OSA (apnea-hypopnea index [AHI] $\geq$ 30) was found to be significantly associated with intubation difficulty. In addition, a review of 50,000 cases of general anesthesia revealed that OSA is anindependent predictor of impossible mask ventilation.Anatomical and positional factors such as increased curvature of the thoracic spine, cephalad movement of the diaphragm, and reduced cross-sectional area of the thorax, in addition to factors such as the decreased ability of the chest wall and lungs to expand, and increased secretion, contribute to the decrease in functional residual capacity (FRC) in the anesthetized patient. Variations in the value of the ventilation-perfusion ratio (VQ) result in impaired CO_2 elimination and oxygenation [3, 4].

Postoperative Pulmonary Changes

Continuing sedation on an obstructed airway floor results in hypoxia and desaturation due to central respiratory depression. Due to the residual effect of neuromuscular blocking drugs and the risk of aspiration resulting from impaired coordination of the pharyngeal and upper esophageal muscles, hypoxia impairs the activity of the genioglossus muscle. Patients with OSA often have accompanying gastroesophageal reflux disease, which may increase the risk of aspiration during induction of general anesthesia. In the postoperative period, the ventilation responses to hypercapnia and hypoxia are blunted. It has been reported that as the degree of obesity increases, the level of hypoxia increases.

Decreased FRC and impaired oxygenation typically return to baseline within a few hours after minor surgery, but hypoxia is present in 90% of patients within 1 hour and in 50% of patients within 24 hours [5, 6].

Perioperative Pulmonary Complications

A spectrum of postoperative pulmonary complications have been described in patients with known or suspected OSA. Perioperative complications result from a combination of ineffective cough, impaired respiratory control, residual atelectasis, and decreased FRC. Postoperative respiratory failure is one of the most serious adverse events. Respiratoryfailure following surgery is one of the mostconcerning complications.

Most Common Perioperative Pulmonary Complications [7, 8].

1) Bronchospasm
2) Acute respiratory distress syndrome
3) Pulmonary embolism
4) Atelectasis
5) Pneumothorax
6) Respiratory failure

7) Pleural effusion
8) Respiratory infection
9) Need for urgent noninvasive ventilation
10) Need for reintubation

Perioperative Cardiac Complications

Undiagnosed obstructive sleep apnea can increase the risks and complications associated with surgery. In patients with OSA, autonomic dysregulation and sympathetic overactivation occur as a result of hypoxemia and hypercapnia. The imbalance between the sympathetic and parasympathetic tonus results in cardiopulmonary dysfunction. In addition to nocturnal blood pressure elevations, OSA patients are more likely to experience a variety of arrhythmias, including bradycardia, prolonged sinus pauses, second-degree heart block, and atrial and ventricular tachyarrhythmias. These mechanisms may play a role in the pattern of nocturnal sudden cardiac death observed in OSA patients.

Common cardiovascular complications are as follows [9, 10].

1) Arrhythmias
2) Ischemia
3) Myocardial infarction
4) Pulmonary edema
5) Cardiac arrest

Additional Postoperative Complications of OSA

The majority of studies indicate that OSA increases the risk of postoperative complications and adverse events. Although some studies find no difference between OSA and control patients in terms of mortality, only isolated studies suggest a mortality benefit. Except for small and retrospective studies, there are insufficient data in the medical literature on complications such as wound healing, gastrointestinal bleeding, impaired kidney function, and postoperative infection in patients with OSA. Be aware that the incidence of postoperative delirium is rising, particularly among older adults [11].

1) Postoperative pain and prolonged use of pain medications
2) Poor wound healing
3) Acute kidney injury
4) Delirium
5) Stroke
6) Gastrointestinal bleeding

Perioperative Management

In the preoperative evaluation of OSA patients, the examination of medical records, the patient interview, and the physical examination are crucial. The evaluation is based on the investigation for the presence of OSA through the patient interview, review of medical records, physical examination, and use of PSG or OSA screening questionnaires. In order to determine the perioperative risk in patients with OSA, the severity of the disease, the invasiveness of the procedure, and the need for postoperative analgesia should be considered.

The patient and family, as well as the surgeon, should be made aware of the potential perioperative consequences of OSA. Before scheduling surgery for patients with an increased perioperative risk due to OSA, it should be determined whether an inpatient or outpatient surgical procedure is more appropriate. In severe OSA or when the associated risk is deemed to be high, preoperative optimization of the patient's health status should be considered [12].

OSA patients; patients with known OSA due to CPAP may present as patients with known OSA who are not dependent on CPAP or have no CPAP experience, and patients with suspected but undiagnosed OSA. After determining the patient's condition and encouraging weight loss and smoking cessation prior to elective surgery, positive airway pressure (PAP) therapy should be initiated in patients who require it, and CPAP therapy should be resumed in patients who have discontinued CPAP therapy. PAP therapy is the mainstay treatment for OSA in adults. Maintaining a positive pharyngeal transmural to keep intraluminal pressure greater than surrounding pressure is the mechanism of CPAP. CPAP also stabilizes the upper airway by increasing the lung volume at the end of exhalation. As a result, respiratory events caused by the collapse of the upper airway are prevented. In cases when CPAP has ineffective, NIPPV treatment should be considered as an option. Uncontrolled systemic or cardiopulmonary comorbidities (such as hypoventilation, pulmonary hypertension, and indefinite resting hypoxemia) may also require further preoperative assessment and management [13].

Recommendations for the perioperative care of patients with obstructive sleep apnea (OSA) have been provided by perioperative societies and expert groups such as the American Society of Anesthesiologists (ASA), the Society of Anesthesia and Sleep Medicine (SASM), and the American Academy of Sleep Medicine, all of which have attempted to base their recommendations on the implementation of scientifically supported management measures. The recommendations are summarized in Tables 1, 2 [14].

Table 1. Recommendations for the intraoperative management of OSA from the Society of Anesthesia and Sleep Medicine and the American Society of Anesthesiologists task force on perioperative management of patients with OSA

Airway management	Known or suspected OSA to be considered an independent risk factor for difficult intubation and mask ventilation. Management according to "The practice guidelines for management of the difficult airway" is recommended.
Hypnotic and sedative medications	Patients at increased perioperative risk from OSA to be considered especially susceptible to the worsening of upper airway collapsibility and depression of central respiratory activity caused by hypnotic medications, including propofol, inhalational agents, and benzodiazepines. Risk for postoperative respiratory compromise to be considered in the determination of medication regimens and drug dosing. Risk for adverse respiratory events to be considered during procedural sedation with propofol or benzodiazepines.
Opioids	Increased risk for opioid-induced respiratory depression to be considered in OSA. Altered pain perception and increased opioid potency to be anticipated in OSA.
Neuromuscular blockade	Increased risk for the impact of postoperative residual neuromuscular blockade, hypoxemia, or respiratory failure to be considered in OSA.

Anesthesia technique	Regional anesthesia is preferable over general anesthesia, whenever applicable. Superficial surgical procedures: use of local anesthesia or peripheral nerve blocks with/without moderate sedation to be considered. Moderate sedation to be continuously monitored by capnography. During sedation, CPAP or oral appliances to be considered in patients with previous use. General anesthesia with a secured airway is preferable over deep sedation without a secure airway in OSA. Neuraxial anesthesia to be considered for peripheral procedures.
Emergence from anesthesia	Patients at increased perioperative risk from OSA to be extubated while awake, in the absence of contraindications. Full reversal of neuromuscular blockade to be verified before extubation. Extubation and recovery recommended in the lateral, semiupright, or other nonsupine positions, whenever feasible.

Abbreviations: ASA, American Society of Anesthesia; CPAP, continuous positive airway pressure; OSA, obstructive sleep apnea.

Table 2. Recommendations for the postoperative management of OSA from the American Society of Anesthesiologists task force on perioperative management of patients with OSA and the Society of Anesthesia and Sleep Medicine

Postoperative analgesia	Regional analgesic techniques should be considered for the reduction of systemic opioid requirements. In the context of neuraxial analgesia, benefits and risks of opioid use versus sole local anesthetic utilization should be considered. Continuous background infusions to be avoided or used with extreme caution in the presence of patient-controlled systemic opioids utilization. Increased risk for respiratory depression and airway obstruction to be considered during concurrent administration of sedative agents. Multimodal analgesia to be considered for the reduction of systemic opioid requirements.

Table 2. (Continued)

Supplemental oxygen	After surgery, supplemental oxygen to be administered continuously, until baseline oxygen saturation can be maintained with room air.
Pulse oximetry	Continuous pulse oximetry to be administered as long as patients remain at increased risk.
Patient positioning	Nonsupine positions are recommended during anesthesia recovery, whenever feasible.
CPAP use	CPAP or noninvasive positive pressure ventilation to be continuously administered throughout the hospitalization in patients with preoperative treatment. Initiation of nasal CPAP or noninvasive positive pressure ventilation to be considered in the event of frequent or severe airway obstruction or hypoxemia during postoperative monitoring.

Abbreviations: ASA, American Society of Anesthesia; CPAP, continuous positive airway pressure; OSA, obstructive sleep apnea.

Conclusion

We purpose of preoperative screening and/or diagnosis for OSA should be to identify patients most likely to develop postoperative complications in hopes of reducing their risk through care pathways. The perioperative community should anticipate difficult airway management in OSA and be prepared for airway complications. Therefore, patients with OSA are urged to develop viable ways and measures that can provide greater patient safety and prevent complications.

References

[1] Singh M, Liao P, Kobah S, Wijeysundera D N, Shapiro C, Chung F. Proportion of surgical patients with undiagnosed obstructive sleep apnoea. *Br. J. Anaesth.* 2013 Apr;110(4):629-36. doi: 10.1093/bja/aes465. Epub 2012 Dec 19. PMID: 23257990.

[2] Fouladpour N, Jesudoss R, Bolden N, Shaman Z, Auckley D. *Perioperative Complications in Obstructive Sleep Apnea Patients Undergoing Surgery: A Review of the Legal Literature.* Anesth Analg. 2016 Jan;122(1):145-51. doi: 10.1213/ANE.0000000000000841.

[3] De Jong A, Rollé A, Souche F R, Yengui O, Verzilli D, Chanques G, Nocca D, Futier E, Jaber S. How can I manage anaesthesia in obese patients? *Anaesth. Crit. Care Pain Med.* 2020 Apr;39(2):229-238. doi: 10.1016/j.accpm.2019.12.009. Epub 2020 Feb 14. PMID: 32068132.

[4] American Society of Anesthesiologists Task Force on Perioperative Management of patients with obstructive sleep apnea. Practice guidelines for the perioperative management of patients with obstructive sleep apnea: an updated report by the American Society of Anesthesiologists Task Force on Perioperative Management of patients with obstructive sleep apnea. *Anesthesiology.* 2014 Feb;120(2):268-86. doi: 10.1097/ALN.0000000000000053. PMID: 24346178.

[5] Bourenne J, Hraiech S, Roch A, Gainnier M, Papazian L, Forel JM. Sedation and neuromuscular blocking agents in acute respiratory distress syndrome. *Ann. Transl. Med.* 2017 Jul;5(14):291. doi: 10.21037/atm.2017.07.19. PMID: 28828366; PMCID: PMC5537113.

[6] Vasu T S, Grewal R, Doghramji K. Obstructive sleep apnea syndrome and perioperative complications: a systematic review of the literature. *J. Clin. Sleep Med.* 2012 Apr 15;8(2):199-207. doi: 10.5664/jcsm.1784. PMID: 22505868; PMCID: PMC3311420.

[7] Peppard P E, Young T, Barnet J H, Palta M, Hagen E W, Hla K M. Increased prevalence of sleep-disordered breathing in adults. *Am. J. Epidemiol.* 2013; 177:1006–14.

[8] Mutter T C, Chateau D, Moffatt M, Ramsey C, Roos L L, Kryger M. A matched cohort study of postoperative outcomes in obstructive sleep apnea: could preoperative diagnosis and treatment prevent complications? *Anesthesiology.* 2014;121:707–18.

[9] Kapur V K, Auckley D H, Chowdhuri S, Kuhlmann D C, Mehra R, Ramar K, Harrod CG. Clinical practice guideline for diagnostic testing for adult obstructive sleep apnea: an American Academy of Sleep Medicine clinical practice guideline. *J. Clin. Sleep Med.* 2017;13:479–504.

[10] Chan M T V, Wang C Y, Seet E, Tam S, Lai H Y, Chew E F F, Wu W K K, Cheng B C P, Lam C K M, Short T G, Hui D S C, Chung F; Postoperative Vascular Complications in Unrecognized Obstructive Sleep Apnea (POSA) Study Investigators. Association of Unrecognized Obstructive Sleep Apnea With Postoperative Cardiovascular Events in Patients Undergoing Major Noncardiac Surgery. *JAMA.* 2019 May 14;321(18):1788-1798. doi: 10.1001/jama.2019.4783. PMID: 31087023; PMCID: PMC6518343.

[11] Nagappa M, Ho G, Patra J, Wong J, Singh M, Kaw R, Cheng D, Chung F. Postoperative Outcomes in Obstructive Sleep Apnea Patients Undergoing Cardiac Surgery: A Systematic Review and Meta-analysis of Comparative Studies. *Anesth. Analg.* 2017 Dec;125(6):2030-2037. doi: 10.1213/ANE.0000000000002558. PMID: 29049073.

[12] Kent D, Stanley J, Aurora R N, Levine C, Gottlieb D J, Spann M D, Torre C A, Green K, Harrod CG. Referral of adults with obstructive sleep apnea for surgical consultation: an American Academy of Sleep Medicine clinical practice guideline.

J. Clin. Sleep Med. 2021 Dec 1;17(12):2499-2505. doi: 10.5664/jcsm.9592. PMID: 34351848; PMCID: PMC8726361.

[13] Lee E, Holt L, Daugherty J, Newsom C. Perioperative management of OSA in the obese patient population. *Int. Anesthesiol. Clin.* 2020 Summer;58(3):47-52. doi: 10.1097/AIA.0000000000000282. PMID: 32282579.

[14] Memtsoudis S G, Cozowicz C, Nagappa M, Wong J, Joshi G P, Wong D T, Doufas A G, Yilmaz M, Stein M H, Krajewski M L, Singh M, Pichler L, Ramachandran S K, Chung F. Society of Anesthesia and Sleep Medicine Guideline on Intraoperative Management of Adult Patients With Obstructive Sleep Apnea. *Anesth. Analg.* 2018 Oct;127(4):967-987. doi: 10.1213/ANE.0000000000003434. PMID: 29944522; PMCID: PMC6135479.

Chapter 25

Telemedicine: Clinical and Practical Implications

Yasuhiro Tomita*

Sleep Center, Toranomon Hospital, Tokyo, Japan

Abstract

Telemedicine offers opportunities to ensure access to healthcare for patients suffering from conditions in specialized fields, which may have few practitioners. The opportunities it offers are particularly significant in sleep-related disorders such as obstructive sleep apnea. The use of telemedicine to treat conditions like obstructive sleep apnea and insomnia became widespread following the publication of a position paper on this topic in 2015 by the American Academy of Sleep Medicine (AASM). Telemedicine allows healthcare providers to consult and provide treatments to patients who are geographically and temporally separated from them. It involves consulting patients over communication platforms like video conferencing and E-messaging. There are two major models in the practice of telemedicine: synchronous and asynchronous. Additionally, based on the location of the healthcare provider and the patient, telemedicine can further be classified as: center-to-center, center-to-home, and out-of-center. The goal of telemedicine is to be able to provide a quality of care that is similar to face-to-face consultations. In many aspects such as conducting interviews to collect medical histories, it has achieved this goal. It is particularly useful for patients who may have difficulty in visiting hospitals for care. This has become particularly relevant since the onset of the COVID-19 pandemic, which has caused fear of contracting infections among many patients. Telemedicine

* Corresponding Author's Email: ytomita.tmy@gmail.com.

In: Obstructive Sleep Apnea in Pulmonary Critical Care
Editors: Antonio M. Esquinas and Takatoshi Kasai
ISBN: 979-8-88697-858-2

additionally allows continued monitoring of patients through frequent interactions. This aids in ensuring adherence to treatment protocols such as Continuous Positive Airway Pressure Therapy. However, despite these advantages, telemedicine has several limitations. It presents barriers to access for those who are not technologically literate and those who have hearing or visual impairments. Additionally, it is unsuited for the treatment of patients who have chronic conditions like heart disease. Nonetheless, it is a valuable tool that can widen access to specialists and enhance the effectiveness of treatment for obstructive sleep apnea.

Keywords: obstructive sleep apnea, telemedicine, continuous positive airway pressure therapy

Introduction

There is a strong affinity between telemedicine and sleep medicine, especially in the diagnosis and treatment of obstructive sleep apnea (OSA). Several studies have reported the usefulness of telemedicine in treating patients with OSA. While many people face sleep-related problems, there are few medical institutions or physicians specializing in sleep. In this situation, the utilization of telemedicine to provide sleep medicine to a large number of people could be beneficial in ensuring wider access to treatment. Notably, most of the patients who seek treatment for sleep-related disorders suffer from OSA and insomnia. The viability of using telemedicine in diagnostic sleep testing and treatment follow-up in the treatment of OSA has been established previously. Additionally, telemedicine is now also increasingly being used in cognitive behavioral therapy for insomnia. Therefore, it is expected that the use of telemedicine in sleep medicine will continue to expand in the future.

The concept of using telemedicine for sleep medicine became widespread when the American Academy of Sleep Medicine (AASM) published a position paper on this topic in 2015 [1]. In addition, many patients also recognized the usefulness and suitability of telemedicine leading to its increased use. The onset of the COVID-19 pandemic in 2020 has accelerated this trend. Consequently, the AASM has updated its position paper for 2021 [2]. This has enabled the provision of sleep medicine through telemedicine more effectively.

This chapter presents an overview of telemedicine in OSA treatment, as using telemedicine requires an understanding of the characteristics of telemedicine, and the technologies and systems required for its use.

Additionally, it is essential to understand the differences between telemedicine and face-to-face care, and the advantages and disadvantages of the two modes of treatment.

Telemedicine is already being used in the treatment of OSA. For example, there are tools to remotely monitor PSG tests, provide education on CPAP treatment, and maintain adherence by monitoring the status of CPAP treatment.

What is Telemedicine?

The term telemedicine refers to providing medical care across time and space. Telemedicine is significant because it improves access to specialists, reduces waiting time for treatment and initiation of therapy, and increases treatment adherence. It includes tele-diagnostics, teleconsultation, teletherapy, telemonitoring, and tele-coaching, which provide diagnosis, consultation, remote initiation of therapy, monitoring of test and therapy data, and remote reinforcement, respectively. It is essential to ensure the quality and value of diagnosis and treatment and protect privacy and safety when providing telemedicine. Furthermore, it is necessary to implement telemedicine in accordance with the standards set by academic societies, medical associations, and the healthcare system in each country and region.

The methodologies of patient-provider interactions are categorized as synchronous and asynchronous. In synchronized live interactive telemedicine visits, patients and health providers are separated by distance alone. For example, one of them may be in a medical institution and the other in their home or office. On the other hand, in asynchronous interactions via telemedicine, patients and providers are separated by both location and time.

Methodology

1. Synchronous Live Interaction

Synchronous live interactive telemedicine visits require an environment where patients and providers in remote locations can communicate in real-time. These telemedicine visits can be achieved by using video conferencing technology for two-way audio and video communication; however, ensuring the security and privacy of patients are essential when exchanging personal and medical information. The technical requirements to ensure this will be discussed later. Therefore, both patients and providers should understand the limitations of telemedicine and have the option of switching to face-to-face care when necessary.

In synchronous live interactions, the patient's location is called the originating site, and the provider's location is called the distant site. The originating site may be the provider's office in the community or a sleep laboratory; the patient's home may also be a potential site if safety can be ensured. The distant site can be anywhere from which the provider can safely perform a clinical assessment.

2. Asynchronous Interactions

There is no real-time communication between patients and providers in asynchronous interactions via telemedicine, and the interactions are separated by both time and space. For example, a system whereby a sleep specialist arrives at their diagnosis without a direct examination, based on test data, or a system that facilitates the exchange of messages between patients and providers. Since the information is more limited than in synchronous interaction, both the patient and the provider must be cognizant of the limitations of this form of telemedicine, and a mechanism to switch to live interactive telemedicine visits or face-to-face office visits must be ensured.

A store-and-forward system is used for the exchange of time-separated information, whereby the medical information provided by the patient or collected in the primary care setting is temporarily stored to be used by the sleep specialist provider. The provider delivers feedback in a written or electronic report; however, the provider does not respond immediately. The data stored may include medical history, interview information, diagnostic imaging, and sleep studies. The store-and-forward system is particularly helpful when consulting primary care physicians and general clinicians.

Another tool commonly used for asynchronous interactions is E-messaging, which is a more familiar mode of communication than real-time communication for most people. It enables two-way conversations that are not in real-time, with e-mail or messaging tools. While a store-and-forward system involves a response to a set of information, E-messaging enables repeated two-way conversations. Despite being unsuitable for urgent medical treatment, it is a viable mode of sleep medicine in many cases. However, it must be ensured that the system can immediately shift to real-time communication in case of an emergency.

In a broader sense, patient education tools that do not involve mutual communication with the provider can also be considered telemedicine. A typical example is a tool that provides online cognitive behavioral therapy for insomnia. Additionally, a system to maintain adherence to CPAP therapy by monitoring and transmitting data on the use of CPAP devices, and by providing regular education can also be considered telemedicine as it aids in improving self-management skills.

2.1. Models of Care

Unlike face-to-face care, in telemedicine, communication takes place between patients and providers across locations. Whether synchronous or asynchronous, telemedicine can be classified into the following three categories according to the location of the providers and patients:

Center-to-Center (C2C)
Center-to-Home (C2H)
Out-of-Center (OOC)

2.1.1. C2C

C2C is a model where the provider is in a medical institution, and the patient is in another medical institution. Patient presenters can be primary care physicians, nurse practitioners, respiratory therapists, sleep technologists, etc., whose roles are limited by their qualifications and national regulations. In addition to taking the patient's history and measuring their blood pressure, the patient presenters can apply a stethoscope and transmit sounds. They also enable the sending of proper projection of images for visual examination of the throat. The necessary devices are essential for utilizing the C2C model.

2.1.2. C2H

In the C2H model, the provider is connected from a medical institution, while the patient is located in a free environment such as their home. While this method disallows the use of medical equipment that can only be accessed from a medical institution, it enables voice and video communication with the provider.

It makes consultation feasible at a low cost and reduces human resource requirements, however, the diagnosis is limited by the need for patients to communicate their condition themselves. Additionally, accessing the service is more straightforward, as patients are free to choose their location as long as they ensure that they are in an environment where their privacy is protected. Diagnosis is also limited by patients needing to secure a means of communication to exchange video and visual images themselves.

2.1.3. OOC

The OOC model is realized when both the provider and the patient are outside the medical institution. The provider is often located in an office that is not in a medical institution. In this model, it is important for providers to ensure that the patients' medical records are stored and accessed securely. The advantages and disadvantages of the patient's side are the same as those of the C2H model. However, it facilitates even more provider access, leading to improved access to specialized care in areas with few specialists, such as sleep medicine.

Use of Telemedicine in OSA Practice

1. Patient Evaluation and Consultation

The medical history can be as detailed as in a face-to-face consultation; thus, telemedicine enables access to quality healthcare services. In the C2H or OOC model, the patient's device, such as a smartphone camera, is used to perform the physical examination. The C2H or OOC model increases access to healthcare for patients with occupations that require them to constantly be on the move, such as truck drivers, as it does not require a patient to come to a specific location. Truck drivers, for example, are at high risk for driving accidents associated with OSA, so it is essential to provide testing and treatment for them. However, it is difficult for transportation companies to provide face-to-face examinations to all truck drivers. Telemedicine can ensure that these truck drivers are diagnosed and thus prevent accidents.

2. Sleep Testing

In the case of a home sleep apnea test (HSAT), the HSAT device and instructions are sent to the patient's home, and the sleep specialist later interprets the results. In the case of home PSG testing, the results can be reported immediately to the sleep specialist by sending the data promptly.

Additionally, the quality of PSG tests performed at home or in non-attendance can be ensured through remote monitoring. Several pilot studies have shown that remote monitoring of PSG is feasible [3].

When testing patients with complications such as heart failure, it is necessary to perform the PSG test in a sleep facility. However, it is possible to use telemedicine for the consultation that should be performed prior to the test. For example, the consulting cardiologist can provide teleconsultation to the sleep specialist, with the sleep specialist acting as a patient presenter to the cardiologist in a C2C model of telemedicine. Prevention of rehospitalization for heart failure through early intervention, for example, can help reduce medical costs.

3. Anatomical Evaluation

In some cases, patients cannot tolerate PAP treatment and require surgery or treatment with an oral appliance, which necessitates an evaluation of the upper airway.

Although telemedicine has limitations in evaluating the anatomy of the upper airway and maxillofacial region, it is possible to evaluate anatomic abnormalities such as micrognathia and retrognathia using a webcam or smartphone camera. Intraoral cameras can be used for proper intraoral observation in the C2C model with the aid of a patient presenter. Additionally, this allows for the assessment of the tonsils and soft tissues, and the classification of the height of the soft palate by Mallampati class.

4. PAP Management and Patient Education

When PAP treatment is initiated, the sleep specialist provides information to the primary care physician in the patient's area. The sleep specialist confirms PAP adherence and efficacy by remote monitoring. Continuous support can be provided to the patient through regular follow-ups using telemedicine.

Providing detailed follow-ups aid in maintaining and improving adherence to CPAP. An RCT conducted in Japan observed that receiving telephone care combined with C2H model telemedicine every month led to a higher level of adherence among patients than only receiving face-to-face follow-ups every three months [4]. In an RCT conducted in Philadelphia, a telemedicine-based OSA evaluation and management pathway showed results similar to a more traditional, in-person care model. However, the telemedicine group improved their mental health scores and positive feedback as well [5]. An RCT in Spain concluded that adherence in an out-of-hospital Virtual Sleep Unit group was similar to that in a hospital routine group. Based on the cost-effectiveness analysis the authors concluded that the use of telemedicine was beneficial [6].

Mechanisms for receiving interactive feedback have also been developed, initially through web-based and automated telephone responses, and more recently, through E-messaging. For example, in an RCT conducted in California, an intervention combining web-based OSA education and CPAP telemonitoring with automated patient feedback was used. Unfortunately, while automated patient feedback improved adherence for up to 90 days, it decreased adherence when feedback messages were terminated prematurely [7]. Adherence was also reported to improve upon the use of the PAP self-management platform, which motivated patients to use the PAP device appropriately every day. For example, in the case of Philips's CPAP, using an App called Dream Mapper [8], and ResMed's CPAP, using an App called myAir [9], it was reported that patients used the CPAP device appropriately every day. Thus, the use of E-messaging apps can improve CPAP usage.

5. Patient Education

Patient education regarding OSA practices, including CPAP use, is expected to be equal in both patients who received face-to-face consultation and teleconsultation. In a study that randomly assigned patients who started CPAP therapy into conventional consultation groups and teleconsultation groups, CPAP adherence was observed to be similar in both groups [10]. In another study on teaching knowledge of OSA and practical skills in CPAP therapy, no significant differences were observed in the responses to the questionnaire between learners that used video conference-based methods and face-to-face practice [11].

Requirement

The most crucial goal of telemedicine is to provide medical care comparable to in-person visits. Therefore, it is necessary to establish appropriate technical specifications; regulations that take into account the characteristics of each country and region; and standards to ensure that the quality and safety of the medical care provided is on par with standard medical care. Furthermore, the technical conditions required should be defined legally as they are related to privacy protection and access to insurance coverage. Concurrently, the laws should be updated to facilitate the use of telemedicine.

1. Technology

A robust communication environment is necessary for telemedicine. A backup communication environment must be prepared to ensure that the communication environment is always available. In the case of the C2H model and the OOC model, the communication environment is dependent on the communication environment on the patient's side as well; thus, the possibilities of the need for a backup communication environment and schedule changes should also be considered.

Privacy and security must be ensured in the data transmission and storage of medical information. In the OOC model, since the provider is outside the consultation room, it is necessary to construct a system for accessing and storing medical records. It is necessary to ensure that the medical records are managed with the same care as for in-person visits.

It is necessary to restrict access to the platform to, for example, patient, provider, and patient presenter, to prevent third parties from accessing the data. A mechanism to authenticate those who access the platform is needed to ensure this. If necessary, the patient must be required to present personal identification and the provider's medical credentials at each visit.

2. Regulations

Laws and regulations exist to maintain safety and fairness in healthcare. Any form of telemedicine must comply with the laws of the country or region from which the patient and provider originate. Additionally, telemedicine practiced across State lines, where the parties may be in different regions, should in principle comply with the laws of both regions.

Similarly, it is necessary to ensure that the requirements for reimbursement are met prior to the provision of telemedicine services. This is necessary as reimbursement requirements may vary depending on the patient's medical insurance and geographic location. For example, in a particular region, the C2C model may be covered, while the OOC model may not; similarly, the provider's job title may be restricted, or there may be stipulations on the qualifications required to provide telemedicine services.

3. Safety

While we set standards for telemedicine to achieve the same quality as in-person visits, we must be cognizant of the limitations of telemedicine. Both the provider and patient should be made aware of these limitations and must take the necessary measures to be able to switch to face-to-face care when necessary. Low levels of digital health literacy among patients may also interfere with care. In addition, language barriers, visual impairments, and hearing impairments may also increase the disadvantages of telemedicine. Therefore, it is essential to ensure that qualified assistants are made available and establish criteria in advance to determine whether telemedicine can be continued or not.

In the C2H and OOC models, patients can access medical services from a variety of locations. While this is an advantage of telemedicine, it is essential to ensure that the patient's location is private and secure. For example, if the patient is accessing the system from a car, then privacy can be maintained, however, it may not be the most appropriate communication environment. Therefore, during their interaction, the provider must ensure that the user has parked the car safely.

Advantages vs. Disadvantages

As described above, telemedicine can be highly effective in the treatment of OSA; and its effectiveness has been demonstrated in actual practice. In this section, we focus on the advantages of using telemedicine, and cover the points to be considered when using telemedicine.

1. Improvement of Health Care Disparities

Telemedicine bridges gaps in time and distance at every step of OSA care. It ensures that patients who had difficulty in accessing healthcare in the traditional medical model due to geographic or socioeconomic constraints could receive appropriate medical care. Thus, telemedicine plays an essential role in reducing healthcare disparities. It is important to note that telemedicine has several disadvantages and may create new disparities in access to healthcare. People with visual or hearing impairments may find it difficult to access telemedicine. Thus, they must be supported to overcome these barriers.

2. Cost-Benefit Analysis

Efforts must be taken to ensure that the same level of safety and accuracy is maintained as in face-to-face practice during every step of OSA practice using telemedicine; this entails a specific cost investment. In today's world of advanced communication technology and infrastructure, some steps of OSA practice may be less costly than others. It is easier to guarantee the accuracy of objective data for evaluation. For example, the results of HSAT are similar if the data can be exchanged safely and quickly.

However, the accuracy of home-PSG testing depends on how the sensor is worn and requires local human resources. This is a limitation of non-attended PSG. According to a cost analysis conducted in 2001 [12], a comparison of the cost of performing TM-PSG and home PSG for OSA diagnosis, concluded that TM-PSG is more effective but costly. It must be noted, however, that this study was conducted when the cost of information and communication was high and may be reduced by using the modern infrastructure.

Compared to tests that deal with objective data, interviews and consultations are more likely to yield different results when using telemedicine, depending on the technological environment. Depending on how much money is invested, it may be possible to create an environment similar to that of face-to-face care. This may be made technically possible in the future; however, it will require investment in human resources and equipment, and its cost-benefit must be evaluated.

The cost-effectiveness of CPAP management has been reported to favor telemedicine. Compared with usual care, telemonitoring and teleconsultation using TM were more cost-effective [13]. In addition, the cost was lower even when the number of interventions was higher in the TM group. Although there was no significant difference in effectiveness, it is possible that at least some of the users benefited from the increased number of interventions. However, another study observed that while telemonitoring was less expensive than standard management, it resulted in lower patient satisfaction [14]. Therefore, it is possible that the frequency of interventions, such as through remote consultation rather than telemonitoring alone, may have increased patient satisfaction.

3. Individualizing Patient Satisfaction

While supporting CPAP management makes sense from a cost-benefit perspective, patient satisfaction must also receive attention. Some studies suggest that patients favor telemonitoring (ref omitted), while others suggest that many find it annoying. Some providers may also find remote monitoring inconvenient. Although the need for frequent monitoring in CPAP management is not high, an appropriate frequency of an intervention is required. Finding the appropriate balance may require immense effort; however, it is necessary to ensure client satisfaction.

Conclusion

Telemedicine has gained widespread acceptance because of the COVID-19 pandemic that started in 2020, which increased the infection risk during face-to-face care. Therefore, the infrastructure for telemedicine has been rapidly developed. Since the threshold for starting telemedicine has been lowered, it will be necessary to reevaluate the advantages and disadvantages of telemedicine in the post-COVID-19 era. Table 1 summarizes the main advantages and disadvantages of using telemedicine for each step of OSA treatment and the target population that should be considered when applying telemedicine.

In addition to C2C and C2H, OOC can also be used for providing healthcare services. However, capital investment is required to ensure that it can offer the same quality in consultation and examination as face-to-face care. Except in the case of trained C2C models, the possibility of a decrease in the quality of the consultation should be recognized. Thus, it is essential to have a mechanism to connect the interview, consultation, and examination phases seamlessly. Patients with visual, speech, or hearing handicaps are at a significant disadvantage when using telemedicine services. However, technological innovations are minimizing these visual and auditory handicaps. Similarly, advancements in making virtual reality and augmented reality more accessible may one day enable us to overcome these handicaps and barriers to consultation. Smartphones, which have become popular among many people, will be the examination device in the C2H and OOC models. Improvements in camera performance are expected to support sufficient coverage to ensure the quality of the examination.

Additionally, HSAT will ensure sufficient quality in delivery services and remote analysis. Logistics and communication technologies, and cloud services infrastructure are already sufficiently widespread. The cost-benefit balance also supports telemedicine models. Remote PSG does not adequately cover the risks posed by complications or guarantee the accuracy of the test and cannot be replaced by HSAT. Currently, the consensus is that telemedicine should be avoided in cases of complications where HSAT should be avoided according to the AASM guidelines. In the future, it will be necessary to evaluate the types of diseases for which remote PSG is feasible in terms of accuracy and safety. This is necessary as it is desirable to correct the disparity in medical care by spreading remote PSG in selected cases.

Table 1. Advantages and disadvantages of using telemedicine for each step of OSA treatment and the target population considerations

Steps	**Advantages**	**Disadvantages**	**Patients who should be given attention**
Medical interview and examination	Correction of healthcare disparities by crossing time and distance	High cost (especially in the C2C model)	People with visual and hearing disadvantages
Diagnostic tests	Correction of healthcare disparities by crossing time and distance	Limitations of accuracy of home PSG	People with complications
CPAP management	Cost reduction and adherence improvement	Management costs for handling huge amounts of data	People who find telemedicine interventions annoying

The instructions for receiving the test results and starting CPAP treatment will be convenient for those who understand the video call. Ideally, it should be possible to tailor the procedure to the patient's wishes. However, only a few people would want to receive an explanation of the procedure in person.

While using the tools to actively continue CPAP therapy can be beneficial, it should be noted that there are patients who do not want to do this. Therefore, it is desirable to develop programs that meet patients' wishes. Additionally, in CPAP management, there are also human-administered online clinics in addition to tools such as app-based, web-based, and telephone autoresponders. It is difficult to define which methods will suit a particular patient. While it may be difficult to scientifically verify the effectiveness of such programs by taking into account each patient's feedback, such programs may eventually be developed.

The practice of telemedicine will continue to evolve with the common goal of promoting a model of care in which sleep specialists, patients, primary care providers, and other healthcare team members can all work together to improve the value of healthcare delivery. Telemedicine is an important field that can ensure access to healthcare through the utilization of technology. Despite its limitations it can enable patients to access quality healthcare in niche fields like sleep disorders, which may otherwise be difficult to obtain.

References

[1] Singh, Jaspal, M. Safwan Badr, Wendy Diebert, Lawrence Epstein, Dennis Hwang, Valerie Karres, Seema Khosla, K. Nicole Mims, Affifa Shamim-Uzzaman, Douglas Kirsch, Jonathan L. Heald, and Kathleen McCann. (2015). "American Academy of Sleep Medicine (AASM) Position Paper for the Use of Telemedicine for the Diagnosis and Treatment of Sleep Disorders." *Journal of Clinical Sleep Medicine*, 11(10), 1187-98.

[2] Shamim-Uzzaman, Qurratul A., Charles J. Bae, Zarmina Ehsan, Arveity R. Setty, Michelle Devine, Swati Dhankikar, Innessa Donskoy, Barry Fields, Hunter Hearn, Dennis Hwang, Vikas Jain, Dennis Kelley, Douglas B. Kirsch, William Martin, Matthew Troester, Lynn Marie Trotti, Christine H. Won, and Lawrence J. Epstein. (2021). "The use of telemedicine for the diagnosis and treatment of sleep disorders: an American Academy of Sleep Medicine update." *Journal of Clinical Sleep Medicine*, 17(5), 1103-1107.

[3] Bruyneel, Marie. (2019). "Telemedicine in the diagnosis and treatment of sleep apnoea" *European Respiratory Review*, 28(151), 180093.

[4] Murase, Kimihiko, Kiminobu Tanizawa, Takuma Minami, Takeshi Matsumoto, Ryo Tachikawa, Naomi Takahashi, Toru Tsuda, Yoshiro Toyama, Motoharu Ohi,

Toshiki Akahoshi, Yasuhiro Tomita, Koji Narui, Hiroshi Nakamura, Tetsuro Ohdaira, Hiroyuki Yoshimine, Tomomasa Tsuboi, Yoshihiro Yamashiro, Shinichi Ando, Takatoshi Kasai, Hideo Kita, Koichiro Tatsumi, Naoto Burioka, Keisuke Tomii, Yasuhiro Kondoh, Hirofumi Takeyama, Tomohiro Handa, Satoshi Hamada, Toru Oga, Takeo Nakayama, Tetsuo Sakamaki, Satoshi Morita, Tomohiro Kuroda, Toyohiro Hirai, and Kazuo Chin. (2020). "A Randomized Controlled Trial of Telemedicine for Long-Term Sleep Apnea Continuous Positive Airway Pressure Management" *Annals of the American Thoracic Society*, 17(3), 329-337.

[5] Fields, Barry, G., Pratima Pathak Behari, Susan McCloskey, Gala True, Diane Richardson, Arwin Thomasson, Danijela Korom-Djakovic, Keith Davies, and Samuel T. Kuna. (2016). "Remote Ambulatory Management of Veterans with Obstructive Sleep Apnea" *Sleep*, 39(3), 501-509.

[6] Lugo, Vera, M., Onintza Garmendia, Monique Suarez-Giron, Marta Torres, Francisco J. Vázquez-Polo, Miguel A. Negrin, Anabel Moraleda, Mariana Roman, Marta Puig, Concepción Ruiz, Carlos Egea, Juan F. Masa, Ramon Farre, and Josep M. Montserrat. (2019). "Comprehensive management of obstructive sleep apnea by telemedicine: Clinical improvement and cost-effectiveness of a Virtual Sleep Unit. A randomized controlled trial." *PLoS One*, 14(10), e0224069.

[7] Hwang, Dennis, Jeremiah W. Chang, Adam V. Benjafield, Maureen E. Crocker, Colleen Kelly, Kendra A. Becker, Joseph B. Kim, Rosa R. Woodrum, Joanne Liang, and Stephen F. Derose. (2018). "Effect of Telemedicine Education and Telemonitoring on Continuous Positive Airway Pressure Adherence. The Tele-OSA Randomized Trial" *American Journal of Respiratory and Critical Care Medicine*, 197(1), 117-126.

[8] Engelman, Heather, Christy Stitt, Lauren Creswick, Nuno Cachada, Matthew Thomas, Jonathan Leahy, Sarah Martin, Neena Derashri, and Tom Kelly. (2018). "Effects on CPAP use of a patient support mobile app." *European Respiratory Journal*, 52, PA2257.

[9] Malhotra, Atul, Maureen E. Crocker, Leslee Willes, Colleen Kelly, Sue Lynch, and Adam V. Benjafield. (2018). "Patient Engagement Using New Technology to Improve Adherence to Positive Airway Pressure Therapy: A Retrospective Analysis." *Chest*, 153(4), 843-850.

[10] Jesús Coma-Del-Corral, Maria, Maria Luz Alonso-Alvarez, Marta Allende, Jose Cordero, Estrella Ordax, Fernando Mosa, and Joaquin Teran-Santos. (2013). "Reliability of telemedicine in the diagnosis and treatment of sleep apnea syndrome." *Telemedicine and e-Health*, 19(1), 7-12.

[11] Isetta, Valentina, Carmen Leon, Marta Torres, Cristina Embid, Josep Roca, Daniel Navajas, Ramon Farre, and Josep M. Montserrat. (2014). "Telemedicine-based approach for obstructive sleep apnea management: building evidence." *Interactive Journal of Medical Research*, 3(1), e6.

[12] Pelletier-Fleury, N., Gagnadoux, F., Philippe, C., Rakotonanahary, D., Lanoé, J. L., and Fleury, B. (2001). "A cost-minimization study of telemedicine. The case of telemonitored polysomnography to diagnose obstructive sleep apnea syndrome." *International Journal of Technology Assessment in Health Care,* 17(4), 604-611.

[13] Isetta, Valentina, Miguel A. Negrín, Carmen Monasterio, Juan F. Masa, Nuria Feu, Ainhoa Álvarez, Francisco Campos-Rodríguez, Concepción Ruiz, Jorge Abad, Francisco J. Vázquez-Polo, Ramon Farré, Marina Galdeano, Patricia Lloberes, Cristina Embid, Mónica de la Peña, Javier Puertas, Mireia Dalmases, Neus Salord, Jaime Corral, Bernabé Jurado, Carmen León, Carlos Egea, Aida Muñoz, Olga Parra, Roser Cambrodi, María Martel-Escobar, Meritxell Arqué, Josep M. Montserrat, and Spanish Sleep Network. (2015). "A Bayesian cost-effectiveness analysis of a telemedicine-based strategy for the management of sleep apnoea: a multicenter randomized controlled trial." *Thorax*, 70(11), 1054-1061.

[14] Winfried Randerath, Johan Verbraecken, Stefan Andreas, Michael Arzt, Konrad E Bloch, Thomas Brack, Bertien Buyse, Wilfried De Backer, Danny Joel Eckert, Ludger Grote, Lars Hagmeyer, Jan Hedner, Poul Jennum, Maria Teresa La Rovere, Carla Miltz, Walter T McNicholas, Josep Montserrat, Matthew Naughton, Jean-Louis Pepin, Dirk Pevernagie, Bernd Sanner, Dries Testelmans, Thomy Tonia, Bart Vrijsen, Peter Wijkstra, and Patrick Levy. (2017). "Definition, discrimination, diagnosis and treatment of central breathing disturbances during sleep." *European Respiratory Journal*, 49(1), 1601128.

Index

A

B

C

D

E

F

H

I

M

N

O

P

About the Editors

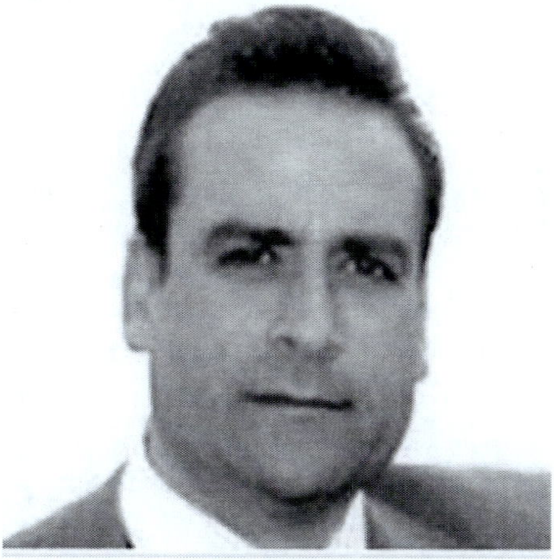

Antonio M. Esquinas, MD, PhD, FCCP, FAARC
Intensive Care Unit, Hospital Morales Meseguer, Murcia, Spain
Director International School of Non-Invasive Ventilation;
Director International Non Invasive Ventilation Expert of College
Email: antmesquinas@gmail.com

Antonio M. Esquinas MD, PhD, FCCP, FAARC is the Director of the International School Noninvasive Mechanical Ventilation and Director of Non-Invasive Ventilation College of Experts. Principal research and academic publications are related acute respiratory failure, noninvasive and invasive mechanical ventilation (weaning mechanical ventilation, COPD exacerbation, hypoxemic respiratory failure and acute cardiac diseases. He has published 667 articles and 60 edited books related with mechanical ventilation and noninvasive mechanical ventilation in pulmonary and critical care.

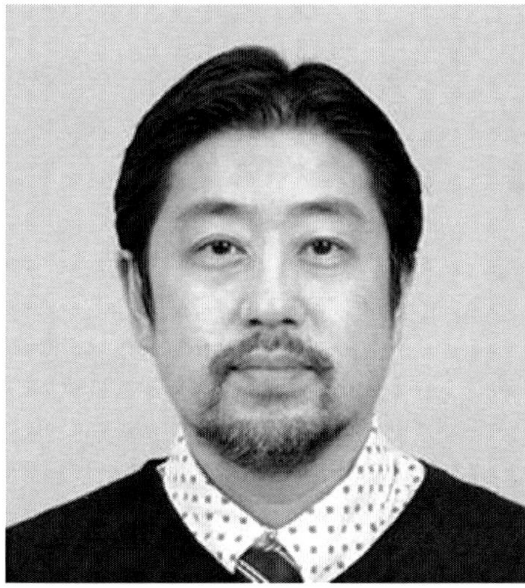

Takatoshi Kasai, MD
Department of Cardiovascular Medicine
Juntendo University Graduate, School of Medicine.
Tokyo, Japan
Email: kasai-t@mx6.nisiq.net

Takatoshi Kasai MD is an international expert in Sleep Medicine. Dr. Kasai is an Associate Professor, Cardio-Respiratory Sleep Medicine, Juntendo University Graduate School of Medicine, 2015-Present Associate Professor, Cardiovascular Respiratory Sleep Medicine, Juntendo University Graduate School of Medicine, 2018-Present Associate Professor, Department of Cardiovascular Medicine, Juntendo University Graduate School of Medicine, 2019-Present Director, Sleep and Sleep Disordered Breathing Center, Juntendo University Hospital 2019-PresentAssociate Professor, Department of Cardiovascular Management and Remote monitoring, Juntendo University Graduate School of Medicine. He conducted a great number of research and clinical contributions for Sleep Medicine and implications in critical care medicine.